Social Behaviors in Childhood: Causes and Consequences

Social Behaviors in Childhood: Causes and Consequences

Guest Editors

Xuechen Ding
Wan Ding

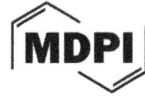 Basel • Beijing • Wuhan • Barcelona • Belgrade • Novi Sad • Cluj • Manchester

Guest Editors

Xuechen Ding
School of Psychology
Shanghai Normal University
Shanghai
China

Wan Ding
School of Psychology
Zhejiang Normal University
Jinhua
China

Editorial Office
MDPI AG
Grosspeteranlage 5
4052 Basel, Switzerland

This is a reprint of the Special Issue, published open access by the journal *Behavioral Sciences* (ISSN 2076-328X), freely accessible at: www.mdpi.com/journal/behavsci/special_issues/0ZA1USY6HF.

For citation purposes, cite each article independently as indicated on the article page online and as indicated below:

Lastname, A.A.; Lastname, B.B. Article Title. *Journal Name* **Year**, *Volume Number*, Page Range.

ISBN 978-3-7258-4062-5 (Hbk)
ISBN 978-3-7258-4061-8 (PDF)
https://doi.org/10.3390/books978-3-7258-4061-8

Contents

About the Editors

Xuechen Ding

Xuechen Ding is a Full Professor at the School of Psychology, Shanghai Normal University. He is the Director of Department of Developmental and Educational Psychology and the Vice President of Shanghai Experimental School. His research interests include peer relationship, social behavior, and socio-emotional adjustment during middle childhood and adolescence. He published over 70 papers in developmental journals such as *Journal of Research on Adolescence*, *School Psychology*, and *Journal of Abnormal Child Psychology*. He is the Associate Editor of *Journal of Applied Developmental Psychology*, the Editorial Board Member of *Child Development* and *Child: Care, Health, and Development*, and the Guest Editor of *Frontiers in Psychiatry* and *Behavioral Sciences*.

Wan Ding

Wan Ding is an Associate Professor at the School of Psychology, Zhejiang Normal University. She serves as the Deputy Director of the Family Education Research Center at Zhejiang Normal University and the Vice President of the 8th Jinhua Women's Federation. Specializing in longitudinal designs and parent–child interactive experimental methods, her research focuses on family education, child development, and mental health in children and adolescents. She has published over 60 papers in leading developmental psychology journals, including *Child Development*, *Journal of Youth and Adolescence*, *Family Process*, and *Journal of Family Psychology*. She is the Guest Editor of *Behavioral Sciences* and *Brain Sciences*, and serves as a peer reviewer for other various academic journals.

Preface

Normative development of children's social, emotional, and school adjustment stems from sources including both family and peer groups. Parent–child and peer interactions have unique and significant implications for children, and these social relationships serve as a foundation for feelings of security and belonging. During the socialization process in family and school contexts, children display a wide variety of social behaviors, including aggressive behavior, social withdrawal, prosocial behavior, antisocial behavior, cooperative behavior, bullying behavior, etc. However, several issues require further exploration. For example, what are the different causal relations that might underlie children's social behaviors? What is the trajectory of these social behaviors at different developmental stages? Could we find a more neural basis for these social behaviors via advanced techniques (e.g., EEG, ERP, fNIRS, and fMRI)? In light of these premises, this Book aims to advance the literature on the development trajectory of children's social behaviors and their cognitive neural mechanisms. The research collated in this Book focuses on predictors and outcomes of children's social behaviors in family and school contexts from early childhood to emerging adulthood, risk/protective factors among these associations, social behaviors in different contexts, or their cognitive neural mechanisms.

Xuechen Ding and Wan Ding
Guest Editors

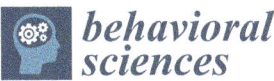

Article

Shyness, Sport Engagement, and Internalizing Problems in Chinese Children: The Moderating Role of Class Sport Participation in a Multi-Level Model

Rumei Zhao [1,†], Xiaoxue Kong [2,†], Mingxin Li [1], Xinyi Zhu [1], Jiyueyi Wang [1], Wan Ding [3,*] and Xuechen Ding [1,4,5,*]

[1] School of Psychology, Shanghai Normal University, Shanghai 200234, China;
    1000546535@smail.shnu.edu.cn (R.Z.); 1000527473@smail.shnu.edu.cn (M.L.);
    1000512181@smail.shnu.edu.cn (X.Z.); 1000514554@smail.shnu.edu.cn (J.W.)
[2] Department of Psychology, Neuroscience and Behaviour, McMaster University, Hamilton, ON L8S 4K1,
    Canada; kongx17@mcmaster.ca
[3] School of Psychology, Parent Education Research Center, Zhejiang Normal University, Jinhua 321004, China
[4] Lab for Educational Big Data and Policymaking, Ministry of Education, Shanghai 200234, China
[5] The Research Base of Online Education for Shanghai Middle and Primary Schools, Shanghai 200234, China
*   Correspondence: dingwan@zjnu.edu.cn (W.D.); dingxuechen@shnu.edu.cn (X.D.)
†   These authors contributed equally to this work.

Abstract: The relations between shyness and internalizing problems have been mainly explored at the individual level, with little known about its dynamics at the group level. This study aims to examine the mediating effect of individual-level sport engagement and the moderating effect of class-level sport participation in the relations between shyness and internalizing problems. The participants were 951 children attending primary and middle school from grade 3 to grade 7 (M_{age} = 11 years, 509 boys) in urban areas of China. Cross-sectional data were collected using self-report assessments. Multi-level analysis indicated that (1) shyness was positively associated with internalizing problems; (2) sport engagement partially mediated the relations between shyness and internalizing problems; and (3) class sport participation was a cross-level moderator in the mediating relations between shyness, sport engagement, and internalizing problems. Shy children in classes with a higher level of sport participation tend to have less sport engagement and more internalizing problems than those in classes with a lower level of sport participation. These findings illuminate implications from a multi-level perspective for shy children's adjustment in a Chinese context. The well-being of shy children could be improved by intervening in sport activity, addressing both individual engagement and group dynamics, such as class participation.

Keywords: shyness; internalizing problems; sport engagement; sport participation; multi-level model

1. Introduction

Shyness refers to excessive wariness, discomfort, and internal anxiety in contexts of social novelty or when perceived social evaluation is present [1]. Shyness is a temperamental trait that is considered moderately inherited and biologically based, demonstrating relative stability throughout personality development [2]. According to the social motivational perspective, social engagement arises from the interplay between two opposing motivational tendencies, social approach and social avoidance [3]. Shyness reflects the underlying approach–avoidance conflict, whereby the desire for engaging with their peers (i.e., high social approach motivation) is simultaneously inhibited by social fear and anxiety (i.e., high social avoidance motivation). This inhibition contributes to the tendency of shy children to withdraw from social interactions and have fewer opportunities to engage with peers, which may lead to negative adjustment outcomes [4]. There is growing evidence indicating shyness is associated with various adjustment difficulties, particularly internalizing problems, such as loneliness, depression, social anxiety, and higher negative affect [5–7]. Research has shown that sport engagement and participation are associated with a variety of positive psychosocial outcomes [8,9]. Class-centered physical education is the primary way for school-aged children to engage in sports activities in the context of Chinese culture [10]. As an important form of team sports activities, physical education class can provide a structured and supportive environment that fosters the development of individual competencies, the formation of social connections, and the expansion of support networks [11]. Thus, participation in and engagement with team sports activities holds the potential to mitigate internalizing problems in shy children. Although extensive research provides evidence linking shyness to internalizing problems, the internal mechanisms that may underlie (i.e., mediators) or modulate (i.e., moderators) these links remain under-investigated. Meanwhile, previous studies on shy children mainly focused on the individual level, with less attention given to the group level influences. Accordingly, the present study aims to fill the gap by exploring the relations between shyness, sport engagement, class sport participation, and internalizing problems among children in mainland China.

1.1. Shyness and Internalizing Problems in China

Shy children tend to withdraw from social interactions, increasing the likelihood of experiencing internalizing problems [12]. In the present study, we particularly focused on loneliness, depression, and social anxiety as indices of internalizing problems, which have a variety of negative consequences for both physical and mental health [13–15].

Peer relationships and friendships are important sources of emotional and social support [16]. Children who interact less with their peers, such as those who are shy, may be at a higher risk of developing emotional problems than their more outgoing counterparts [17]. Shy children often feel uncomfortable in social situations, making it difficult to establish deep friendships with peers. As a result, they are perceived to be sad and anxious and may even be intentionally excluded by peers, which leads to loneliness [18]. Moreover, shyness can disconnect children from peer play, contributing to feelings of loneliness [19]. It has also been reported that low levels of peer acceptance and approval in shy children result in higher levels of loneliness [20]. Empirical support from the Chinese sample has shown that shyness is associated with feelings of loneliness [21–25]. For example, Tan et al. found Chinese children with greater level of shyness were not conducive to developing close relationships, resulting in insufficient social support and greater feelings of loneliness [26].

Similarly, shyness interferes with the healthy development of satisfying interpersonal relationships in children. Interpersonal failures and concomitant anxiety can produce negative affect, which may cause an increase in depression [27]. Meanwhile, shy children may develop negative self-perceptions and other psychological problems such as depression when they realize their difficulties in social situations [28]. Numerous studies have shown that shyness is linked to depression [6,29–32].

According to the cognitive model of social anxiety, anxiety arises from the negative cognitive processing bias towards self and external information [33]. Shy children, who often focus on themselves with fear of negative judgment, are particularly prone to experiencing social anxiety [28]. Furthermore, shy individuals tend to have relatively pessimistic perceptions of their social performance, influenced by previous negative social experiences [34], which consequently leads to the development of social anxiety [35]. Previous studies have also shown that shyness is related to social anxiety in China [6,36,37]. For example, Ran et al. found that shy individuals were more likely to have low self-esteem, resulting in high social anxiety [38].

Research has also highlighted differences in the interpretation and implications of shyness across cultural contexts [39]. In Western societies, where assertiveness and expressiveness are strongly encouraged [40], shyness is likely to be perceived as socially immature and inappropriate [7]. However, the definition and development of shyness in China is not exactly the same as in the Western context. On the one hand, shyness from the Chinese perspective involves self-conscious avoidance of public attention and social restraint in behavior that presents as modesty and maintains social harmony, in line with traditional Chinese culture and the collectivist orientation [37,41]. On the other hand, in China, which has experienced large-scale economic and social reforms in the past 30 years, the evaluation and perception of shyness have undergone great changes from positive to negative. Specifically, in the traditional Chinese culture, shyness is often valued as a positive behavioral trait that reflects social maturity, mastery, and understanding [42]. Now, new behavioral qualities such as initiative-taking and self-expression are increasingly appreciated by individuals in the competitive urban environment [43]. Thus, shyness may be perceived as a negative quality in the current social evaluation system and has been proven to be increasingly associated with the internalizing dimension of adjustment difficulties among children and adolescents in urban China [36,44,45]. In summary, shy children's internalizing problems deserve more attention.

1.2. Shyness and Internalizing Problems: Mediating Role of Sport Engagement

As mentioned above, shyness is directly related to internalizing problems, such as loneliness, depression, and social anxiety. In addition to the direct relations, the present study focused on the underlying process from shyness to these internalizing problems. Ryan and Deci's self-determination theory [46] suggests that shy children often experience diminished feelings of competence, autonomy, and connectedness with peers, which, in turn, contributes to the development of internalizing problems like anxiety and depression. These basic human behavioral needs, particularly the sense of connection with others, coincide with the concept of sport engagement proposed by positive psychologists [47]. Ramey et al. proposed that sport engagement could be conceptualized as comprising three elements: (a) an affective component, including positive and negative responses (e.g., enjoyment, excitement, and stress) to a sport activity; (b) a cognitive component, including thoughtfulness and knowledge about the sport activity; and (c) a relational component indicating the connection to others or group (e.g., relatedness, belongingness, etc.) [47]. Drawing upon this perspective, this study proposed that sport engagement would mediate the relations between shyness and internalizing problems.

Shy children may avoid sport engagement. They were less likely to list sports activity as their primary activity as compared to other activities [48] and reported less involvement in sports activities than their more sociable peers [49]. From a motivational perspective, shy students may feel anxious or uncomfortable [7], which can lead to a lack of interest or engagement in team sports activities. In fact, there is some evidence to suggest that shy children are less likely to be involved in sports activities [48,50]. For example, Miller suggested that shy children may hesitate to become involved in team sports because of fear of negative evaluation from peers and coaches [51].

Furthermore, lack of sport engagement may be related to shy children's internalizing problems. Positive sport engagement (e.g., enjoyment, competence, and relatedness) may be uniquely important in promoting well-being [9], as it enhances peer relations, increases self-esteem, fosters a sense of security, and reduces anxiety [52]. On the contrary, shy children tend to be more concerned with others' evaluations [1], leading to less enjoyment and more negative experiences during sports activities. This preoccupation negatively impacts their happiness and increases their likelihood of developing internalizing problems. In fact, previous studies have explored the role of sport engagement in internalizing problems [53,54]. For example, Fletcher et al. found that sport engagement was related to lower social anxiety in elementary school children [53]. Page et al. found that children aged 6 to 11 years with higher sport activity engagement reported lower scores on loneliness [55]. Moreover, a longitudinal study showed that sport engagement was related to lowered depression across two years (from 10 to 12 years of age) [56]. Taken together, shy children could experience internalizing problems through less sport engagement.

1.3. Moderating Role of Class Sport Participation

According to ecological systems theory [57], the class, as an important part of the micro-system, is a direct environment for individual activities and social interaction. Sport participation, as an aspect of the class environment, is also critical for the establishment of peer relationships and the shaping of their own behavior, which has a profound impact on children's mental health and socialization [58]. Class sport participation refers to an organized, class-centered physical activity that is characterized by regular time schedules, specified locations, coach supervision, and a group setting and usually includes goals for performance or skill development [59]. A growing body of research has demonstrated that class sport participation is negatively associated with internalizing problems among samples of general individuals or non-shy children [8,60]. However, for shy children with social withdrawal, there are different explanations. Salmivalli's healthy context paradox may provide new insight into the relation between class sport participation and internalizing problems [61]. This paradox proposes that an improved social environment can be detrimental for some children. For example, Bellmore et al. found that the negative impact of victimization may be especially damaging in contexts where the overall level of aggression or victimization is low [62]. Their findings were interpreted in terms of social misfit and attribution theories. Specifically, being victimized in a context where very few others share this plight, one is a social misfit deviating from what is normative. In such a context, attributing the cause of victimization to oneself is likely [61]. Similarly, for shy children, they play the role of social misfits and deviants in a class with more active sport participation, and they then believe they possess personal inadequacies due to the negative self-attribution tendency [63,64]. Thus, they may suffer more negative impacts from sport participation. Therefore, we hypothesized that shy children in high-class-sport-participation environments would develop more internalizing problems than shy children in low-class-sport-participation environments.

In addition, class sport participation is also reasonable as a moderator in the relation between shyness and sport engagement. Shy children often undergo feelings of self-consciousness, worry, and anxiety when engaging in high social interactions [7]. For example, in group play activities, shy children may behave by hovering, onlooking, and avoiding approaching [3,65]. When shy children partake in class sports activities, they may derive less enjoyment from the experience, which means less sport engagement based on the affective component of sport engagement [48]. Meanwhile, shy children are less likely to be included in class sports activities, which may lead to less bonding with other participants in class sports, meaning less relational sport engagement [51]. Therefore, we hypothesized that shy children in high-class-sport-participation environments would have less sport engagement than shy children in low-class-sport-participation environments.

1.4. The Present Study

This study aimed to evaluate a model linking shyness, sport engagement, class sport participation, and internalizing problems among Chinese children. Based on the relevant theories and empirical literature, the following hypotheses were forwarded: (a) shyness would be positively related to internalizing problems (depression, loneliness, and social anxiety); (b) sport engagement would mediate the relations between shyness and internalizing problems; and (c) the relations between shyness and internalizing problems as well as shyness and sport engagement would be moderated by class sport participation. It should be mentioned that the amount of time spent with peers develops steadily from middle childhood through to early adolescence [66], and peers become increasingly significant in children's daily lives throughout this developmental stage [67]. Consequently, withdrawing from social interactions may be considered as particularly unfavorable and undesirable during this stage. In the context of traditional culture in China, social interactions have become increasingly crucial; disengagement from social settings could potentially lead to increased distress for socially withdrawn individuals, such as shy children [25]. Accordingly, we focused on children in middle childhood and early adolescence.

2. Materials and Methods

2.1. Participants

The participants were N = 951 students (509 boys, age range = 8.75 to 13.34 years old, Mage = 11.29 years, SD = 1.47 years) in grades 3 to 7 from public primary and middle schools in the urban areas of Shanghai, China. The participants included 181 third graders (Mage = 9.38 years, SD = 0.49 years), 240 fourth graders (Mage = 10.26 years, SD = 0.46 years), 169 fifth graders (Mage = 11.30 years, SD = 0.47 years), 180 sixth graders (Mage = 12.31 years, SD = 0.46 years), and 181 seventh graders (Mage = 13.41 years, SD = 0.49 years), respectively. The sample was drawn from 21 classes in total, with an average of approximately 45 students per class. All children in this sample were of the Han ethnicity, which is the predominant ethnic group in China.

2.2. Measures

2.2.1. Shyness

The Chinese version of the Children's Shyness Questionnaire (CSQ) was used to measure shyness [1], which consists of 19 items related to shyness (e.g., "I find it difficult to talk to people I don't know", "I feel nervous when I am with important people", etc.). Children were asked to rate each item on a 3-point scale, ranging from 1 = no to 3 = yes. Higher average scores indicated greater levels of shyness. This measure has demonstrated good psychometric properties and reliability in previous studies with Chinese children [36], with a Cronbach's alpha of 0.88 in the present study.

2.2.2. Sport Engagement and Class Sport Participation

Sport engagement and class sport participation were assessed using the Chinese version of the Snapshot Survey of Engagement tool—Revised (The Snapshot Survey of Engagement tool—Revised was validated among Chinese individuals ($n = 535$). A confirmatory factors analysis (CFA) indicated that the data fit well, $\chi^2 = 163.31$, $df = 38$, $p < 0.001$, CFI = 0.97, TLI = 0.95, RMSEA = 0.06, and SRMR = 0.03, and all loadings for items ranged from 0.66 to 0.89), which includes 11 items and has a reliability of $\alpha = 0.91$ [68–70]. Nine of these items assess three aspects of sport engagement—cognitive engagement, affective engagement, and relational engagement —on a 4-point scale ranging from 1 (not at all) to 4 (a lot). For example, cognitive engagement includes items like "I really focus on sports activities when I am doing it", affective engagement includes items like "I enjoy sports activities and have fun when I am involved", and relational engagement includes items like "Sports activities help me connect to something greater than myself". Higher average scores reflect greater sport engagement. The remaining two items measure sport participation by asking children how often they participate in sports activities (e.g., "How often do you participate in sports activities?") and how long they have been involved (e.g., "How long have you been involved in sports activities?"). The responses for frequency range from 1 (achieved it just once) to 6 (several times a week), and for duration from 1 (just started) to 6 (more than 5 years) [9]. These frequency and duration scores are multiplied to create an individual sport participation score, which is then averaged to calculate the class sport participation score. Higher scores indicate greater class sport participation.

2.2.3. Depression

A 14-item measure of the Children's Depression Inventory (CDI) was used to assess children's depressive symptoms [71]. Each item offers three possible responses to capture the frequency and intensity of depressive feelings, such as "I feel like crying every day", "I feel like crying most days", and "I feel like crying once in a while". Children were asked to choose the statement that best represented their feelings over the past two weeks. An average score was then calculated for each child, with higher scores indicating more severe depressive symptoms. This tool has been validated and shown to be reliable in previous research involving Chinese children [72], with the present study reporting a Cronbach's alpha of 0.87.

2.2.4. Social Anxiety

The Social Anxiety Scale for Children—Revised, developed by La Greca and Stone [73], was used to measure children's social anxiety. Children completed the Chinese version of this scale, adapted by Liu et al. [74], which consists of 15 items rated on a 5-point scale ranging from 1 (never) to 5 (always). An example item is "Kids are making fun of me". Higher average scores on this scale indicate greater levels of social anxiety. This scale has demonstrated reliability and validity in studies with Chinese students [74], with the current study reporting a Cronbach's alpha of 0.92.

2.2.5. Loneliness

Loneliness was measured using the Children's Loneliness Scale, a self-report measure adapted from Asher [75]. This scale includes 16 items, such as "I don't have any friends", which are rated on a 5-point scale from 1 (not at all true) to 5 (always true). An average loneliness score was calculated for each child, with higher scores indicating greater feelings of loneliness. This measure has been validated and shown to be reliable in previous research with Chinese children [76], with the current study reporting a Cronbach's alpha of 0.92.

2.3. Procedure

Children completed self-report measures that were group-administered during class time on a school day. The administration of the measures was carried out by trained researchers (i.e., graduate students). The Research Ethics Committee of Shanghai Normal University (No. 2023026) approved this study in 2021, which was carried out in compliance with the standards of the Declaration of Helsinki. Written informed consent was obtained from all students and their parents through the school beforehand. Extensive explanations of the procedure were provided during the administration. No evidence was found that the children had difficulties understanding the procedure or the items in the measures. Recruitment and data collection were all completed at the end of semester.

2.4. Plan of Data Analysis

Two-level hierarchical linear modeling (HLM) was conducted to examine the main effect, the mediating effect of sport engagement, and the moderating effect of class sport participation [77]. The analyses were conducted by SPSS 23.0 and Mplus 8.0. Drawing on previous studies [47,48,78,79], two latent variables were created as follows: sport engagement (cognitive engagement, affective engagement, and relational engagement) and internalizing problems (depression, loneliness, and social anxiety). Shyness, sport engagement, and internalizing problems were included as individual-level predictors, and child gender and individual sport participation were included as control variables at the individual level. Class sport participation was included as a group-level predictor, and class size and grade were included as control variables at the class level. As suggested by Enders and Tofighi [80], the selection of centering should not be based on statistical evidence but instead depends on substantive research questions. Group-mean centering is appropriate when the primary substantive interest involves a Level 1 (i.e., individual level) predictor, while grand-mean centering is suitable for interactions involving Level 2 (i.e., class level) variables. Thus, shyness was group-mean centered, and class sport participation was grand-mean centered.

3. Results

3.1. Descriptive Statistics

A MANOVA was conducted to test the effect of gender on all study variables. A significant effect of gender was found: Wilk's $\lambda = 0.90$, $F (7, 897) = 13.82$, $p < 0.001$, and $\eta^2 = 0.10$. Follow-up univariate analysis indicated that girls had higher scores on shyness and social anxiety and lower scores on individual sport participation and sport engagement (including cognitive engagement, affective engagement, and relational engagement) than boys. Detailed descriptive statistics are presented in Table 1. The magnitudes of the intercorrelations among the variables ranged from low to moderate, indicating that these variables measured different but related aspects of child adjustment. Pearson correlations among variables are presented in Table 2.

Table 1. Means and standard deviations of study variables.

Variable	Boys	Girls
Shyness	1.44 (0.45)	1.56 (0.41)
Cognitive engagement	3.25 (0.77)	2.87 (0.81)
Affective engagement	3.28 (0.81)	2.93 (0.92)
Relational engagement	3.20 (0.84)	2.97 (0.91)
Social anxiety	1.99 (0.84)	2.20 (0.91)
Depression	1.40 (0.33)	1.42 (0.38)
Loneliness	1.92 (0.71)	1.90 (0.75)
Individual sport participation	24.28 (11.52)	22.68 (12.08)

Note: standard deviations are in parenthesis.

Table 2. Pearson correlations among study variables.

Variable	1	2	3	4	5	6	7
1. Shyness	-						
2. Cognitive engagement	−0.31 **	-					
3. Affective engagement	−0.32 **	0.79 **	-				
4. Relational engagement	−0.30 **	0.74 **	0.77 **	-			
5. Depression	0.53 **	−0.37 **	−0.39 **	−0.41 **	-		
6. Loneliness	0.47 **	−0.35 **	−0.36 **	−0.40 **	0.64 **	-	
7. Social anxiety	0.74 **	−0.30 **	−0.32 **	−0.33 **	0.65 **	0.54 **	-
8. Class sport participation	0.11 **	−0.15 **	−0.11 **	−0.08 *	0.14 **	−0.02	0.14 **

Note: * $p < 0.05$. ** $p < 0.01$.

3.2. Testing Cross-Level Moderated Mediation Model

The HLM results regarding the main effects of the individual- and class-level variables and the cross-level interactions between shyness and class sport participation are presented in Table 3 and Figure 1. For within-group associations, shyness was positively associated with internalizing problems and negatively associated with sport engagement. Sport engagement was negatively associated with internalizing problems. For between-group associations, the results showed that after controlling for shyness, sport engagement, and internalizing problems, class sport participation was positively associated with internalizing problems and negatively associated with sport engagement.

Table 3. Results of hypotheses testing.

	Model 1		Model 2		Model 3
Variables	Internalizing Problems	Sport Engagement	Internalizing Problems	Sport Engagement	Internalizing Problems
Individual level					
Gender	−0.03 (0.03)	−0.15 *** (0.03)	−0.08 ** (0.03)	0.35 *** (0.08)	0.28 *** (0.07)
ISP	−0.09 *** (0.03)	0.26 *** (0.04)	−0.03 (0.03)	0.04 *** (0.01)	−0.01 ** (0.01)
Shyness	0.79 *** (0.02)	−0.31 *** (0.03)	0.71 *** (0.03)	−0.77 *** (0.12)	0.67 *** (0.26)
Sport engagement			−0.24 *** (0.04)		−0.32 *** (0.07)
Class level					
Class size				−0.01 (0.14)	−0.03 (0.09)
CSP				−0.30 *** (0.03)	0.10 *** (0.03)
Shyness × CSP				−0.06 ** (0.03)	0.09 * (0.04)

Notes. ISP = individual sport participation; CSP = class sport participation. Standard errors are in parenthesis. * $p < 0.05$. ** $p < 0.01$. *** $p < 0.001$.

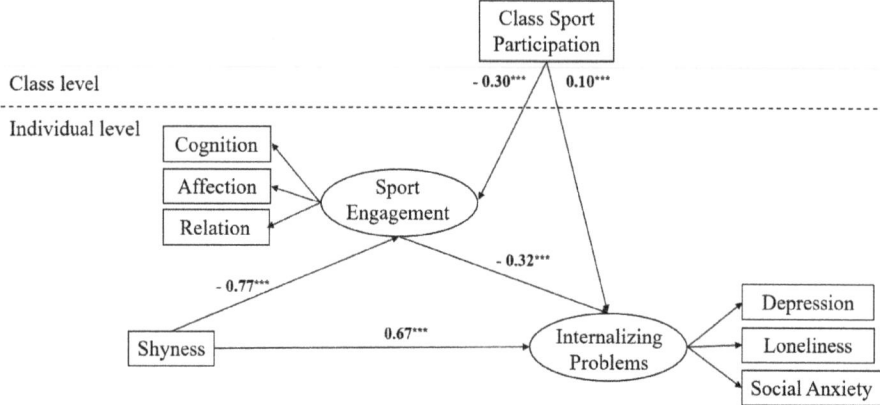

Figure 1. Estimates of moderated mediation model for shyness on internalizing problems.
*** $p < 0.001$.

For the mediating effect, we found that shyness was negatively associated with sport engagement ($\beta = -0.31$, $p < 0.001$, Model 2) and, in turn, sport engagement was negatively associated with internalizing problems ($\beta = -0.24$, $p < 0.001$, Model 2). The positive relations between shyness and internalizing problems were significant when sport engagement entered in the same model ($\beta = 0.71$, $p < 0.001$, Model 2). These results suggest that sport engagement partially mediated the relations between shyness and internalizing problems.

For the moderating effects, there were significant shyness × class sport participation interactions on sport engagement ($\gamma = -0.06$, $p < 0.05$, Model 3) and internalizing problems ($\gamma = 0.09$, $p < 0.05$, Model 3). Follow-up simple slope tests were conducted to understand the moderating effects of class sport participation following the approaches suggested by Aiken and West [81]. Specifically, the associations of internalizing problems–shyness and sport engagement–shyness were plotted at a high value (1 *SD* above the mean) and a low value (1 *SD* below the mean) of class sport participation, respectively. The results are presented in Figures 2 and 3. As illustrated in the figures, the associations between shyness and internalizing problems were stronger in classes with higher class sport participation (*simple slope* = 1.02, $p < 0.001$) than in classes with lower class sport participation (*simple slope* = 0.31, $p < 0.001$). In addition, the associations between shyness and sport engagement were stronger in classes with higher class sport participation (*simple slope* = −1.03, $p < 0.001$) than in classes with lower class sport participation (*simple slope* = −0.51, $p < 0.001$). In summary, higher class sport participation made children with high shyness have less sport engagement than lower class sport participation. Additionally, higher class sport participation made children with high shyness have more internalizing problems than lower class sport participation.

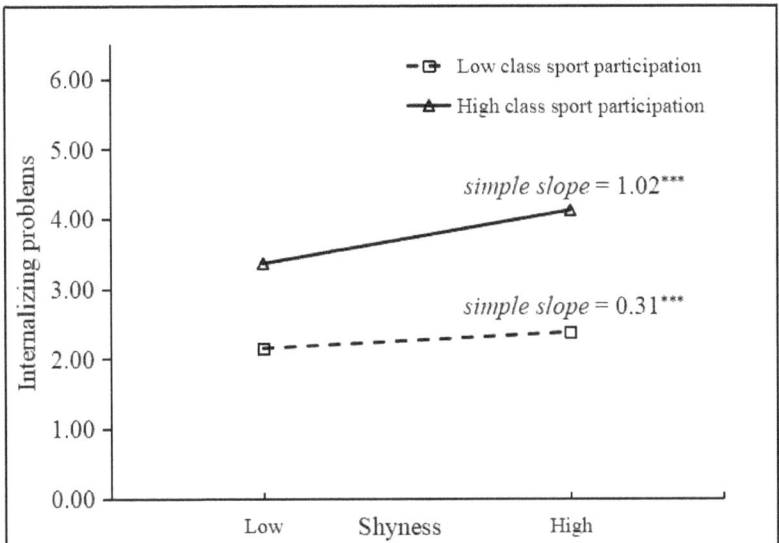

Figure 2. Moderating effect of class sport participation on the relations between shyness and internalizing problems. ($\gamma = 0.09$, $p < 0.05$). *** $p < 0.001$.

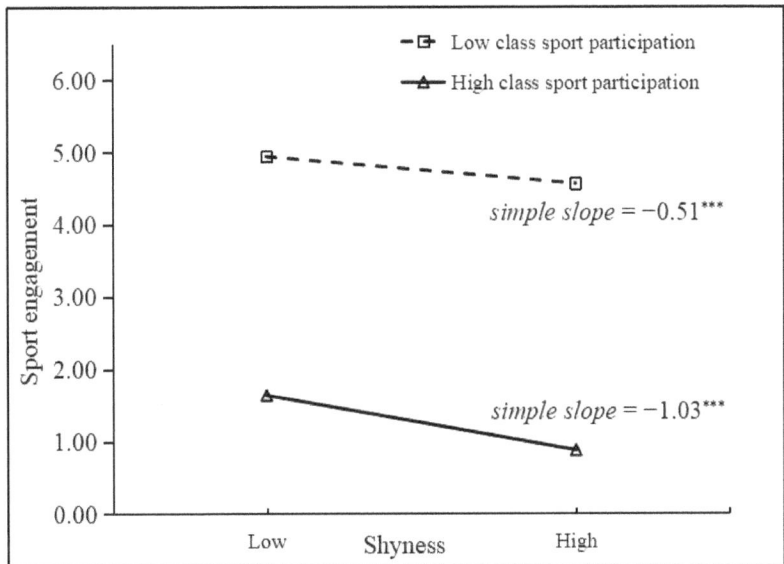

Figure 3. Moderating effect of class sport participation on the relations between shyness and sport engagement. ($\gamma = -0.06$, $p < 0.05$). *** $p < 0.001$.

4. Discussion

Previous studies have demonstrated that shyness is associated with internalizing problems among Chinese children [6,22]. However, the underlying mechanisms are not well understood. Therefore, we investigated a model linking shyness, sport engagement, class sport participation, and internalizing problems among Chinese children. Our findings demonstrate that sport engagement mediated the relations between shyness and internalizing problems. In addition, our result also indicated that class sport participation plays a moderating role between shyness and internalizing problems, as well as between shyness and sport engagement.

4.1. Shyness, Sport Engagement, and Internalizing Problems

We found evidence that shyness is negatively associated with sport engagement, which, in turn, was negatively associated with internalizing problems. To the best of our knowledge, this is the first study to demonstrate that sport engagement mediates the relations between shyness and internalizing problems among Chinese youth. Consistent with previous research, shyness has consistent links with indices of internalizing problems from early childhood through adolescence (e.g., loneliness, anxiety, and depressive symptoms) [82–84]. Shy children may experience heightened feelings of worry, anxiety, and rumination, especially when facing stressful situations, such as sports with peers [7]. They may not like engaging in sports due to the social interaction and communication, leading to negative thoughts about the sport and unwillingness to invest in the sport. Indeed, previous findings suggest that shy children reported less engagement in sports activities [49,85]. Sport engagement may be a salient factor for internalizing outcomes associated with shyness [86]. Individuals may experience a sense of belonging, intimate friendships, fellowship, and positive peer relationships through engaging in sports activities, all of which are linked to better mental health [60,87]. The need to belong is thought to be most important in terms of buffering against perceptions of loneliness. Intimate relationships also provide an important source of emotional support and happiness, which is beneficial to relieve depression and social anxiety [88]. Positive social contact within the context of valued relationships with people is seen as essential for greater emotional well-being [59]. In contrast, when individuals experience lower levels of sport engagement, negative thoughts may arise and feelings of connection with others may diminish, which, in turn, was associated with higher levels of internalizing problems. Take together, in our study, the less sports shy children were involved in, the more internalizing problems they experienced.

4.2. Role of Class Sport Participation

We further found that class sport participation played a moderating role in the relations between shyness and internalizing problems as well as shyness and sport engagement. Specifically, a stronger sports environment in class is likely to lead to less sport engagement and more internalizing problems among shy children. Sports for children and adolescents are frequently performed within group settings such as classes [89]. Feeling of social wariness and self-consciousness may cause shy children to withdraw from opportunities to participate in class sports, resulting in their inability to enjoy and engage in sports activities. Shy children may constitute a minority group in classes where sports are popular, making them more prone to being overlooked by peers, leading to a significant psychological disparity. The team collaboration and competitive atmosphere of class sports competitions may be related to experiences of stress, which would exacerbate anxiety and tension in shy children [90]. Moreover, due to their negative attribution and poor emotion regulation ability, shy children may experience more internalizing problems [91]. In addition, according to the "healthy environment paradox" theory, despite an overall positive or healthy environment, certain individuals or groups may still experience significant difficulties, leading to negative outcomes within that context [61]. In the present study, in classes with a stronger sports environment, children who are shy and dislike sports may feel increased pressure to deal with the group activities. Due to the peer pressure and the fear of their performance in sports, shy children may disengage from sports activities, which, in turn, exacerbates the internalizing problems [92].

4.3. Limitations and Implications

The present study explored the internal mechanism and factors between shyness and internalizing problems. However, there are several limitations that must be considered. The first limitation arises from the cross-sectional, single-source research design of this study. Although we theoretically delineated the causal relations among variables, the design features increase the possibility that the results are influenced by common method variance and limit our ability to establish causal relations [93–95]. Thus, future research could use longitudinal or experimental approaches to examine the causal nature of these relations. Second, we used a multi-level modeling approach to analyze hierarchical data in this study, which may risk underestimating the effects. The method of Multi-level Structural Equation Modeling (MSEM) is recommended to produce more accurate estimated effects and confidence intervals [96]. Despite this, there are some challenges of using MSEM; serious convergence issues may be encountered with MSEM estimates based on fewer than 80 groups [97]. Due to its accuracy and precision in latent variable models, MSEM is still recommended for further studies, which should consider enlarging the sample size at the school level. Third, we conducted the study in urban China where the sociocultural context is different from other Chinese contexts, which limits the generalizability of the findings to other suburban or rural areas of China. Given that there are significant geographical differences in terms of social and cultural values within China, these results should be interpreted with caution when generalizing to other regions and cultures. Fourth, the measurement of sport engagement in this study was limited to the school context, without distinguishing between individual sports and team sports. Future studies could employ more detailed and effective measurements to differentiate between these types of sports activities. Finally, there are potential effects of other mediating variables that have not been discovered, such as perceived positive effects of exercise and exercise efficacy [98]. These are also considered as important variables, which are affected by individual cognition and exercise experience and deserve further attention. Future research should investigate other potential pathways to gain a more comprehensive understanding of the complex interplay between these variables.

Despite these limitations, by exploring the underlying mechanism of the relations between shyness and internalizing problems, this study extends existing research by uncovering the mediating role of sport engagement and expanding the mediation model to include the cross-level moderating effect of class sport participation. Our findings provide educational guidelines and suggestions about how to alleviate internalization problems among shy children. First, our findings have demonstrated that sport engagement is a mediator linking shyness to internalizing problems. This finding implies that wider sport engagement within the school can be essential in reducing loneliness, depression, and social anxiety among shy students. In this regard, more accessible, inclusive, and diverse sports activities should be available for students to choose from, especially for shy individuals. Second, it was found that class sport participation moderates the relations between shyness and internalizing problems as well as shyness and sport engagement. It means that the plight of shy children should be improved not only from an individual perspective but also from a group perspective such as the class. For example, teachers or coaches could build an autonomic and relaxed class sport atmosphere, which could promote shy students to establish more positive self-evaluation of their social capacity. Finally, professionals or coaches could help shy students by creating more sport programs that meet their individual needs and interests. These programs could involve sports that enhance engagement, participation, social skills, and self-esteem, and, more importantly, can be delivered in a supportive and inclusive sport environment.

5. Conclusions

Our study tested a multi-level moderated mediation model of sport engagement as a mediator and class sport participation as a moderator between shyness and internalizing problems among Chinese children. The results suggest that shyness is related to lower levels of sport engagement, which, in turn, is associated with lower levels of internalizing problems. A higher level of class sport participation is associated with lower sport engagement and higher internalizing problems among shy children in China. The mechanisms of these relations may inform prevention and early intervention programs for internalizing problems through the strength of class sport participation. This highlights the importance of considering individual experiences and needs within broader social contexts, rather than assuming that a positive environment guarantees positive outcomes for everyone.

Author Contributions: Conceptualization, X.D. and W.D.; methodology, X.Z. and R.Z.; software, X.Z.; validation, M.L., J.W. and X.D.; formal analysis, R.Z. and X.K.; investigation, M.L. and J.W.; resources, X.D.; data curation, X.Z.; writing—original draft preparation, R.Z., X.K. and M.L.; writing—review and editing, X.D. and W.D.; supervision, X.D. and W.D.; project administration, X.D.; funding acquisition, X.D. All authors have read and agreed to the published version of the manuscript.

Funding: This research was supported by the National Natural Science Foundation of China (32000756).

Institutional Review Board Statement: The study was conducted in accordance with the Declaration of Helsinki, and approved by the Institutional Review Board of Shanghai Normal University (No. 2023026, 1 January 2021).

Informed Consent Statement: Informed consent was obtained from all subjects involved in the study.

Data Availability Statement: The data presented in this study are available on request from the corresponding author.

Conflicts of Interest: The authors declare no conflicts of interest.

References

1. Crozier, W.R. Shyness and self-esteem in middle childhood. *Br. J. Educ. Psychol.* **1995**, *65*, 85–95. [CrossRef]
2. Goldsmith, H.H.; Lemery, K.S.; Aksan, N.; Buss, K.A. Temperamental substrates of personality development. In *Temperament and Personality Development across the Life Span*; Molfese, V.J., Molfese, D.L., Eds.; Lawrence Erlbaum Associates: Mahwah, NJ, USA, 2000; pp. 1–32.
3. Asendorpf, J.B. Beyond social withdrawal: Shyness, unsociability, and peer avoidance. *Hum. Dev.* **1990**, *33*, 250–259. [CrossRef]
4. Coplan, R.J.; DeBow, A.; Schneider, B.H.; Graham, A.A. The social behaviors of extremely inhibited children in and out of preschool. *Br. J. Dev. Psychol.* **2009**, *27*, 891–905. [CrossRef] [PubMed]
5. Baardstu, S.; Coplan, R.J.; Karevold, E.B.; Laceulle, O.M.; von Soest, T. Longitudinal pathways from shyness in early childhood to personality in adolescence: Do peers matter? *J. Res. Adolesc.* **2020**, *30*, 362–379. [CrossRef]
6. Ding, X.; Zhang, W.; Ooi, L.L.; Coplan, R.J.; Zhu, X.; Sang, B. Relations between social withdrawal subtypes and socio-emotional adjustment among Chinese children and early adolescents. *J. Res. Adolesc.* **2023**, *33*, 774–785. [CrossRef]
7. Rubin, K.H.; Coplan, R.J.; Bowker, J.C. Social withdrawal in childhood. *Annu. Rev. Psychol.* **2009**, *60*, 141–171. [CrossRef]
8. Guilmette, M.; Mulvihill, K.; Villemaire-Krajden, R.; Barker, E.T. Past and present participation in extracurricular activities is associated with adaptive self-regulation of goals, academic success, and emotional well-being among university students. *Learn. Individ. Differ.* **2019**, *73*, 8–15. [CrossRef]
9. Ramey, H.L.; Busseri, M.A.; Khanna, N.; Hamilton, Y.N.; Ottawa, Y.N.; Rose-Krasnor, L. Youth engagement and suicide risk: Testing a mediated model in a Canadian community sample. *J. Youth Adolesc.* **2010**, *39*, 243–258. [CrossRef]
10. Liang, Y.; Guo, H.; Yi, H. Use IoT in physical education and sport in China schools. *Wirel. Commun. Mob. Comput.* **2022**, *2022*, 8133279. [CrossRef]
11. Busseri, M.A.; Rose-Krasnor, L.; Mark Pancer, S.; Pratt, M.W.; Adams, G.R.; Birnie-Lefcovitch, S.; Polivy, J.; Gallander Wintre, M. A longitudinal study of breadth and intensity of activity involvement and the transition to university. *J. Adolesc. Res.* **2011**, *21*, 512–518. [CrossRef]
12. Ladd, G.W.; Kochenderfer-Ladd, B.; Eggum, N.D.; Kochel, K.P.; McConnell, E.M. Characterizing and comparing the friendships of anxious-solitary and unsociable preadolescents. *Child Dev.* **2011**, *82*, 1434–1453. [CrossRef] [PubMed]
13. Hawkley, L.C.; Capitanio, J.P. Perceived social isolation, evolutionary fitness and health outcomes: A lifespan approach. *Philos. Trans. R. Soc. B Biol. Sci.* **2015**, *370*, 20140114. [CrossRef]
14. Ollendick, T.H.; Hirshfeld-Becker, D.R. The developmental psychopathology of social anxiety disorder. *Biol. Psychiatry* **2002**, *51*, 44–58. [CrossRef] [PubMed]
15. Thapar, A.; Collishaw, S.; Pine, D.S.; Thapar, A.K. Depression in adolescence. *Lancet* **2012**, *379*, 1056–1067. [CrossRef]
16. Hodges, E.V.; Boivin, M.; Vitaro, F.; Bukowski, W.M. The power of friendship: Protection against an escalating cycle of peer victimization. *Dev. Psychol.* **1999**, *35*, 94–101. [CrossRef]
17. Rubin, K.H.; LeMare, L.J.; Lollis, S. Social withdrawal in childhood: Developmental pathways to peer rejection. In *Peer Rejection in Childhood*; Asher, S.R., Coie, J.D., Eds.; Cambridge University Press: Cambridge, UK, 1990; pp. 217–249.
18. Bowker, J.C.; Raja, R. Social withdrawal sub-types during early adolescence in India. *J. Abnorm. Child Psychol.* **2011**, *39*, 201–212. [CrossRef]

19. Jahng, K.E.; Kim, Y. Relationships between children' s shyness, play disconnection, and loneliness: Moderating effect of children' s perceived child-teacher intimate relationship. *Child Psychiatry Hum. Dev.* **2021**, *52*, 829–840. [CrossRef]
20. Hwang, J.E.; Lee, K.H. The mediating effect of friendship quality sub-factors on the relationship of shyness and loneliness: With a focus on 5th, 6th grade boys and girls. *Stud. Korean Youth* **2009**, *53*, 65–89.
21. Coplan, R.J.; Rose-Krasnor, L.; Weeks, M.; Kingsbury, A.; Kingsbury, M.; Bullock, A. Alone is a crowd: Social motivations, social withdrawal, and socioemotional functioning in later childhood. *Dev. Psychol.* **2013**, *49*, 861–875. [CrossRef] [PubMed]
22. Ding, X.; Chen, X.; Fu, R.; Li, D.; Liu, J. Relations of shyness and unsociability with adjustment in migrant and non-migrant children in urban China. *J. Abnorm. Child Psychol.* **2020**, *48*, 289–300. [CrossRef]
23. Sang, B.; Ding, X.; Coplan, R.J.; Liu, J.; Pan, T.; Feng, X. Assessment and implications of social avoidance in Chinese early adolescents. *J. Early Adolesc.* **2018**, *38*, 554–573. [CrossRef]
24. Yang, P.; Xu, G.; Zhao, S.; Li, D.; Liu, J.; Chen, X. Shyness and psychological maladjustment in Chinese adolescents: Selection and influence processes in friendship networks. *J. Youth Adolesc.* **2021**, *50*, 2108–2121. [CrossRef] [PubMed]
25. Zhang, S.; Xiao, B.; Zhang, Y.; Zhu, X.; Dong, Q.; Ding, X. Relation between social avoidance and loneliness in urban Chinese children: A moderated-mediation model. *Eur. J. Dev. Psychol.* **2024**, *21*, 171–187. [CrossRef]
26. Tan, J.; Ai, Y.; Wu, Y.; Wen, X.; Wang, W. Relationship between shyness and loneliness among Chinese adolescents: Social support as mediator. *Soc. Behav. Personal. Int. J.* **2016**, *44*, 201–208. [CrossRef]
27. Dill, J.C.; Anderson, C.A. Loneliness, shyness, and depression: The etiology and interrelationships of everyday problems in living. In *The Interactional Nature of Depression: Advances in Interpersonal Approaches*; Joiner, T., Coyne, J.C., Eds.; American Psychological Association: Washington, DC, USA, 1999; pp. 93–125.
28. Coplan, R.J.; Prakash, K.; O' Neil, K. Do you "want" to play? Distinguishing between conflicted shyness and social disinterest in early childhood. *Dev. Psychol.* **2004**, *40*, 244–258. [CrossRef] [PubMed]
29. Coplan, R.J.; Arbeau, K.A.; Armer, M. Don't fret, be supportive! Maternal characteristics linking child shyness to psychosocial and school adjustment in kindergarten. *J. Abnorm. Child Psychol.* **2008**, *36*, 359–371. [CrossRef] [PubMed]
30. Chen, X.; Yang, F.; Wang, L. Relations between shyness-sensitivity and internalizing problems in Chinese children: Moderating effects of academic achievement. *J. Abnorm. Child Psychol.* **2013**, *41*, 825–836. [CrossRef] [PubMed]
31. Eggum-Wilkens, N.D.; Valiente, C.; Swanson, J.; Lemery-Chalfant, K. Children's shyness, popularity, school liking, cooperative participation, and internalizing problems in the early school years. *Early Child. Res. Q.* **2014**, *29*, 85–94. [CrossRef]
32. Yang, P.; Coplan, R.J.; Zhang, Y.; Ding, X.; Zhu, Z. Assessment and implications of aloneliness in Chinese children and early adolescents. *J. Appl. Dev. Psychol.* **2023**, *85*, 101514. [CrossRef]
33. Clark, D.M.; Wells, A. A cognitive model of social phobia. In *Social Phobia: Diagnosis, Assessment, and Treatment*; Heimberg, R.G., Liebowitz, M., Hope, D., Scheier, F., Eds.; The Guilford Press: New York, NY, USA, 1995; pp. 69–93.
34. Weeks, M.; Ooi, L.L.; Coplan, R.J. Cognitive biases and the link between shyness and social anxiety in early adolescence. *J. Early Adolesc.* **2016**, *36*, 1095–1117. [CrossRef]
35. Blöte, A.W.; Miers, A.C.; Van den Bos, E.; Westenberg, P.M. Negative social self-cognitions: How shyness may lead to social anxiety. *J. Appl. Dev. Psychol.* **2019**, *63*, 9–15. [CrossRef]
36. Ding, X.; Liu, J.; Coplan, R.J.; Chen, X.; Li, D.; Sang, B. Self-reported shyness in Chinese children: Validation of the children' s shyness questionnaire and exploration of its links with adjustment and the role of coping. *Personal. Individ. Differ.* **2014**, *68*, 183–188. [CrossRef]
37. Kong, X.; Brook, C.A.; Li, J.; Li, Y.; Schmidt, L.A. Shyness sub-types and associations with social anxiety: A comparison study of Canadian and Chinese children. *Dev. Sci.* **2023**, e13369. [CrossRef]
38. Ran, G.; Zhang, Q.; Huang, H. Behavioral inhibition system and self-esteem as mediators between shyness and social anxiety. *Psychiatry Res.* **2018**, *270*, 568–573. [CrossRef]
39. Chen, X. Culture and shyness in childhood and adolescence. *New Ideas Psychol.* **2019**, *53*, 58–66. [CrossRef]
40. Greenfield, P.M.; Suzuki, L.K.; Rothstein-Fisch, C. Cultural pathways through human development. In *Handbook of Child Psychology*; Renninger, K.A., Sigel, I.E., Damon, W., Lerner, R.M., Eds.; John Wiley & Sons, Inc: New York, NY, USA, 2006; pp. 655–699.
41. Xu, Y.; Farver, J.A.M.; Chang, L.; Zhang, Z.; Yu, L. Moving away or fitting in? Understanding shyness in Chinese children. *Merrill. Palmer. Q.* **2007**, *53*, 527–556. [CrossRef]
42. Chen, X. Shyness-inhibition in childhood and adolescence: A cross-cultural perspective. In *The Development of Shyness and Social Withdrawal*; Rubin, K.H., Coplan, R.J., Eds.; The Guilford Press: New York, NY, USA, 2010; pp. 213–235.
43. Liu, J.; Bowker, J.C.; Coplan, R.J.; Yang, P.; Li, D.; Chen, X. Evaluating links among shyness, peer relations, and internalizing problems in Chinese young adolescents. *J. Res. Adolesc.* **2019**, *29*, 696–709. [CrossRef]
44. Chen, X.; Cen, G.; Li, D.; He, Y. Social functioning and adjustment in Chinese children: The imprint of historical time. *Child Dev.* **2005**, *76*, 182–195. [CrossRef] [PubMed]
45. Liu, J.; Chen, X.; Li, D.; French, D. Shyness-sensitivity, aggression, and adjustment in urban Chinese adolescents at different historical times. *J. Res. Adolesc.* **2012**, *22*, 393–399. [CrossRef]
46. Ryan, R.M.; Deci, E.L. Self-determination theory and the facilitation of intrinsic motivation, social development, and well-being. *Am. Psychol.* **2000**, *55*, 68–78. [CrossRef]

47. Ramey, H.L.; Rose-Krasnor, L.; Busseri, M.A.; Gadbois, S.; Bowker, A.; Findlay, L. Measuring psychological engagement in youth activity involvement. *J. Adolesc.* **2015**, *45*, 237–249. [CrossRef]
48. Xiao, B.; Bullock, A.; Coplan, R.J. Shyness, extracurricular activity engagement, and internalizing problems among emerging adults in university. *Canadian J. Behav. Sci.* **2023**. [CrossRef]
49. Schneider, B.H.; Younger, A.J.; Smith, T.; Freeman, P. A longitudinal exploration of the cross-contextual stability of social withdrawal in early adolescence. *J. Early Adolesc.* **1998**, *18*, 374–396. [CrossRef]
50. Prakash, K.; Coplan, R.J. Shy skaters? Shyness, coping, and adjustment outcomes in female adolescent figure skaters. *Athl. Insight* **2003**, *5*, 1–19.
51. Miller, S.R. I don't want to get involved: Shyness, psychological control, and youth activities. *J. Soc. Pers. Relat.* **2012**, *29*, 908–929. [CrossRef]
52. Findlay, L.C.; Coplan, R.J. Come out and play: Shyness in childhood and the benefits of organized sports participation. *Can. J. Behav. Sci.* **2008**, *40*, 153–161. [CrossRef]
53. Fletcher, A.C.; Nickerson, P.; Wright, K.L. Structured leisure activities in middle childhood: Links to well-being. *J. Community Psychol.* **2003**, *31*, 641–659. [CrossRef]
54. Schumacher, A.; Dimech, A.; Seiler, R. Extra-curricular sport participation: A potential buffer against social anxiety symptoms in primary school children. *Psychol. Sport Exerc.* **2011**, *12*, 347–354. [CrossRef]
55. Page, R.M.; Frey, J.; Talbert, R.; Falk, C. Children's feelings of loneliness and social dissatisfaction: Relationship to measures of physical fitness and activity. *J. Teach. Phys. Educ.* **1992**, *11*, 211–219. [CrossRef]
56. McHale, S.M.; Crouter, A.C.; Tucker, C. Free-time activities in middle childhood: Links with adjustment in early adolescence. *Child Dev.* **2001**, *72*, 1764–1778. [CrossRef]
57. Bronfebrenner, U. *The Ecology of Human Development: Experiments by Nature and Design*; Harvard University Press: Boston, MA, USA, 1979.
58. Chang, L. The role of classroom norms in contextualizing the relations of children's social behaviors to peer acceptance. *Dev. Psychol.* **2004**, *40*, 691–702. [CrossRef]
59. Haugen, T.; Säfvenbom, R.; Ommundsen, Y. Sport participation and loneliness in adolescents: The mediating role of perceived social competence. *Curr. Psychol.* **2013**, *32*, 203–216. [CrossRef]
60. Viau, A.; Denault, A.S.; Poulin, F. Organized activities during high school and adjustment one year post high school: Identifying social mediators. *J. Youth Adolesc.* **2015**, *44*, 1638–1651. [CrossRef]
61. Salmivalli, C. Peer victimization and adjustment in young adulthood: Commentary on the special section. *J. Abnorm. Child Psychol.* **2018**, *46*, 67–72. [CrossRef]
62. Bellmore, A.; Witkow, M.; Graham, S.; Juvonen, J. Beyond the individual: The impact of ethnic context and classroom behavioral norms on victims' adjustment. *Dev. Psychol.* **2004**, *40*, 1159–1172. [CrossRef]
63. Alden, L.E.; Phillips, N. An interpersonal analysis of social anxiety and depression. *Cognit. Ther. Res.* **1990**, *14*, 499–513. [CrossRef]
64. Bruch, M.A.; Belkin, D.K. Attributional style in shyness and depression: Shared and specific maladaptive patterns. *Cognit. Ther. Res.* **2001**, *25*, 247–259. [CrossRef]
65. Bekkhus, M.; McVarnock, A.; Coplan, R.J.; Ulset, V.; Kraft, B. Developmental changes in the structure of shyness and internalizing symptoms from early to middle childhood: A network analysis. *Child Dev.* **2023**, *94*, 1078–1086. [CrossRef]
66. Coplan, R.J.; Ooi, L.L.; Baldwin, D. Does it matter when we want to be alone? Exploring developmental timing effects in the implications of unsociability. *New Ideas Psychol.* **2019**, *53*, 47–57. [CrossRef]
67. Rubin, K.H.; Bukowski, W.M.; Bowker, J.C. Children in peer groups. In *Handbook of Child Psychology and Developmental Science*; Lerner, R.M., Bornstein, M.H., Leventhal, T., Eds.; John Wiley & Sons, Inc.: New York, NY, USA, 2015; pp. 175–222.
68. Busseri, M.A.; Rose-Krasnor, L. Subjective experiences in activity involvement and perceptions of growth in a sample of first-year female university students. *J. Coll. Stud. Dev.* **2008**, *49*, 425–442. [CrossRef]
69. Hu, L.T.; Bentler, P.M. Cutoff criteria for fit indexes in covariance structure analysis: Conventional criteria versus new alternatives. *Struct. Equ. Model. A Multidiscip. J.* **1999**, *6*, 1–55. [CrossRef]
70. Kline, R.B. *Principles and Practice of Structural Equation Modeling*, 2nd ed.; The Guilford Press: New York, NY, USA, 2005.
71. Kovacs, M. *The Children's Depression Inventory (CDI) Manual*, 1st ed.; Multi-Health Systems: Oppenheim, Germany, 1992.
72. Ding, X.; Coplan, R.J.; Deng, X.; Ooi, L.L.; Li, D.; Sang, B. Sad, scared, or rejected? A short-term longitudinal study of the predictors of social avoidance in Chinese children. *J. Abnorm. Child Psychol.* **2019**, *47*, 1265–1276. [CrossRef] [PubMed]
73. La Greca, A.M.; Stone, W.L. Social Anxiety Scale for Children-Revised: Factor structure and concurrent validity. *J. Clin. Child Psychol.* **1993**, *22*, 17–27. [CrossRef]
74. Liu, J.; Coplan, R.J.; Ooi, L.L.; Chen, X.; Li, D. Examining the implications of social anxiety in a community sample of Chinese mainland children. *J. Clin. Psychol.* **2015**, *71*, 979–993. [CrossRef] [PubMed]
75. Asher, S.R.; Hymel, S.; Renshaw, P.D. Loneliness in children. *Child Dev.* **1984**, *55*, 1456–1464. [CrossRef]
76. Li, M.; Jin, G.; Ren, T.; Haidabieke, A.; Chen, L.; Ding, X. Relations between Prosociality and Psychological Maladjustment in Chinese Elementary and Secondary School Students: Mediating Roles of Peer Preference and Self-Perceived Social Competence. *Behav. Sci.* **2023**, *13*, 547. [CrossRef]
77. Bryk, A.S.; Raudenbush, S.W. *Hierarchical Linear Models: Applications and Data Analysis Methods*; Sage Publications, Inc.: Thousand Oaks, CA, USA, 1992.

78. Liu, J.; Coplan, R.J.; Chen, X.; Li, D.; Ding, X.; Zhou, Y. Unsociability and shyness in Chinese children: Concurrent and predictive relations with indices of adjustment. *Soc. Dev.* **2014**, *23*, 119–136. [CrossRef]
79. Qualter, P.; Rouncefield-Swales, A.; Bray, L.; Blake, L.; Allen, S.; Probert, C.; Crook, K.; Carter, B. Depression, anxiety, and loneliness among adolescents and young adults with IBD in the UK: The role of disease severity, age of onset, and embarrassment of the condition. *Qual. Life Res.* **2021**, *30*, 497–506. [CrossRef]
80. Enders, C.K.; Tofighi, D. Centering predictor variables in cross-sectional multilevel models: A new look at an old issue. *Psychol. Methods* **2007**, *12*, 121–138. [CrossRef]
81. Aiken, L.S.; West, S.G. *Multiple Regression: Testing and Interpreting Interactions*; Sage Publications, Inc.: Thousand Oaks, CA, USA, 1991.
82. Coplan, R.J.; Closson, L.; Arbeau, K. Gender differences in the behavioral associates of loneliness and social dissatisfaction in kindergarten. *J. Child Psychol. Psychiatry* **2007**, *48*, 988–995. [CrossRef]
83. Hughes, K.; Coplan, R.J. Exploring the processes linking shyness and academic achievement in childhood. *Sch. Psychol. Q.* **2010**, *25*, 213–222. [CrossRef]
84. Volbrecht, M.M.; Goldsmith, H.H. Early temperamental and family predictors of shyness and anxiety. *Dev. Psychol.* **2010**, *46*, 1192–1205. [CrossRef] [PubMed]
85. Page, R.M.; Zarco, E.P. Shyness, physical activity, and sports team participation among Philippine high school students. *Child Study J.* **2001**, *31*, 193–204.
86. Miller, S.R.; Coll, E. From social withdrawal to social confidence: Evidence for possible pathways. *Curr. Psychol.* **2007**, *26*, 86–101. [CrossRef]
87. Bohnert, A.M.; Aikins, J.W.; Edidin, J. The role of organized activities in facilitating social adaptation across the transition to college. *J. Adolesc. Res.* **2007**, *22*, 189–208. [CrossRef]
88. Harkins, C.; Menezes, M.; Sadikova, E.; Mazurek, M. Friendship and anxiety/depression symptoms in boys with and without autism spectrum disorder. *Am. J. Intellect. Dev. Disabil.* **2023**, *128*, 119–133. [CrossRef] [PubMed]
89. Jekauc, D.; Reimers, A.K.; Wagner, M.O.; Woll, A. Physical activity in sports clubs of children and adolescents in Germany: Results from a nationwide representative survey. *Z. Gesundh. Wiss.* **2013**, *21*, 505–513. [CrossRef]
90. Larson, R.W.; Hansen, D.M.; Moneta, G. Differing profiles of developmental experiences across types of organized youth activities. *Dev. Psychol.* **2006**, *42*, 849–863. [CrossRef]
91. Hipson, W.E.; Coplan, R.J.; Séguin, D.G. Active emotion regulation mediates links between shyness and social adjustment in preschool. *Soc. Dev.* **2019**, *28*, 893–907. [CrossRef]
92. Lu, K.; Brown, C. Susceptibility to peer pressure among adolescents: Biological, demographic, and peer-related determinants. *J. Stud. Res.* **2023**, *11*, 1576. [CrossRef]
93. Evans, M.G. A Monte Carlo study of the effects of correlated method variance in moderated multiple regression analysis. *Organ. Behav. Hum. Decis. Process.* **1985**, *36*, 305–323. [CrossRef]
94. Podsakoff, P.M.; MacKenzie, S.B.; Lee, J.Y.; Podsakoff, N.P. Common method biases in behavioral research: A critical review of the literature and recommended remedies. *J. Appl. Psychol.* **2003**, *88*, 879–903. [CrossRef] [PubMed]
95. Siemsen, E.; Roth, A.; Oliveira, P. Common method bias in regression models with linear, quadratic, and interaction effects. *Organ. Res. Methods* **2010**, *13*, 456–476. [CrossRef]
96. MacKinnon, D.P.; Valente, M.J. Mediation from multilevel to structural equation modeling. *Ann. Nutr. Metab.* **2014**, *65*, 198–204. [CrossRef] [PubMed]
97. Li, X.; Beretvas, S.N. Sample size limits for estimating upper level mediation models using multilevel SEM. *Struct. Equ. Model.* **2013**, *20*, 241–264. [CrossRef]
98. Bang, H.; Won, D.; Park, S. School engagement, self-esteem, and depression of adolescents: The role of sport participation and volunteering activity and gender differences. *Child. Youth Serv. Rev.* **2020**, *113*, 105012. [CrossRef]

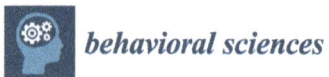

Article

The Risks of Being a Wallflower: Exploring Links Between Introversion, Aspects of Solitude, and Indices of Well-Being in Adolescence

Anna Stone [1], Megan DeGroot [1], Alicia McVarnock [1], Tiffany Cheng [1], Julie C. Bowker [2] and Robert J. Coplan [1,*]

[1] Department of Psychology, Carleton University, Ottawa, ON K1S 5B6, Canada; annastone@cmail.carleton.ca (A.S.); megandegroot@cmail.carleton.ca (M.D.); aliciamcvarnock@cmail.carleton.ca (A.M.); tiffanycheng@cmail.carleton.ca (T.C.)
[2] Department of Psychology, University at Buffalo, Buffalo, NY 14068, USA; jcbowker@buffalo.edu
* Correspondence: robert.coplan@carleton.ca

Abstract: The aim of the current study was to examine the unique relations between introversion and indices of well-being while accounting for aspects of solitude (i.e., time spent alone, shyness, affinity for solitude, and negative thinking while alone). Participants were $n = 1036$ adolescents (15–19 years of age, $M = 16.19$ years, $SD = 0.58$; 67% girls) who completed a series of self-report measures assessing introversion, time spent alone, negative thinking while alone, motivations for solitude (shyness, affinity for solitude), and indices of well-being (i.e., loneliness, positive/negative affect, general well-being). Overall, results from correlational analyses indicated that introversion was associated with poorer functioning across all indices of well-being. However, when controlling for aspects of solitude, results from hierarchical regression analyses indicated a complex set of associations that varied across indices of well-being. Introversion remained associated significantly and negatively with well-being and positive affect, was no longer related significantly to loneliness, and became related significantly and negatively to negative affect. Findings are discussed in terms of how personality characteristics and aspects of solitude can impact the well-being of adolescents.

Keywords: adolescence; solitude; introversion; well-being

1. Introduction

1.1. Adolescence

Adolescence is a transitional developmental period between late childhood and early adulthood characterized by increased time spent alone, identity development, the navigation of new intimate relationships, and the shaping of personality traits that will become more stable over the course of one's life (Klimstra et al., 2013; Weinstein et al., 2021). As a result, personality traits are particularly important to study in adolescence (De Fruyt & Karevold, 2021), a developmental period with important implications for mental health and well-being implications (Gale et al., 2013; Roberts et al., 2006; Steinmayr et al., 2019).

The *extroversion-introversion* dimension of personality may be particularly impactful on well-being during adolescence (Steinmayr et al., 2019). Extroverted individuals are bold, outgoing, and lively compared to their introverted counterparts, who are more reflective, thoughtful, and reserved (Briggs Myers, 2022; Eysenck, 1991). Whereas extroverts tend to prefer social environments and avoid being alone, introverts are more prone to seeking solitude (Card & Skakoon-Sparling, 2023; Teppers et al., 2013). Importantly, although there are happy introverts (Hills & Argyle, 2001), there is a large and robust empirical literature indicating that, overall, introversion is negatively related to aspects of psychological well-being (Anglim et al., 2020; Buecker et al., 2020; Zelenski et al., 2021). However, introversion is also related to other characteristics and behaviors that may also impact well-being (Zelenski et al., 2021).

For example, in terms of behaviors, evidence indicates that introverts tend to spend more time alone than their more extroverted counterparts (Srivastava et al., 2008), which may reduce opportunities for social interactions that serve to boost positive mood (Sandstrom & Dunn, 2014; Sprecher et al., 2023). Introversion is also positively associated with both an affinity for solitude (i.e., the tendency to enjoy spending time alone; Borg & Willoughby, 2022) and shyness (i.e., a personality trait characterized by fear and self-consciousness in social situations; Cheek et al., 1986). Being highly motivated to seek solitude may undermine adolescents' abilities to build meaningful bonds with others, which are conducive to promoting and of paramount importance to well-being during adolescence (Bagwell et al., 2021; Coplan et al., 2019). Notwithstanding solitude motivations, spending time alone can also promote engagement in negative patterns of thinking, such as rumination, which is negatively associated with indices of well-being (i.e., negative affect, loneliness; Hipson et al., 2021).

Although there are many theories that attempt to account for why extroverts are generally happier than introverts, additional empirical research is required to better understand the unique contributions of extroversion-introversion that account for this association (Zelenski et al., 2021). Importantly, there have only been a handful of studies that have specifically explored the correlates of introversion in adolescence (e.g., Suldo et al., 2015). Accordingly, the goal of the current study was to examine associations between introversion, aspects of solitude, and indices of well-being in the under-studied developmental period of adolescence. In particular, we sought to assess the unique associations between introversion and well-being (loneliness, positive/negative affect, general well-being) after accounting for factors related to aspects of solitude, including time spent alone, motivations for seeking solitude (e.g., shyness, affinity for solitude), and negative thinking in solitude.

1.2. Overview of Introversion-Extroversion

Extraversion-introversion is a core personality trait that is part of the predominant contemporary models of personality (McCrae & John, 1992; Zelenski et al., 2021). At one end of the continuum, extraversion is broadly characterized as reflecting a desire for gratification from sources outside of the self, whereas introversion denotes interest in one's internal mental faculties (Briggs Myers, 2022; Petric, 2022). Jung (1921) first proposed that introversion-extroversion describes individual differences in energy among people, which drive behavior. He argued that introverts gain energy from *inward*-focused endeavors (e.g., reflection), whereas extroverts receive energy by engaging *outwards* with others (e.g., social encounters). Eysenck later asserted that introversion-extroversion is a singular dimension of personality and individual differences in the trait are dependent on need for cortical arousal (Eysenck, 1967). Extraverts require more arousal than introverts and, in turn, may be more likely to seek stimulation through spending time with others or engaging in exciting activities (Hills & Argyle, 2001). Introverts have a lower threshold for arousal and are more likely to engage in activities that have little stimulation, such as reading a book (Eysenck & Eysenck, 1985).

Although Jung (1921) argued that people are either dichotomously introverts or extroverts, the introversion-extroversion personality trait is a continuous dimension of personality, and people usually fall between the two extremes (Petric, 2022; Zelenski et al., 2021). The introversion-extroversion dimension of personality has been conceptualized as a *super trait*, which includes additional narrower facets that could provide a further understanding of the intricacies of the dimension (Zelenski et al., 2021). Facets of extroversion-introversion include sociability/unsociability, assertiveness/passivity, gregariousness/shyness, and risk-taking/cautiousness (Costa & McCrae, 1992; Eysenck & Eysenck, 1985; Zelenski et al., 2021).

Introversion/extroversion is a robust predictor of well-being (Busseri & Erb, 2024; Zelenski et al., 2021). For example, as compared to their more introverted counterparts, extroverts tend to experience more positive emotions, which last longer and are more intense (Hemenover, 2003; Rusting, 2001). Across studies of adults, extroversion has been found to be negatively associated with loneliness (Cacioppo et al., 2006; Vanhalst et al., 2012) and robustly positively related to happiness, resilience, subjective well-being, job satisfaction, and other indices of well-being (Anglim et al., 2020; Lun & Yeung, 2019; Soto & Tackett, 2015). Although the trait of extroversion has some overlap with the greater experience of positive emotions, there are other aspects of extroversion that are associated with happiness outside the measure of emotionality (Steel et al., 2008). Moreover, in experimental manipulations, being assigned to act in more extroverted ways (e.g., being more talkative) can make people happier compared to when they are assigned to act in introverted ways (e.g., being quiet or reserved; Margolis & Lyubomirsky, 2020). Of note, relative to knowledge about the concomitants of introversion during adulthood, considerably less is known about the implications of introversion during the adolescent developmental period.

Adolescence, typically studied as the ages of 10–18 years, is often described as a tumultuous time, characterized by a plethora of biological, cognitive, behavioral, and social developmental changes (D. Wood et al., 2018). Adolescence is a critical time for pubertal and brain development, cultivating peer relationships and avoiding peer rejection, and identity formation (Corsano et al., 2006; Griffin, 2017; Luyckx & Robitschek, 2014). It is also a time associated with developing advanced reasoning skills and agency to formulate autonomous goals and engage in task-specific endeavors, which may in turn promote positive psychological development (Napolitano et al., 2021; Wehmeyer & Shogren, 2017). Personality traits are an important contributor to shaping social, biological, and health outcomes in adolescence (Carvalho & Novo, 2014; Tackett, 2006). For example, Suldo et al. (2015) found that personality accounted for 47% of an adolescent's total life satisfaction.

As aforementioned, little is known about the psychological concomitants of introversion during adolescence. However, consistent with findings among adults, there is some indication that introverted adolescents tend to be less happy than their more extroverted counterparts (Cheng & Furnham, 2003; Young & Bradley, 1998). Moreover, introversion during adolescence has been related negatively to general well-being, as well as self-esteem, life satisfaction, and positive affect (Butkovic et al., 2012; Ho et al., 2008; Steinmayr et al., 2019). For example, in one study of younger (M_{age} = 14.6 years) and older adolescents (M_{age} = 17.4 years), introversion was significantly and negatively related to indices of well-being (i.e., positive attitudes, self-esteem, joy in life, lack of depressed mood) and positively associated with indices of ill-being (i.e., problems/worrying, somatic complaints), even after controlling for other personality traits such as neuroticism (Lampropoulou, 2018). Introverted adolescents are also more likely to report both peer-related and parent-related loneliness (Teppers et al., 2013).

1.3. Introversion, Solitude, and Well-Being: Considering Conceptual Mechanisms

Several possible explanations for the negative relation between introversion and indices of well-being have been proposed. For example, it has been suggested that introverts are less likely to possess positive traits (e.g., positive emotions, energy) and skills (e.g., social competence; Argyle & Lu, 1990a, 1990b), which in turn may interfere with psychological well-being. They may also be less prone to engage in social activities, which are conducive to fostering positive relationships that promote well-being (Lampropoulou, 2018; Suldo et al., 2015; Teppers et al., 2013). However, to date, there has been limited direct empirical support for these relations (Zelenski et al., 2021), particularly in adolescence. Given the well-established linkages between introversion and solitude-seeking (Burger, 1995; Thomas et al., 2021; Thomas & Nelson, 2024; Yuan & Grühn, 2023), in the current study, we considered several plausible factors related to aspects of *solitude* that may help to account for the negative association between introversion and well-being.

1.4. Time Spent Alone

A relatively simple explanation for why introverts report lower well-being is that they spend too much *time alone*. Time alone can be problematic in adolescence because it limits opportunities for positive interactions with peers, which are particularly important in the face of growing social expectations and norms during this developmental period (Borg & Willoughby, 2021; Bowker et al., 2020; Coplan et al., 2015). Engaging in more social interactions also promotes the obtainment of social capital, which may open doors for future opportunities to pursue endeavors perceived as rewarding (Card & Skakoon-Sparling, 2023; Zelenski et al., 2021). Results from several studies indicate a positive association between introversion and solitude in adulthood (e.g., Burger, 1995; Thomas et al., 2021; Thomas & Nelson, 2024; Yuan & Grühn, 2023). Research indicates that introverted adolescents show less aversion to being alone (Teppers et al., 2013), but, somewhat surprisingly, our review of the literature did not uncover any studies directly examining the link between introversion and time spent alone in adolescence. Limited research has examined time spent alone in adolescence (McVarnock et al., 2023). Although solitude emerges as a context for positive development in later adolescence (Larson, 1990), generally, time spent alone appears to be associated with socio-emotional difficulties, including symptoms of anxiety and depression, low self-esteem, and lower quality friendships, during adolescence (Borg & Willoughby, 2022; Coplan et al., 2019; Hipson et al., 2021; Sette et al., 2024). However, additional research is needed to establish what role, if any, the tendency to spend time in solitude plays in the links between introversion and well-being.

1.5. Motivations for Seeking Solitude

Just as time alone is important, it is also important to consider introverts' underlying motivations for seeking solitude. For example, some introverts may report lower well-being because they also tend to be *shy*. In adolescence, the personality trait of shyness is characterized by feelings of wariness and self-consciousness in social contexts, particularly in situations involving perceived social evaluation (Cheek et al., 1986). Shyness is positively associated with the personality trait of neuroticism, which is likely a result of the worrying associated with neuroticism accompanying shyness (Bratko et al., 2002). However, introversion is also strongly associated with shyness in adolescents (Kwiatkowska & Rogoza, 2019). Shyness in adolescence is associated with heightened negative affect and loneliness, lower positive affect, and a negative view of the self (Coplan et al., 2021; Zhao et al., 2018). Further, shy adolescents often have both fewer social relationships overall and fewer close relationships and are more prone to peer victimization than their more sociable counterparts (Kwiatkowska & Rogoza, 2019; Ojanen et al., 2017).

Adolescents may also seek time alone due to an affinity for solitude (Borg & Willoughby, 2022). Adolescents high in an affinity for solitude seek solitude because they enjoy and value spending time alone (Coplan et al., 2019). Results from numerous studies have indicated a positive association between introversion and affinity for solitude (and related constructs) in samples of adults (e.g., Burger, 1995; Thomas & Azmitia, 2019) and adolescents (e.g., Corsano et al., 2019; Teppers et al., 2013). Of note, affinity for solitude is typically conceptualized as a relatively 'benign' reason for seeking solitude in adolescence, particularly when compared to shyness (Coplan et al., 2015; Daly & Willoughby, 2020). Having an affinity for solitude can be considered adaptive in adolescence, and depending on motivations, it can be associated with psychosocial benefits (Borg & Willoughby, 2022). However, results from several studies suggest that affinity for solitude often demonstrates associations with indices of socio-emotional difficulties (e.g., symptoms of anxiety and depression, low self-esteem, emotion dysregulation, loneliness) in adolescence (Borg & Willoughby, 2022; Endo et al., 2017; Wang et al., 2013), perhaps due to cascading negative social consequences of seeking solitude, for any reason, during adolescence. Mixed findings regarding affinity for solitude emphasize the need for more research during this important developmental period. Thus, motivations for solitude, such as shyness and affinity for solitude, should be considered in conjunction with introversion due to their associations with introversion and potential differential impacts on how time alone affects adolescents.

1.6. Negative Thinking While Alone

Finally, we considered what introverted adolescents might do during their time alone. Adolescents engage in a variety of activities while alone, which are differentially associated with adjustment (Hipson et al., 2021). One particularly maladaptive solitary activity appears to be engaging in patterns of *negative thinking*, such as worrying (Borkovec et al., 1983), rumination (Constantin et al., 2018), and procrastination (Flett et al., 2012). Introverts are characterized as individuals who spend time engaged with their inner thoughts, which may promote introspection but also patterns of negative thinking (Thomas & Nelson, 2024). In support of this notion, introversion has been positively (and moderately) associated with rumination (Conway et al., 2000; Oral & Arslan, 2017; Thomas & Nelson, 2024). However, findings pertaining to the links between introversion and negative thinking styles have been more mixed (Hui et al., 2024; Vélez et al., 2024). Results from two recent studies found that adolescents (Hipson et al., 2021) and adults (McVarnock et al., 2023) who frequently engage in thinking (e.g., rumination, daydreaming, planning) *when alone* were more likely to experience negative affect and loneliness. There is also some preliminary evidence to indicate that negative thinking styles (i.e., brooding and reflection) mediate the association between introversion and depressive symptoms (Lyon et al., 2021).

2. The Current Study

The goal of this research was to examine the links between introversion, aspects of solitude, and indices of well-being in the under-studied developmental period of adolescence. Further, we sought to examine whether introversion remained negatively associated with well-being after accounting for the postulated explanatory factors related to solitude, including time spent alone, motivations for seeking solitude (i.e., shyness, affinity for solitude), and negative thoughts while alone. It was hypothesized that introversion would be negatively related to general well-being and positive affect, as well as positively related to loneliness and negative affect. In terms of aspects of solitude, time alone, shyness, and negative thinking were each expected to be negatively associated with well-being. Given the aforementioned mixed findings, affinity for solitude was tentatively expected to be non-significantly (or even positively) associated with well-being. Finally, we sought to test whether associations between introversion and indices of well-being remain significant after controlling for aspects of solitude to determine whether introversion, or its known correlates, best explains variability in well-being during adolescence.

3. Method

3.1. Participants

Participants were n = 1036 adolescents (n = 304 boys, n = 692 girls, n = 40 did not specify) ages 15–19 years (M = 16.19, SD = 0.58) attending public high schools in Eastern Ontario, Canada. Participants were students in an elective *Introduction to Psychology, Sociology, and Anthropology* course. The initial sample consisted of 1140 participants. Participants who did not provide written consent (n = 29) or did not indicate their age (n = 75) were removed.

Although school boards did not permit the collection of individual data on ethnicity or socioeconomic status, the participating schools were from a mix of urban, suburban, and rural neighborhoods. In addition, the most recent publicly available data for the 2019–2020 academic year indicated that: (1) 73% of secondary school students lived in homes where English was the primary language; (2) 20% came from a lower-income home, 14% from a middle-income home, 38% from an upper-income home, and 19% preferred not to answer; and (3) 58% identified as White, with a variety of racial/ethnic identities represented (e.g., 14% Middle Eastern, 9% Black, 8% South Asian, 11% East Asian, 4% Southeast Asian, 3% Latino/Latina/Latinx, 2% Indigenous, 1% Other; Ottawa-Carleton District School Board OCDSB, 2020).

3.2. Procedure

Following approval from the university ethics board and public School boards, written parental consent and online adolescent participant consent were obtained. Participants completed the online survey during class time on a laptop or smartphone. Surveys were completed independently, but graduate students and trained research assistants were available for questions and clarification of survey items. Survey responses were anonymous. Data were collected in two cohorts: Cohort 1 (October 2022–April 2023) and Cohort 2 (November 2023–May 2024).

3.3. Measures

3.3.1. Introversion

Introversion was assessed using the extraversion/introversion subscale of the *Big Five Personality Inventory* (John & Srivastava, 1999). The subscale contains 8 items that ask participants to rate how much each statement reflects them as a person (e.g., "generates a lot of enthusiasm", "tends to be quiet"). Items are rated on a 5-point scale (from 1 = "disagree strongly" to 5 = "agree strongly"). Of note, to ease presentation and interpretation, extraversion scores were reverse-coded such that higher scores reflect *higher* introversion. The extraversion/introversion subscale was found to have good internal reliability in the current sample (α = 0.84).

3.3.2. Time Alone

Time alone was measured by aggregating two items assessing the average number of times during the last 7 days they spent at least 15 min alone (1 = "not at all", 6 = "more than 3 times a day") and hours they spent alone in the last seven days (1 = "<1 h [<15 min per day]", 6 = "more than 15 h [more than 2 h per day]" (Coplan et al., 2019, 2021). Time spent alone was defined for participants as being alone or doing something alone, not including sleeping. The items of time alone were highly correlated with each other (r = 0.61, p < 0.001).

3.3.3. Affinity for Solitude

Affinity for solitude was examined using the *Affinity for Solitude Scale* (AFS; Coplan et al., 2019), which was adapted from the original *Preference for Solitude Scale* (PSS; Burger,

1995). The AFS contains 9 items (e.g., "I try to structure my day so that I always have some time to myself"; I often have a strong desire to get away by myself") rated on a 7-point scale (from 1 = "strongly disagree" to 7 = "strongly agree"). AFS is calculated by using a composite score, where higher scores indicate greater affinity for solitude, and it was found to have had good internal reliability ($\alpha = 0.86$) in the current sample.

3.3.4. Shyness

Shyness was assessed using the *Cheek and Buss Shyness Scale* (Cheek & Buss, 1981). The scale contains 12 items (e.g., "I feel tense when I'm with people I don't know well"; "It is hard for me to act natural when I am meeting new people") rated on a 5-point scale (from 1 = "very uncharacteristic or untrue" to 5 = "very characteristic or true"). Items were averaged to create a composite score, and higher scores indicated greater shyness. The shyness scale was found to have good internal reliability in the current sample ($\alpha = 0.88$).

3.3.5. Negative Thinking While Alone

Finally, participants' negative thoughts while alone were measured using a single item created for the current study. Participants were asked to indicate how often they engaged in "negative thoughts (e.g., worrying, rumination, bored, procrastinating)" while they were alone (defined as "by yourself or doing something by yourself—not including sleeping") on a 5-point scale (from 1 = "never" to 5 = "most of the time").

3.3.6. Positive and Negative Affect

Affect was measured using the *positive and negative affect schedule* (PANAS; Watson et al., 1988). This measure includes a 10-item subscale for both positive affect (e.g., "interested", "enthusiastic") and negative affect (e.g., "distressed", "guilty"). Participants could indicate their agreement using a 5-point scale (from 1 = "not at all" to 5 = "extremely"). The scales are calculated using a sum, where higher scores indicate greater positive or negative affect. Both subscales were found to have good internal reliability in the current sample ($\alpha = 0.80$ for positive affect; $\alpha = 0.86$ for negative affect).

3.3.7. Loneliness

Loneliness was assessed using the *UCLA Loneliness Scale Short Form* (Russell, 1996). The scale includes 8 items (e.g., "I lack companionship", "I am unhappy being so withdrawn") that tap into how often participants experience feelings of loneliness (from 1 = "never" to 4 = "often"). The scale was found to have good internal reliability in the current sample ($\alpha = 0.83$).

3.3.8. Well-Being

Well-being was measured using the *EPOCH Measure of Adolescent Well-Being* (Kern et al., 2016). This measure taps into five aspects of well-being (i.e., engagement, perseverance, optimism, connectedness, and happiness). The scale contains 20 items (e.g., "I am optimistic about my future", "there are people in my life who really care about me") and asks participants to rate how much they believe each statement describes them (from 1 = "almost never" to 5 = "almost always"). Items were aggregated to create a general index of well-being. The scale was found to have excellent internal reliability in the current sample ($\alpha = 0.90$).

4. Results

4.1. Preliminary Analyses

Descriptive statistics and inter-correlations among the main study variables are presented in Table 1. Of note, introversion was significantly related to all aspects of solitude and indices of well-being in expected directions. Specifically, introversion was positively associated with loneliness, negative affect, time alone, shyness, affinity for solitude, and negative thinking, as well as negatively associated with general well-being and positive affect.

Table 1. Descriptive Statistics and Intercorrelations Among Study Variables.

Variables	M	SD	1	2	3	4	5	6	7	8	9	10
1. Age	16.190	0.583	-									
2. Loneliness	2.619	0.492	0.048	-								
3. Shyness	3.081	0.796	−0.025	0.299 ***	-							
4. Well-Being	3.171	0.695	0.061	−0.403 ***	−0.421 ***	-						
5. AFS	4.688	1.231	−0.029	0.013	0.268 ***	0.060	-					
6. Positive Affect	31.536	6.560	0.053	−0.198 ***	−0.396 ***	0.610 ***	0.024	-				
7. Negative Affect	27.457	8.133	−0.021	0.398 ***	0.361 ***	−0.275 ***	0.075 *	−0.019	-			
8. Time Alone	4.340	1.384	0.001	0.093 **	0.142 ***	−0.176 ***	0.195 ***	−0.164 ***	0.063 *	-		
9. Negative Thinking	3.780	1.018	−0.037	0.375 ***	0.344 ***	−0.321 ***	0.066 *	−0.205 ***	0.562 ***	0.108 ***	-	
10. Introversion	2.922	0.804	−0.010	0.165 ***	0.644 ***	−0.399 ***	0.292 ***	−0.439 ***	0.111 ***	0.172 ***	0.185 ***	-

Note: * $p < 0.05$, ** $p < 0.01$, *** $p < 0.001$. AFS = Affinity for Solitude.

Additionally, aspects of solitude were also generally associated with indices of well-being in the expected directions. Notably (and supporting its validity), the single-item assessment of negative thinking was positively associated with loneliness and negative affect, as well as negatively associated with well-being and positive affect. Finally, introversion was not significantly related to age, and there was no significant gender difference in introversion ($t = -0.682$, $p = 0.496$).

4.2. Hierarchical Regression Analyses

A series of hierarchical regressions was computed to explore the unique relations between introversion and indices of well-being (i.e., loneliness, well-being, positive affect, negative affect), while accounting for gender, time alone, motivations for seeking solitude (i.e., shyness, affinity for solitude), and negative thinking while alone. Separate equations were computed to predict each index of well-being. For each equation, gender was entered at Step 1, all aspects of solitude (shyness, affinity for solitude, time alone, negative thinking while alone) were entered at Step 2, and introversion was entered at Step 3.

Results predicting *well-being* are displayed in Table 2. At Step 2, aspects of solitude added a significant amount of explained variance in predicting well-being. Examination of individual beta values suggested that time alone, shyness, and negative thinking were negatively associated with well-being, whereas AFS was positively related to well-being. At Step 3, after accounting for these variables, introversion still displayed a significant and negative relation to general well-being.

Table 2. Multiple Regression Predicting Well-Being.

Variable	Model 1			Model 2			Model 3		
	B	SE B	β	B	SE B	β	B	SE B	β
Gender	−0.099	0.051	−0.066	0.012	0.046	0.008	−0.027	0.045	−0.018
Shyness				−0.339	0.028	−0.387 ***	−0.186	0.034	−0.212 ***
AFS				0.112	0.017	0.199 ***	0.132	0.017	0.234 ***
Time Alone				−0.069	0.015	−0.136 ***	−0.063	0.015	−0.123 ***
Negative Thinking				−0.125	0.022	−0.184 ***	−0.129	0.021	−0.190 ***
Introversion							−0.240	0.033	−0.279 ***
Adj. R^2		0.003			0.247			0.290	
F for ΔR^2		3.853			72.466 ***			54.114 ***	

Note: * $p < 0.05$, ** $p < 0.01$, *** $p < 0.001$. Gender was coded Males = 1, Females = 2. AFS = Affinity for Solitude.

Results predicting *positive affect* are displayed in Table 3. At Step 2, aspects of solitude added a significant amount of variance to the prediction of positive affect. Similarly to well-being, individual beta values suggested that time alone and shyness were negatively associated with positive affect, and AFS was positively related to positive affect. At Step 3, after accounting for control variables, introversion still displayed a significant and negative relation to positive affect.

Table 3. Multiple regression predicting positive affect.

Variable	Model 1			Model 2			Model 3		
	B	SE B	β	B	SE B	β	B	SE B	β
Gender	−1.683	0.465	−0.120	−1.088	0.443	−0.077 *	−1.560	0.425	−0.111 ***
Shyness				−3.247	0.271	−0.396 ***	−1.362	0.324	−0.166 ***
AFS				0.880	0.167	0.167 ***	1.111	0.161	0.211 ***
Time Alone				−0.580	0.146	−0.123 ***	−0.503	0.139	−106 ***
Negative Thinking				−0.244	0.209	−0.038	−0.294	0.199	−0.046
Introversion							−2.942	0.307	−0.365 ***
Adj. R^2		0.013			0.190			0.264	
F for ΔR^2		13.116 ***			50.263 ***			91.765 ***	

Note: * $p < 0.05$, ** $p < 0.01$, *** $p < 0.001$. *Gender was coded Males = 1, Females = 2. AFS = Affinity for Solitude.*

Results predicting *negative affect* are displayed in Table 4. At Step 2, aspects of solitude added a significant amount of variance to the prediction of negative affect. Examination of individual beta values suggested that shyness and negative thinking most strongly predicted negative affect. However, at Step 3, after accounting for these variables, introversion demonstrated a significant *negative* association with negative affect.

Table 4. Multiple regression predicting negative affect.

Variable	Model 1			Model 2			Model 3		
	B	SE B	β	B	SE B	β	B	SE B	β
Gender	5.068	0.562	0.287 ***	2.449	0.492	0.139 ***	2.189	0.490	0.124 ***
Shyness				1.788	0.301	0.170 ***	2.828	0.375	0.275 ***
AFS				−0.045	0.186	−0.006	0.082	0.186	0.012
Time Alone				−0.063	0.162	−0.010	−0.021	0.161	−0.003
Negative Thinking				3.769	0.232	0.479 ***	3.742	0.230	0.468 ***
Introversion							−1.623	0.355	−0.160 ***
Adj. R^2		0.083			0.366			0.380	
F for ΔR^2		81.319 ***			100.548 ***			20.898 ***	

Note: * $p < 0.05$, ** $p < 0.01$, *** $p < 0.001$. *Gender was coded Males = 1, Females = 2. AFS = Affinity for Solitude.*

Finally, results predicting *loneliness* are displayed in Table 5. At Step 2, aspects of solitude added a significant amount of variance to the prediction of loneliness. Examination of individual beta values suggested that both shyness and negative thinking most strongly predicted loneliness. However, after accounting for these variables, at Step 3, introversion was not significantly associated with loneliness.

Table 5. Multiple regression predicting loneliness.

Variable	Model 1			Model 2			Model 3		
	B	SE B	β	B	SE B	β	B	SE B	β
Gender	0.146	0.035	0.137 ***	0.045	0.034	0.042	0.042	0.034	0.040
Shyness				0.130	0.021	0.209 ***	0.139	0.026	0.223 ***
AFS				−0.024	0.013	−0.061	−0.023	0.013	−0.058
Time Alone				0.018	0.011	0.050	0.018	0.011	0.051
Negative Thinking				0.139	0.016	0.285 ***	0.138	0.016	0.285 ***
Introversion							−0.013	0.025	−0.022
Adj. R^2		0.018			0.172			0.171	
F for ΔR^2		17.126 ***			42.644 ***			0.295	

Note: * $p < 0.05$, ** $p < 0.01$, *** $p < 0.001$. *Gender was coded Males = 1, Females = 2. AFS = Affinity for Solitude.*

5. Discussion

A large body of research has shown that introversion is negatively related to aspects of well-being across domains, time points, and cultures (Anglim et al., 2020; Gale et al., 2013; Lun & Yeung, 2019). However, only a few studies have examined the implications of introversion among samples of adolescents (e.g., Suldo et al., 2015). Moreover, it remains unclear whether introversion is associated with negative outcomes after accounting for its known correlates. Finding solace in solitude is one of the defining characteristics of introverts (Zelenski et al., 2021), but several aspects of solitude may negatively impact well-being. Accordingly, the goal of this current study was to examine the unique relation between introversion and indices of well-being in adolescence after accounting for conceptually relevant aspects of solitude (i.e., time alone, motivations for solitude, negative thinking while alone).

Overall, results from correlational analyses indicated that introversion was associated with poorer functioning across all indices of well-being. However, when controlling for aspects of solitude, results from hierarchical regression analyses indicated a complex set of associations that varied across indices of well-being. Introversion remained significantly and negatively associated with well-being and positive affect, was no longer significantly related to loneliness, and became significantly and *negatively* related to negative affect. The results from the current study speak to the complex and unique links between introversion and indices of well-being and indicate that there are other factors beyond solitary motivations, negative thinking, and time alone that account for these links in adolescence.

5.1. Aspects of Solitude and Well-Being in Adolescence

Although not the primary focus of the study, our results add to our understanding of how different aspects of solitude are related to well-being in adolescence. For example, shyness was positively related to loneliness and negative affect, as well as negatively related to general well-being and positive affect. These findings are consistent with previous research (Sette et al., 2024) and suggest that shyness remains a risk factor for internalizing problems in adolescence. For affinity for solitude, results supported the notion that this motivation for solitude is more benign in adolescence (Borg & Willoughby, 2021; Coplan et al., 2019). Overall, affinity for solitude was not significantly related to well-being, positive affect, or loneliness, although it did demonstrate a significant (albeit modest) positive relation with negative affect. Of note, in regressions that controlled for other aspects of solitude (i.e., shyness, time alone, negative thinking while alone), affinity for solitude demonstrated a significant and *positive* association with both general well-being and positive affect.

Both time spent alone and negative thinking while alone were positively related to loneliness and negative affect and negatively related to general well-being and positive affect. The association between time alone and indices of well-being remains relatively unexplored in adolescents, but the results are in line with previous research in adolescents (e.g., Hipson et al., 2021; R. Larson & Csikszentmihalyi, 1978), indicating that spending too much time alone can have negative implications in adolescence. Similarly, previous research has found that negative thinking in solitude can exacerbate negative emotions and lead to feelings of loneliness in adolescents (e.g., Hipson et al., 2021) and young adults (e.g., J. Lay et al., 2019; Vanhalst et al., 2012). This finding supports the notion that thinking in solitude can be an uncomfortable experience (Wilson et al., 2014).

5.2. Introversion, Solitude, and Well-Being

Overall, in line with predictions, results from correlational analyses indicated that introversion was significantly associated with poorer well-being indices. Specifically, introversion was negatively associated with general well-being and positive affect, as well as positively related to loneliness and negative affect. These findings are in line with results from considerable research in adults (Anglim et al., 2020; Card & Skakoon-Sparling, 2023) and add to the few studies demonstrating such effects among adolescents (Suldo et al.,

2015; Teppers et al., 2013). However, when controlling aspects of solitude, results were more complex and appeared to vary across domains of well-being.

To begin, after accounting for aspects of solitude, introversion remained significantly and negatively related to adolescent general well-being and positive affect. These results suggest that aspects of solitude play a role in impacting adolescent well-being outcomes but do not account for why introverts tend to report poorer well-being. That is, our findings suggest that introverts are not less happy *because* they also tend to be more shy or spend more time alone. Rather, there seem to be aspects of the introversion-extraversion dimension of personality that explain adolescent well-being outcomes beyond aspects of solitude.

Several other potential explanations as to why introverts might experience less happiness than extroverts have been postulated (Zelenski et al., 2021). For example, extroverts may perceive ambiguous events as more positive than introverts or may have a higher set point for positive emotions (Hemenover, 2003; J. C. Lay et al., 2017). Introverts are less likely to engage in social situations and have more high-quality friendships than extroverts, which is conducive to promoting happiness (Waldinger & Schulz, 2023). Introverts may also have neurological differences in reward sensitivity, which make seeking out social situations perceived as less worthwhile (Card & Skakoon-Sparling, 2023).

Findings were more nuanced in terms of the relation between introversion and both loneliness and negative affect. After accounting for aspects of solitude, the relation between introversion and loneliness was no longer significant, and introversion evidenced a significant and *negative* association with negative affect. These findings suggest that aspects of solitude do play a potentially significant explanatory role in the links between introversion and these specific indices of adolescent ill-being.

For example, our findings indicate that the tendency to seek solitude—and spending more time alone—may help to explain why introversion displays a positive association with loneliness. Navigating new social challenges and pressures is a fundamental characteristic of adolescence; however, retreating to solitude as a respite from these stresses can lead to feelings of loneliness (Matthews et al., 2023). Our findings can be interpreted to suggest this may be particularly true for introverts (Teppers et al., 2013). Despite the belief that introverts require less social interaction than extroverts to fulfill their *need to belong* (Baumeister & Leary, 1995), emerging research indicates that social connection is equally as important for the well-being of both introverts and extroverts (Card & Skakoon-Sparling, 2023). However, this begs the question, if introverts need social connection similarly to extroverts, why are they more likely to seek solitude over spending time with others? It has been argued that introverts may *perceive* themselves to derive less benefit from spending time with others than extroverts and, in turn, find it less appealing than spending time alone (T. T. Nguyen et al., 2022; Thomas & Azmitia, 2019). However, this perception is a forecasting error, and introverts derive similar levels of happiness as extroverts from social interactions (Zelenski et al., 2013).

Forecasting errors may also be related to neurotic tendencies during solitude (i.e., shyness, negative thinking). Having a positive social mindset (i.e., motivation to engage in social interactions) is key to establishing and maintaining social relationships conducive to reducing feelings of loneliness (Turner et al., 2024). However, perceptions of having inadequate social competencies (e.g., shyness) and engaging in maladaptive coping strategies (e.g., ruminating) may negatively impact one's mindset and, in turn, lead to feelings of loneliness (Turner et al., 2024). Importantly, the neurotic tendencies associated with aspects of solitude may have negative implications for introversions down the line. Vanhalst et al. (2012) found that at age 15, participants with the highest levels of introversion were more likely to be in a moderate decreasing trajectory of loneliness, which was associated with high levels of anxiety and social phobia at age 20. As such, it may be important to promote the use of positive solitary reappraisal strategies (e.g., highlight the benefits of solitude; Rodriguez et al., 2020; Turner et al., 2024) to buffer the negative impacts that loneliness can have on introverts.

Introversion was significantly and positively correlated with negative affect. However, after controlling for aspects of solitude in regression analyses, introversion evidenced a significant and *negative* relation with negative affect. It is possible that this result is a statistical artifact known as a suppression effect (Akinwande et al., 2015). The suppression effect is when a predictor variable increases predictive validity in other variables in a model, which impacts the ability to appropriately interpret the regression coefficients (Ludlow & Klein, 2014). As such, this finding should be interpreted with caution. Suppression effects are less replicable (Wiggins, 1973). The strong bivariate correlation between introversion and shyness suggests that the suppression effect may be present.

However, it may also be that the *neurotic* tendencies associated with aspects of solitude (i.e., shyness, negative thinking) contribute most strongly to adolescent ill-being. It is possible that when accounting for an introvert's neurotic solitary tendencies, spending time alone reduced the negative emotions for introverts, as opposed to exacerbating them. This is in line with research that found having a capacity for solitude (i.e., feeling comfortable in solitude) is negatively related to neuroticism, suggesting that people with neurotic tendencies may experience frequent negative emotions and discomfort in solitude (Lin et al., 2020). This goes back to the notion that solitude is not inherently bad—solitude is what you make of it, which is dependent on various individualistic characteristics (Weinstein et al., 2023). Although solitude offers adolescents a place to engage in growth, self-regulation, identity development, and self-reflection (Larson, 1990; T. V. T. Nguyen et al., 2018), it may also be a place for individuals to socially withdraw and engage in rumination (Li et al., 2021).

5.3. Limitations and Future Directions

Although this study is relatively novel in its focus on the outcomes of introversion among adolescents, it is not without its limitations. For one, this research was cross-sectional, and thus alternative causal explanations of the relations between variables cannot be discounted—nor can the influence of other variables. For example, lonely introverts may seek out solitude because of their experiences of being ostracized (Ren et al., 2021). The cross-sectional design also prevented us from conducting formal tests of mediation, which would have allowed us to more specifically test mechanisms of influence. Understanding how aspects of solitude may impact the well-being of introverted adolescents provides initial statistical evidence of how aspects of solitude play meaningfully impact introverted adolescent's well-being. However, future research should examine the mediating role of aspects of solitude towards further uncovering *why* introversion is associated with negative outcomes in adolescence and beyond. Also, we considered the particular developmental stage of adolescence. It is important to further examine the development and implications of introversion and aspects of solitude across the lifespan and longitudinally over time. The current study only examined individuals between mid-to-late adolescence. However, it has been argued that introversion may pose a greater risk for well-being in *early* adolescence (10–14 years), when friendships are still forming and cultivating, as opposed to late adolescence and early adulthood, when spending time alone becomes more comfortable (Vanhalst et al., 2012; Steinmayr et al., 2019) and viewed as more normative (Bowker et al., 2020; K. R. Wood et al., 2021).

From a methodological perspective, the use of a single item to assess negative thinking while alone substantially reduces the validity of this measure (Allen et al., 2022). We were

Behav. Sci. **2025**, *15*, 108

also not able to consider different types of negative thinking patterns. Notwithstanding, this item did correlate in expected directions with theoretically relevant variables (e.g., shyness, negative affect), providing at least some initial support for its construct validity. However, future research will need to further explore how negative thinking impacts the relation between personality characteristics and adolescent well-being.

Finally, the current study did not include assessments of other personality traits. Previous research has suggested that the *combination* of specific traits may have heightened associations with aspects of well-being (Lynn & Steel, 2006; Steinmayr et al., 2019). For example, Young and Bradley (1998) found in a sample of adolescents that, overall, emotionally stable (i.e., less neurotic) introverts were less happy than emotionally stable extraverts. However, emotionally stable introverts were happier than emotionally unstable extraverts and introverts. As such, neurotic tendencies seem to explain some of the variance between introversion and well-being. Results from other studies also suggest that heightened neuroticism may exacerbate the negative associations between introversion and well-being (Fadda & Scalas, 2016). As such, future research will need to further explore the interactions between neuroticism and introversion (as well as other personality traits) in the prediction of well-being in adolescence.

6. Conclusions

A growing body of evidence has indicated the potential negative impacts that introversion can have on well-being (Butkovic et al., 2012; Ho et al., 2008; Steinmayr et al., 2019). Adolescence is a developmental time period surrounding immense transition and growth, and as such, introversion may be particularly consequential during this milestone (Corsano et al., 2006; Griffin, 2017; Luyckx & Robitschek, 2014). Yet, few studies have examined the role of introversion in adolescence. Considering that enjoyment of solitude is marked as a defining feature of introversion (Zelenski et al., 2021), the current study considered aspects of solitude as contributing factors in the relation between introversion and well-being in adolescence. Initial support was found to suggest that aspects of solitude do not play a significant role in impacting adolescent well-being or negative affect. However, the neurotic tendencies associated with aspects of solitude, such as rumination and shyness, were found to meaningfully minimize the relation between introversion and loneliness. These results highlight that while solitude may negatively impact an adolescent's need to belong, the mechanisms that are reducing the happiness of introverts beyond aspects of solitude are still unclear. Future research will need to further explore the complex relations between personality, aspects of solitude, and well-being in adolescence to further understand under what conditions and for whom spending time alone will help versus hinder development.

Author Contributions: Conceptualization, R.J.C.; Methodology, M.D. and A.S.; Software, A.S. and R.J.C.; Validation, A.S., M.D., and R.J.C.; Formal Analysis, A.S. and R.J.C.; Investigation, R.J.C., A.M., T.C., A.S., and M.D.; Resources, R.J.C.; Data Curation, R.J.C. and A.S.; Writing—Original Draft Preparation, A.S., M.D., and R.J.C.; Writing—Review and Editing, R.J.C., A.S., M.D., A.M., T.C., and J.C.B.; Visualization, A.S., M.D., and R.J.C.; Supervision, R.J.C.; Project Administration, R.J.C., A.S., and M.D.; Funding Acquisition, R.J.C. All authors have read and agreed to the published version of the manuscript.

Funding: This study was funded by a SSHRC Insight Grant (435-2017-0849).

Institutional Review Board Statement: This study has been approved by the Ottawa-Carleton Research Advisory Committee, the principal of the high school, as well as the Carleton University Research Ethics Board—B (CUREB-B) (Study # 107297, 3 August 2022).

Informed Consent Statement: Informed consent was obtained from all subjects involved in the study.

Data Availability Statement: Data is available upon request from the author.

Conflicts of Interest: The authors declare no conflicts of interest.

References

Akinwande, M. O., Dikko, H. G., & Samson, A. (2015). Variance inflation factor: As a condition for the inclusion of suppressor variable(s) in regression analysis. *Open Journal of Statistics, 5*(07), 754. [CrossRef]

Allen, M. S., Iliescu, D., & Greiff, S. (2022). Single item measures in psychological science: A call to action [Editorial]. *European Journal of Psychological Assessment, 38*(1), 1–5. [CrossRef]

Anglim, J., Horwood, S., Smillie, L. D., Marrero, R. J., & Wood, J. K. (2020). Predicting psychological and subjective well-being from personality: A meta-analysis. *Psychological Bulletin, 146*(4), 279. [CrossRef] [PubMed]

Argyle, M., & Lu, L. (1990a). Happiness and social skills. *Personality and Individual Differences, 11*, 1255–1261. [CrossRef]

Argyle, M., & Lu, L. (1990b). The happiness of extraverts. *Personality and Individual Differences, 11*, 1011–1017. [CrossRef]

Bagwell, C. L., Bowker, J. C., & Asher, S. R. (2021). Back to the dyad: Future directions for friendship research. *Merrill-Palmer Quarterly, 67*(4), 457–484. [CrossRef]

Baumeister, R. F., & Leary, M. R. (1995). The need to belong: Desire for interpersonal attachments as a fundamental human motivation. *Psychological Bulletin, 117*(3), 497–529. [CrossRef] [PubMed]

Borg, M. E., & Willoughby, T. (2021). A latent class examination of affinity for aloneness in late adolescence and emerging adulthood. *Social Development, 31*(3), 587–602. [CrossRef]

Borg, M. E., & Willoughby, T. (2022). Affinity for solitude and motivations for spending time alone among early and mid-adolescents. *Journal of Youth and Adolescence, 51*(1), 156–168. [CrossRef] [PubMed]

Borkovec, T. D., Robinson, E., Pruzinsky, T., & DePree, J. A. (1983). Preliminary exploration of worry: Some characteristics and processes. *Behavior Research and Therapy, 21*, 9–16. [CrossRef] [PubMed]

Bowker, J. C., Ooi, L. L., Coplan, R. J., & Etkin, R. G. (2020). When is it okay to be alone? Gender differences in normative beliefs about social withdrawal. *Sex Roles, 82*(7–8), 482–492. [CrossRef]

Bratko, D., Vukosav, Ž., Zarevski, P., & Vranić, A. (2002). The relations of shyness and assertiveness traits with the dimensions of the five-factor model in adolescence. *Review of Psychology, 9*(1–2), 17–24.

Briggs Myers, I. (2022). *Extraversion or introversion*. The Myers & Briggs Foundation. Available online: https://www.myersbriggs.org/my-mbti-personality-type/mbti-basics (accessed on 10 July 2024).

Buecker, S., Maes, M., Denissen, J. J. A., & Luhmann, M. (2020). Loneliness and the big five personality traits: A meta-analysis. *European Journal of Personality, 34*(1), 8–28. [CrossRef]

Burger, J. M. (1995). Individual differences in preference for solitude. *Journal of Research in Personality, 29*(1), 85–108. [CrossRef]

Busseri, M. A., & Erb, E. M. (2024). The happy personality revisited: Re-examining associations between Big Five personality traits and subjective well-being using meta-analytic structural equation modeling. *Journal of Personality, 92*(4), 968–984. [CrossRef] [PubMed]

Butkovic, A., Brkovic, I., & Bratko, D. (2012). Predicting well-being from personality in adolescents and older adults. *Journal of Happiness Studies, 13*, 455–467. [CrossRef]

Cacioppo, J. T., Hawkley, L. C., Ernst, J. M., Burleson, M., Berntson, G. G., Nouriani, B., & Spiegel, D. (2006). Loneliness within a nomological net: An evolutionary perspective. *Journal of Research in Personality, 40*(6), 1054–1085. [CrossRef]

Card, K. G., & Skakoon-Sparling, S. (2023). Are social support, loneliness, and social connection differentially associated with happiness across levels of introversion-extraversion? *Health Psychology Open, 10*(1), 20551029231184034. [CrossRef] [PubMed]

Carvalho, R. G., & Novo, R. F. (2014). The relationship between structural dimensions of personality and school life in adolescence. *Psicologia: Reflexão e Crítica, 27*(02), 368–376. [CrossRef]

Cheek, J. M., & Buss, A. H. (1981). Shyness and sociability. *Journal of Personality and Social Psychology, 41*(2), 330–339. [CrossRef]

Cheek, J. M., Carpentieri, A. M., Smith, T. G., Rierdan, J., & Koff, E. (1986). Adolescent shyness. In W. H. Jones, J. M. Cheek, & S. R. Briggs (Eds.), *Emotions, personality, and psychotherapy* (pp. 108–115). Springer. [CrossRef]

Cheng, H., & Furnham, A. (2003). Personality, self-esteem, and demographic predictions of happiness and depression. *Personality and Individual Differences, 34*(6), 921–942. [CrossRef]

Constantin, K., English, M. M., & Mazmanian, D. (2018). Anxiety, depression, and procrastination among students: Rumination plays a larger mediating role than worry. *Journal of Rational-Emotive and Cognitive-Behavior Therapy, 36*(1), 15–27. [CrossRef]

Conway, M., Csank, P. A. R., Holm, S. L., & Blake, C. K. (2000). On assessing individual differences in rumination on sadness. *Journal of Personality Assessment, 75*(3), 404–425. [CrossRef] [PubMed]

Coplan, R. J., Hipson, W. E., & Bowker, J. C. (2021). Social withdrawal and aloneliness in adolescence: Examining the implications of too Much and not enough solitude. *Journal of Youth and Adolescence, 50*(6), 1219–1233. [CrossRef]

Coplan, R. J., Ooi, L. L., & Baldwin, D. (2019). Does it matter when we want to be alone? Exploring developmental timing effects in the implications of unsociability. *New Ideas in Psychology, 53*, 47–57. [CrossRef]

Coplan, R. J., Ooi, L. L., & Nocita, G. (2015). When one is company and two is a crowd: Why some children prefer solitude. *Child Development Perspectives, 9*, 133–137. [CrossRef]

Corsano, P., Grazia, V., & Molinari, L. (2019). Solitude and loneliness profiles in early adolescents: A person-centered approach. *Journal of Child and Family Studies, 28*, 3374–3384. [CrossRef]

Corsano, P., Majorano, M., & Champretavy, L. (2006). Psychological well-being in adolescence: The contribution of interpersonal relations and experience of being alone. *Adolescence, 41*, 341–353. [PubMed]

Costa, P. T., & McCrae, R. R. (1992). The five-factor model of personality and its relevance to personality disorders. *Journal of Personality Disorders, 6*(4), 343–359. [CrossRef]

Daly, O., & Willoughby, T. (2020). A longitudinal person-centered examination of affinity for aloneness among children and adolescents. *Child Development, 91*(6), 2001–2018. [CrossRef] [PubMed]

De Fruyt, F., & Karevold, E. B. (2021). Personality in adolescence. In O. P. John, & R. W. Robins (Eds.), *Handbook of personality: Theory and research* (pp. 303–321). Guilford Press.

Endo, K., Ando, S., Shimodera, S., Yamasaki, S., Usami, S., Okazaki, Y., Sasaki, T., Richards, M., Hatch, S., & Nishida, A. (2017). preference for solitude, social isolation, suicidal ideation, and self-harm in adolescents. *Journal of Adolescent Health, 61*(2), 187–191. [CrossRef] [PubMed]

Eysenck, H. J. (1967). *The biological basis of personality* (pp. 100–117). Thomas.

Eysenck, H. J. (1991). Dimensions of personality: The biosocial approach to personality. In J. Strelau, & A. Angleitner (Eds.), *Explorations in temperament: International perspectives on theory and measurement* (pp. 87–103). Springer US.

Eysenck, H. J., & Eysenck, M. W. (1985). *Personality and individual differences: A natural science approach.* Plenum Press.

Fadda, D., & Scalas, L. F. (2016). Neuroticism as a moderator of direct and mediated relationships between introversion-extraversion and well-being. *Europe's Journal of Psychology, 12*(1), 49–67. [CrossRef] [PubMed]

Flett, G. L., Stainton, M., Hewitt, P. L., Sherry, S. B., & Lay, C. (2012). Procrastination automatic thoughts as a personality construct: An analysis of the Procrastinatory Cognitions Inventory. *Journal of Rational-Emotive & Cognitive-Behavior Therapy, 30*(4), 223–236. [CrossRef]

Gale, C. R., Booth, T., Mõttus, R., Kuh, D., & Deary, I. J. (2013). Neuroticism and extraversion in youth predict mental wellbeing and life satisfaction 40 years later. *Journal of Research in Personality, 47*(6), 687–697. [CrossRef] [PubMed]

Griffin, A. (2017). Adolescent neurological development and implications for health and well-being. *Healthcare, 5*(4), 62. [CrossRef] [PubMed]

Hemenover, S. H. (2003). Individual differences in the rate of affect change: Studies in affective chronometry. *Journal of Personality and Social Psychology, 85*, 121–131. [CrossRef] [PubMed]

Hills, P., & Argyle, M. (2001). Happiness, introversion–extraversion and happy introverts. *Personality and individual Differences, 30*(4), 595–608. [CrossRef]

Hipson, W. E., Coplan, R. J., Dufour, M., Wood, K. R., & Bowker, J. C. (2021). Time alone well spent? A person-centered analysis of adolescents' solitary activities. *Social Development, 30*(4), 114–1130. [CrossRef]

Ho, M. Y., Cheung, F. M., & Cheung, S. F. (2008). Personality and life events as predictors of adolescents' life satisfaction: Do life events mediate the link between personality and life satisfaction? *Social Indicators Research, 89*, 457–471. [CrossRef]

Hui, W., Haiqing, W., & Qiu, W. (2024). Understanding rumination thinking from the perspectives of psychological control source and personality traits. *Academic Journal of Humanities & Social Sciences, 7*(2), 176–184. [CrossRef]

John, O. P., & Srivastava, S. (1999). The Big Five Trait taxonomy: History, measurement, and theoretical perspectives. In L. A. Pervin, & O. P. John (Eds.), *Handbook of personality: Theory and research* (2nd ed., pp. 102–138). Guilford Press.

Jung, C. G. (1921). Psychological Types. In G. Ardler, & R. F. C. Hull (Eds.), *The collected works of C.G. Jung.* Complete Digital Edition. Available online: https://www.jungiananalysts.org.uk/wp-content/uploads/2018/07/C.-G.-Jung-Collected-Works-Volume-6_-Psychological-Types.pdf (accessed on 21 July 2024).

Kern, M. L., Benson, L., Steinberg, E. A., & Steinberg, L. (2016). The EPOCH measure of adolescent well-being. *Psychological Assessment, 28*(5), 586–597. [CrossRef] [PubMed]

Klimstra, T. A., Luyckx, K., Branje, S., Teppers, E., Goossens, L., & Meeus, W. H. (2013). Personality traits, interpersonal identity, and relationship stability: Longitudinal linkages in late adolescence and young adulthood. *Journal of Youth and Adolescence, 42*, 1661–1673. [CrossRef] [PubMed]

Kwiatkowska, M. M., & Rogoza, R. (2019). Shy teens and their peers: Shyness in respect to basic personality traits and social relations. *Journal of Research in Personality, 79*, 130–142. [CrossRef]

Lampropoulou, A. (2018). Personality, school, and family: What is their role in adolescents' subjective well-being. *Journal of Adolescence, 67*, 12–21. [CrossRef] [PubMed]

Larson, R., & Csikszentmihalyi, M. (1978). Experiential correlates of time alone in adolescence 1. *Journal of Personality, 46*(4), 677–693. [CrossRef]

Larson, R. W. (1990). The solitary side of life: An examination of the time people spend alone from childhood to old age. *Developmental Review*, *10*, 155–183. [CrossRef]

Lay, J., Pauly, T., Graff, J., Biesanz, J. C., & Hoppmann, C. (2019). By myself and liking it? Predictors of distinct types of solitude experiences in daily life. *Journal of Personality*, *87*, 633–647. [CrossRef] [PubMed]

Lay, J. C., Gerstorf, D., Scott, S. B., Pauly, T., & Hoppmann, C. A. (2017). Neuroticism and extraversion magnify discrepancies between retrospective and concurrent affect reports. *Journal of Personality*, *85*, 817–829. [CrossRef] [PubMed]

Li, S., Chen, X., Ran, G., Zhang, Q., & Li, R. (2021). Shyness and internalizing problems among Chinese adolescents: The roles of independent interpersonal stress and rumination. *Children and Youth Services Review*, *128*, 106151. [CrossRef]

Lin, P. H., Wang, P. Y., Lin, Y. L., & Yang, S. Y. (2020). Is it weird to enjoy solitude? Relationship of solitude capacity with personality traits and physical and mental health in junior college students. *International Journal of Environmental Research and Public Health*, *17*(14), 5060. [CrossRef] [PubMed]

Ludlow, L., & Klein, K. (2014). Suppressor variables: The difference between 'is' versus 'acting as'. *Journal of Statistics Education*, *22*(2), 1–28. Available online: https://jse.amstat.org/v22n2/ludlow.pdf (accessed on 15 September 2024). [CrossRef]

Lun, V. M.-C., & Yeung, J. C. (2019). Elaborating on the effect of culture on the relations of extraversion and neuroticism to life satisfaction. *Personality and Individual Differences*, *142*, 79–84. [CrossRef]

Luyckx, K., & Robitschek, C. (2014). Personal growth initiative and identity formation in adolescence through young adulthood: Mediating processes on the pathway to well-being. *Journal of Adolescence*, *37*(7), 973–981. [CrossRef]

Lynn, M., & Steel, P. (2006). National differences in subjective well-being: The interactive effects of extraversion and neuroticism. *Journal of Happiness Studies: An Interdisciplinary Forum on Subjective Well-Being*, *7*(2), 155–165. [CrossRef]

Lyon, K. A., Elliott, R., Brown, L. J. E., Eszlari, N., & Juhasz, G. (2021). Complex mediating effects of rumination facets between personality traits and depressive symptoms. *International Journal of Psychology*, *56*(5), 721–728. [CrossRef]

Margolis, S., & Lyubomirsky, S. (2020). Experimental manipulation of extraverted and introverted behavior and its effects on well-being. *Journal of Experimental Psychology. General*, *149*(4), 719–731. [CrossRef]

Matthews, T., Qualter, P., Bryan, B. T., Caspi, A., Danese, A., Moffitt, T. E., Odgers, C. L., Strange, L., & Arseneault, L. (2023). The developmental course of loneliness in adolescence: Implications for mental health, educational attainment, and psychosocial functioning. *Development and Psychopathology*, *35*(2), 537–546. [CrossRef] [PubMed]

McCrae, R. R., & John, O. P. (1992). An introduction to the five-factor model and its applications. *Journal of Personality*, *60*(2), 175–215. [CrossRef] [PubMed]

McVarnock, A., Cheng, T., Polakova, L., & Coplan, R. J. (2023). Are you alone? Measuring solitude in childhood, adolescence, and emerging adulthood. *Frontiers in Psychiatry*, *14*, 1179677. [CrossRef] [PubMed]

Napolitano, C. M., Sewell, M. N., Yoon, H. J., Soto, C. J., & Roberts, B. W. (2021). Social, emotional, and behavioral skills: An integrative model of the skills associated with success during adolescence and across the life span. *Frontiers in Education*, *6*, 679561. [CrossRef]

Nguyen, T. T., Weinstein, N., & Ryan, R. M. (2022). Who enjoys solitude? autonomous functioning (but not introversion) predicts self-determined motivation (but not preference) for solitude. *PLoS ONE*, *17*(5), e0267185. [CrossRef] [PubMed]

Nguyen, T. V. T., Ryan, R. M., & Deci, E. L. (2018). Solitude as an approach to affective self-regulation. *Personality and Social Psychology Bulletin*, *44*(1), 92–106. [CrossRef] [PubMed]

Ojanen, T., Findley-Van Nostrand, D., Bowker, J. C., & Markovic, A. (2017). Examining the distinctiveness and the socio-emotional correlates of anxious-withdrawal and unsociability during early adolescence in Finland. *The Journal of Early Adolescence*, *37*(3), 433–446. [CrossRef]

Oral, T., & Arslan, C. (2017). The investigation of university students' forgiveness levels in terms of self-compassion, rumination and personality traits. *Universal Journal of Educational Research*, *5*(9), 1447–1456. [CrossRef]

Ottawa-Carleton District School Board (OCDSB). (2020). *Valuing voices–identity matters!* Survey results. OCDSB Student Survey Results (Report). Available online: https://cdnsm5-ss13.sharpschool.com/UserFiles/Servers/Server_55394/File/News/OCDSB%20News/2020/June/Valuing%20Voices%20Final%20Tech%20Rpt%20%20Jun19%20v2.pdf#page=2.09 (accessed on 9 November 2024).

Petric, D. (2022). The introvert-ambivert-extrovert spectrum. *Open Journal of Medical Psychology*, *11*(3), 103–111. [CrossRef]

Ren, D., Wesselmann, E. D., & van Beest, I. (2021). Seeking solitude after being ostracized: A replication and beyond. *Personality & Social Psychology Bulletin*, *47*(3), 426–440. [CrossRef]

Roberts, B. W., Walton, K. E., & Viechtbauer, W. (2006). Patterns of mean-level change in personality traits across the life course: A meta-analysis of longitudinal studies. *Psychological Bulletin*, *132*, 1–25. [CrossRef] [PubMed]

Rodriguez, M., Bellet, B. W., & McNally, R. J. (2020). Reframing Time Spent Alone: Reappraisal Buffers the Emotional Effects of Isolation. *Cognitive Therapy and Research*, *44*(6), 1052–1067. [CrossRef]

Russell, D. W. (1996). UCLA loneliness scale (Version 3): Reliability, validity, and factor structure. *Journal of Personality Assessment*, *66*(1), 20–40. [CrossRef] [PubMed]

Rusting, C. L. (2001). Personality as a moderator of affective influences on cognition. In J. P. Forgas (Ed.), *Handbook of affect and social cognition* (pp. 163–183). Erlbaum.

Sandstrom, G. M., & Dunn, E. W. (2014). Is efficiency overrated? Minimal social interactions lead to belonging and positive affect. *Social Psychological and Personality Science*, *5*(4), 437–442. [CrossRef]

Sette, S., Brunetti, M., Pecora, G., Laghi, F., Longobardi, E., & Coplan, R. J. (2024). Examining links between motivations for social withdrawal, time spent alone, and indices of internalizing problems in childhood and early adolescence. *The Journal of Early Adolescence*. Advanced on-line publication. [CrossRef]

Soto, C. J., & Tackett, J. L. (2015). Personality traits in childhood and adolescence: Structure, development, and outcomes. *Current Directions in Psychological Science*, *24*(5), 358–362. [CrossRef]

Sprecher, S., Miller, R., Fehr, B., Kanter, J. B., Perlman, D., & Felmlee, D. (2023). Enhanced mood after a getting-acquainted interaction with a stranger: Do shy people benefit too? *Journal of Social and Personal Relationships*, *40*(7), 2110–2126. [CrossRef]

Srivastava, S., Angelo, K. M., & Vallereux, S. R. (2008). Extraversion and positive affect: A day reconstruction study of person–environment transactions. *Journal of Research in Personality*, *42*(6), 1613–1618. [CrossRef]

Steel, P., Schmidt, J., & Shultz, J. (2008). Refining the relationship between personality and subjective well-being. *Psychological Bulletin*, *134*(1), 138–161. [CrossRef] [PubMed]

Steinmayr, R., Wirthwein, L., Modler, L., & Barry, M. M. (2019). Development of subjective well-being in adolescence. *International Journal of Environmental Research and Public Health*, *16*(19), 3690. [CrossRef] [PubMed]

Suldo, S. M., Minch, D., & Hearon, B. V. (2015). Adolescent life satisfaction and personality characteristics: Investigating relationships using a five factor model. *Journal of Happiness Studies*, *16*(4), 965–983. [CrossRef]

Tackett, J. L. (2006). Evaluating models of the personality-psychopathology relationship in children and adolescents. *Clinical Psychology Review*, *26*, 584–599. [CrossRef] [PubMed]

Teppers, E., Klimstra, T. A., Damme, C. V., Luyckx, K., Vanhalst, J., & Goossens, L. (2013). Personality traits, loneliness, and attitudes toward aloneness in adolescence. *Journal of Social and Personal Relationships*, *30*(8), 1045–1063. [CrossRef]

Thomas, V., & Azmitia, M. (2019). Motivation matters: Development and validation of the motivation for solitude scale–short form (MSS-SF). *Journal of adolescence*, *70*, 33–42. [CrossRef] [PubMed]

Thomas, V., Carr, B. B., Azmitia, M., & Whittaker, S. (2021). Alone and online: Understanding the relationships between social media, solitude, and psychological adjustment. *Psychology of Popular Media*, *10*(2), 201–211. [CrossRef]

Thomas, V., & Nelson, P. A. (2024). The effects of multifaceted introversion and sensory processing sensitivity on solitude-seeking behavior. *Journal of Personality*, *93*(1), 51–66. [CrossRef] [PubMed]

Turner, S., Fulop, A., & Woodcock, K. A. (2024). Loneliness: Adolescents' perspectives on what causes it, and ways youth services can prevent it. *Children and Youth Services Review*, *157*, 107442. [CrossRef]

Vanhalst, J., Klimstra, T. A., Luyckx, K., Scholte, R. H. J., Engels, R., & Goossens, L. (2012). The interplay of loneliness and depressive symptoms across adolescence: Exploring the role of personality traits. *Journal of Youth and Adolescence*, *41*, 776–787. [CrossRef] [PubMed]

Vélez, C. E., Hoang, K. N., Krause, E. D., & Gillham, J. E. (2024). The Rumination on Problems Questionnaire: Broadening our understanding of rumination and its links to depression, anxiety, and stress in young adults. *Journal of Psychopathology and Behavioral Assessment*, *46*(1), 191–204. [CrossRef]

Waldinger, R., & Schulz, M. (2023). *The good life: Lessons from the world's longest scientific study of happiness*. Simon and Schuster.

Wang, J. M., Rubin, K. H., Laursen, B., Booth-LaForce, C., & Rose-Krasnor, L. (2013). Preference-for-solitude and adjustment difficulties in early and late adolescence. *Journal of Clinical Child and Adolescent Psychology*, *42*(6), 834–842. [CrossRef] [PubMed]

Watson, D., Clark, L. A., & Tellegen, A. (1988). Development and validation of brief measures of positive and negative affect: The PANAS scales. *Journal of Personality and Social Psychology*, *54*(6), 1063–1070. [CrossRef] [PubMed]

Wehmeyer, M. L., & Shogren, K. A. (2017). The development of self-determination during adolescence. In M. L. Wehmeyer, K. A. Shogren, T. D. Little, & S. J. Lopez (Eds.), *Development of self-determination through the life-course* (pp. 89–98). Springer Science+Business Media. [CrossRef]

Weinstein, N., Hansen, H., & Nguyen, T. V. (2023). Who feels good in solitude? A qualitative analysis of the personality and mindset factors relating to well-being when alone. *European Journal of Social Psychology*, *53*(7), 1443–1457. [CrossRef]

Weinstein, N., Nguyen, T. V., & Hansen, H. (2021). What time alone offers: Narratives of solitude from adolescence to older adulthood. *Frontiers in Psychology*, *12*, 714518. [CrossRef] [PubMed]

Wiggins, J. S. (1973). *Personality and prediction: Principles of personality assessment*. Addison-Wesley.

Wilson, T. D., Reinhard, D. A., Westgate, E. C., Gilbert, D. T., Ellerbeck, N., Hahn, C., Brown, C. L., & Shaked, A. (2014). Just think: The challenges of the disengaged mind. *Science*, *345*(6192), 75–77. [CrossRef]

Wood, D., Crapnell, T., Lau, L., Bennett, A., Lotstein, D., Ferris, M., & Kuo, A. (2018). Emerging adulthood as a critical stage in the life course. In *Handbook of life course health development* (pp. 123–143). Springer. [CrossRef]

Wood, K. R., Coplan, R. J., Hipson, W. E., & Bowker, J. C. (2021). Normative beliefs about social withdrawal in adolescence. *Journal of Research on Adolescence*, *32*(1), 372–381. [CrossRef] [PubMed]

Young, M. R., & Bradley, M. T. (1998). Social withdrawal: Self-efficacy, happiness, and popularity in introverted and extroverted adolescents. *Canadian Journal of School Psychology*, *14*(1), 21–35. [CrossRef]

Yuan, J., & Grühn, D. (2023). Preference and motivations for solitude in established adulthood: Antecedents, consequences, and adulthood phase differences. *Journal of Adult Development*, *30*(1), 64–77. [CrossRef]

Zelenski, J. M., Sobocko, K., & Whelan, D. C. (2021). Introversion, solitude, and happiness. In R. J. Coplan, J. C. Bowker, & L. J. Nelson (Eds.), *The handbook of solitude: Psychological perspectives on social isolation, social withdrawal, and being alone* (2nd ed., pp. 311–324). Wiley Blackwell. [CrossRef]

Zelenski, J. M., Whelan, D. C., Nealis, L. J., Besner, C. M., Santoro, M. S., & Wynn, J. E. (2013). Personality and affective forecasting: Trait introverts underpredict the hedonic benefits of acting extraverted. *Journal of Personality and Social Psychology*, *104*(6), 1092–1108. [CrossRef] [PubMed]

Zhao, J., Song, F., Chen, Q., Li, M., Wang, Y., & Kong, F. (2018). Linking shyness to loneliness in Chinese adolescents: The mediating role of core self-evaluation and social support. *Personality and Individual Differences*, *125*, 140–144. [CrossRef]

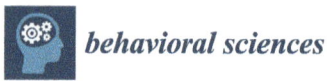

Article

Observed Shyness-Related Behavioral Responses to a Self-Presentation Speech Task: A Study Comparing Chinese and Canadian Children

Xiaoxue Kong [1,2,*], Taigan L. MacGowan [3], Shumin Wang [4], Yan Li [4] and Louis A. Schmidt [2]

[1] Department of Psychology, University of Northern British Columbia, Prince George, BC V2N 4Z9, Canada
[2] Department of Psychology, Neuroscience & Behaviour, McMaster University, Hamilton, ON L8S 4L8, Canada; schmidtl@mcmaster.ca
[3] Department of Psychology, Queen's University, Kingston, ON K7L 3N6, Canada; macgowat@mcmaster.ca
[4] Shanghai Institute of Early Childhood Education, Shanghai Normal University, Shanghai 201418, China; 1000529027@smail.shnu.edu.cn (S.W.); liyan@shnu.edu.cn (Y.L.)
* Correspondence: xiaoxue.kong@unbc.ca

Abstract: Past research suggests that expressions of shyness are associated with several distinct behaviors that may differ between Eastern and Western cultures. However, this evidence has largely been derived from subjective ratings, such self-, teacher-, and parent-report measures. In this study, we examined between-country differences on measures of directly observed shyness-related behaviors during a speech task in children. Participants were 74 Chinese (M_{age} = 4.76 years old, SD_{age} = 0.62 years old; 77.0% male) and 189 Canadian (M_{age} = 4.80 years old, SD_{age} = 0.82 years old; 48.1% male) children aged 4–6 years. As predicted, the results reveal that Chinese children exhibit a higher frequency of gaze aversion and lower total time speaking compared to Canadian children. Additionally, significant interactions between country and gender were found for fidgeting and smiling behaviors, indicating that cultural expectations and norms influence how boys and girls express some shyness-related behaviors in social situations. These preliminary findings extend prior cross-cultural research on shyness-related behaviors indexed using subjective report measures to directly observed measures, highlighting the importance of cultural context in shaping children's responses to social evaluation.

Keywords: shyness-related behaviors; gender differences; cross-cultural comparison; cultural norms

1. Introduction

Shyness is a characteristic of personality that reflects a tendency to feel anxious and inhibited in anticipation of or during social situations [1]. Shyness is perceived differently across Western and Eastern cultures due to varying cultural norms and values. In Western cultures, which emphasize individualism and personal freedom, shyness is often associated with social withdrawal and is linked to negative outcomes, such as low social status, peer victimization, and academic underachievement [2–4]. On the other hand, Eastern cultures, which prioritize group harmony and respect for authority, may view shyness more positively. In societies like traditional China, shyness is seen as a reflection of humility and respect for others, and is often considered an acceptable and adaptive behavior [5,6]. Although many previous articles have focused on the differences in shyness between Western and Eastern cultures [7], most studies have primarily measured shyness using subjective scales, with very few cross-cultural studies examining the expression of shyness-related behaviors.

Shyness-related behavioral responses occur when a person is in a situation that elicits perceived social evaluation, such as during a public performance or when meeting new people. Some of these behaviors include fidgeting, avoidance, gaze aversion, limited time spent speaking, and smiling [8–11]. The expression of shyness-related behaviors may vary by culture. For example, during a free-play laboratory session, Rubin and colleagues found that young children from East Asian countries (e.g., South Korea and China) exhibited more inhibitory behaviors, such as more time spent in contact with the mother and long latency to approach strangers and touch unfamiliar objects than young children from individualistic cultures (e.g., Italy and Australia) [12]. In addition, a study examined behavioral differences in trait measures of social anxiety, which is conceptually and empirically linked to shyness between Asian Americans and White Americans [13]. The responses of both groups of participants to social stimuli could be behaviorally coded in a speech task (e.g., avoidance of gaze and fidgeting), and the results indicate that Asian Americans reported more anxiety than White Americans on trait measures and mood rating scales.

Another important factor related to different manifestations of shyness in different cultures might be the social expectations of shyness vary across cultures [14]. Many Western studies consider shyness as a negative personality characteristic and consistently observe that young children lacked social initiation and exhibited more social withdrawal and inhibitory behaviors [15,16]. Since shyness may affect children's interaction with their peers, a lack of social initiation may result in peer rejection and refusal [17], as well as deficits in long-term social competence [18]. In contrast, Chinese cultures value personal interdependence, focusing on group harmony associated with modesty, self-control, and unassuming behaviors [7,19]. These different social expectations influence the prevalence of shyness and how others treat shy people [7]. To gain social acceptance, connectedness, and a sense of belonging, children need to maintain or change their behavior in accordance with social views and expectations [12]. Additionally, China has experienced large-scale economic and social reforms in the past 30 years; different evaluations and perceptions of shyness are beginning to emerge [20]. In traditional Chinese culture, shyness has been viewed more positively than in Western cultures. However, in recent decades, as China has become more globalized and individualistic traits have gained prominence, perceptions of shyness have shifted [21,22]. Researchers found that shyness is increasingly seen as a social hindrance in urban China, and shyness may lead to more negative peer relations and psychological challenges compared to their rural counterparts [22]. Due to the sociocultural changes and shifts in attitudes toward shyness, the expression of shyness in both Eastern and Western contexts in the new era needs more attention and research.

Collectively, in addition to those behaviors associated with shyness and related constructs, such as social anxiety, which have been mentioned above, a question remains: Are there other behaviors (fidgeting, avoidance, gaze aversion, smiling, and length of speech) associated with shyness across countries? Whether these behaviors manifest with different intensities in different cultures is still in need of study. An investigation of these issues will help developmental researchers better understand the similarities and differences in the process of social interaction in different cultures. Additionally, most existing studies on cultural differences regarding the expression of shyness focus exclusively on toddlers and subjective measures of shyness (e.g., self-, parent, and teacher reports), leaving a gap in our understanding of whether these differences persist in preschoolers and early school-aged children in both Western and Eastern cultural contexts, and whether the effects are present on more objective behavioral measures of shyness. The preschool and early school-age periods are particularly critical for examining shyness, as these time periods are when key features of shyness, such as self-awareness and self-consciousness, begin to develop and crystallize [23].

While some cultural differences in shyness-related behaviors have been explored, it is also important to consider how these differences interact with gender, particularly given the varied social norms and expectations that shape behavior in different cultural contexts. Although there has been a general lack of consistent gender differences reported in observed shyness-related behaviors in early and middle childhood [15,24–26], cultural norms regarding gender roles may influence these behaviors differently across cultures. For example, Chinese culture has more traditional attitudes toward girls [27]. In traditional Chinese culture, compared to boys, girls are typically expected to be quieter, more modest, and gentler and softer [28]. These expectations can lead to greater demands on girls' behavior, such as maintaining a proper posture, displaying good manners, and minimizing outward emotional expressions [29]. Research suggests that girls are often encouraged to be more compliant and to conform to social norms within family and social environments [30]. These cultural expectations may contribute to differences in how shyness is expressed and perceived across genders in different cultural contexts.

The Present Study

The purpose of the current study was to examine whether expressions of shyness-related behaviors in response to a self-presentation birthday speech differed between preschoolers and early school-aged children in China and Canada. This task, in which children speak about their most recent birthday, is commonly used to elicit self-presentation anxiety and expressions of shyness-related behaviors in the lab in children [31–33]. Here, we coded five shyness-related behaviors in response to the task, including fidgeting, avoidance, gaze aversion, time spent speaking, and smiling. Based on previous findings regarding behavioral inhibition (a shyness-related construct) across different countries [18], we predicted that there would be between-country differences in observed shyness-related behaviors during the speech task. Specifically, we expected that Chinese children would exhibit more fidgeting, avoidance, gaze aversion, and would speak and smile less than Canadian children.

Although gender differences regarding shyness appear during early and middle childhood in the Western context [15,24], we know relatively little about the interaction between culture and gender in shyness-related behaviors. However, based on the previous literature and cultural differences, we hypothesized that the interaction between culture and gender may have a more noticeable impact on behaviors like fidgeting and smiling, as these are more influenced by gender-specific social norms [25,26]. In contrast, behaviors like avoidance, gaze aversion, and speaking duration reflect more general cultural expectations and may be less likely to show an interaction between culture and gender.

The practical implications of this study are relevant for understanding the socialization processes and cultural expectations that shape early childhood development across different societies. Insights from this research could inform culturally responsive approaches in educational and developmental settings, allowing caregivers and educators to support diverse expressions of shyness in constructive and culturally sensitive ways.

2. Materials and Methods

2.1. Participants

Chinese participants included 74 children (M_{age} = 4.76 years old, SD_{age} = 0.62 years old; 77.0% male) between four and six years of age and their parents who were recruited from preschools in Shanghai, the People's Republic of China. The annual income of the Chinese sample, who were predominantly from the middle class in China, was approximately CAD 29,500. Procedures for the Chinese sample were conducted in a quiet extracurricular activity room in the kindergarten with a portable camera.

Canadian participants included 189 children (M_{age} = 4.80 years old, SD_{age} = 0.82 years old; 48.1% male) between four and six years of age and their parents who were recruited from a Child Database at McMaster University. The majority of the participants (81.9%) was White, and more than half (57.3%) had a total annual family income more than CAD 100,000 (in Canadian dollars). The Canadian sample was tested in a quiet playroom at McMaster University equipped with two closed-circuit TV (CCTV) cameras mounted on the walls.

Written informed consent was obtained from all children and their parents in both countries. In the consent form and prior to the study, both children and parents were informed about the entire study procedure and were told that they could withdraw from the experiment at any time for any reason during or after the study. If the parents chose to provide a debriefing to their children, the researchers would provide a debriefing of the study afterward. The Shanghai Normal University and McMaster University Research Ethics Boards approved the study procedures for both samples.

2.2. Self-Presentation Task

2.2.1. Procedures

The procedures and measures were identical across the two countries. For both country samples, a self-presentation task was used to elicit shy behavior in preschool-aged children [31–33]. The children were asked to stand in front of a video camera, then to look into the camera and talk about their most recent birthday. They were informed that the videotape of their speech would be shown to other children later, so that other children could know all about what they did on their last birthday.

If children were silent for more than 20 s, experimenters prompted the child with open-ended questions about their last birthday (e.g., "Did you have a birthday cake?"). The speech was videotaped, and behavioral responses to the task were coded offline by research assistants who were naive to the study hypotheses.

2.2.2. Behavioral Coding and Measures

Five shyness-related behaviors were coded based on coding schemes previously used with similar tasks [32,34,35]: fidgeting, avoidance, gaze aversion, time spent speaking, and smiling. These behaviors were coded across 6 10 s epochs (i.e., the first 60 s of the speech task), and average scores were calculated for each child's behavior. The mean values reported represent the average individual 10 s epoch.

2.2.3. Fidgeting

Intensity of nervous fidgeting was coded on a 4-point scale: 0 = *no evidence of fidgeting or very small incidences of fidgeting* to 3 = *highly repetitive and large bodily movements* (e.g., big arm swinging, kicking, and swiveling body back and forth). Intensity of avoidance behavior was coded on a 4-point scale: 0 = *no avoidance behavior* (e.g., the child stands in a designated place, no bodily avoidance) to 3 = *high avoidance behavior* (e.g., the child refuses to stand in a designated place or turns more than 90 degrees, covers their face, and articulates fearfulness).

2.2.4. Gaze Aversion

Gaze aversion was assessed by the extent to which children avoided the gaze of the experimenter and/or the camera over the course of 6 10 s epochs. Each epoch was coded in accordance with either a majority (6 s or more out of 10 s) gaze aversion or social gaze: *gaze aversion* was coded when children averted their gaze from the researcher or camera for at least 6 s within the 10 s epoch; *social gaze* was coded when children sustained their gaze with either the researcher or the camera for at least 6 s within the 10 s epoch. The proportion of epochs in which each child was considered to have been engaging in gaze aversion was then calculated.

2.2.5. Time Spent Speaking

Time spent speaking was assessed by recording the time (in seconds) that the child spent speaking during each 10 s epoch. An average time speaking scare was then calculated across all six epochs.

2.2.6. Smiling

Smiling was coded for each 10 s epoch, and the proportion of epochs in which smiling was present was calculated.

2.2.7. Behavioral Reliability

The Chinese coders who were fluent in both English and Chinese coded behaviors in the Chinese sample. These coders were trained to reach inter-coder reliability with the first author. The coders were naive to the study hypotheses and completed a subset of 20% of participant videos within the Chinese sample to establish inter-rater reliability. The inter-rater reliability was computed on this 20% subset across 2 raters. Inter-rater reliability was established (avoidance: $\kappa = 0.83$; fidgeting: $\kappa = 0.82$; gaze aversion $\kappa = 0.78$;

time spent speaking: $r = 92$; smiles: $r = 0.98$). Similarly, two English-speaking RAs coded videos for the Canadian sample on a subset of 19% of the participants (15% subset for time spent speaking). Inter-rater reliability was then established (avoidance: $\kappa = 0.69$; fidgeting: $\kappa = 0.73$; gaze aversion $\kappa = 0.70$; time spent speaking: $r = 84$; smiles: $r = 0.83$).

2.3. Data Analysis

A series of Pearson correlations was computed to examine the relations among the five coded shyness-related measures in the country. A repeated measures ANCOVA was conducted to examine the effects of country (China vs. Canada) and gender (boys vs. girls) on five z-scored shyness-related behaviors (gaze aversion, time spent speaking, fidgeting, smiling, and avoidance), while controlling for children's age. All analyses were performed using SPSS Version 24.

3. Results

3.1. Descriptive Statistics

Descriptive statistics and between-country differences of the five shyness-related behaviors coded from the birthday speech task are presented in Table 1. The mean values for each behavior measure represent the average per each 10 s coded epoch. Skewness and kurtosis values for these items in both samples were well within the cutoff levels of ± 2.

Table 1. Means and standard deviations and between-group differences on the five expressions of children's shyness-related behaviors by country.

Variable	China (N = 74)				Canada (N = 189)				Df	t	p
	M	SD	Skewness	Kurtosis	M	SD	Skewness	Kurtosis			
Gaze aversion	0.740	0.278	−0.754	−0.529	0.472	0.306	0.049	−0.984	250	6.504	<0.001
Time spent speaking	3.449	2.232	0.659	−0.251	4.985	2.206	−0.290	−0.543	250	−5.017	<0.001
Fidgeting	1.639	0.770	0.101	−0.935	1.900	0.664	−0.554	0.084	119.420	−2.528	0.013
Smiling	0.232	0.326	1.285	0.370	0.578	0.388	−0.315	−1.479	161.566	−7.216	<0.001
Avoidance	1.667	0.586	0.257	−0.591	1.557	0.753	−0.226	−0.867	174.885	1.234	>0.05

Notes. Mean values represent the mean value in an average 10 s coded epoch. Between country differences are evaluated at $p = 0.01$ to correct for multiple comparisons (i.e., $p < 0.05/5 = p = 0.01$).

Pearson correlations among the five shyness-related measures for each country are presented in Table 2. Of note, there were significant correlations between gaze aversion and avoidance in both countries, suggesting that these two shyness-related measures were associated with self-presentation in children, regardless of their country. However, the other observed behavioral measures during their speech were not inter-related in either country, suggesting that the individual behavioral measures may have presented different, unrelated, behavioral aspects of shyness.

Table 2. Correlations among the five expressions of children's shyness-related behaviors by country.

Item	1	2	3	4	5
1. Gaze aversion	-	−0.026	−0.208	−0.102	0.498 **
2. Time spent speaking	0.106	-	−0.018	0.021	−0.034
3. Fidgeting	−0.045	0.013	-	0.199	0.203
4. Smiling	−0.157 *	−0.002	0.256 **	-	0.140
5. Avoidance	0.262 **	−0.021	0.272 **	−0.021	-

Notes. Correlations above the diagonal are for the Chinese sample, and correlations below the diagonal are for the Canadian sample. All behaviors are standardized. Chinese $N = 74$; Canadian $N = 189$. * $p < 0.05$; ** $p < 0.01$.

3.2. Country by Gender

A significant interaction was found between country and gender for shyness-related behaviors, $F (3.660, 867.521) = 2.850$, $p = 0.027$, indicating that the pattern of these shyness-related behaviors differs significantly when considering the interaction of country and gender. In order to understand this interaction, we computed a series of separate two-way

ANCOVAs to examine how the interaction between country (China vs. Canada) and gender (boys vs. girls) affected each of the five shyness-related behaviors separately, while controlling for the children's age (Table 3).

Table 3. Results of repeated measures ANCOVA for the effects of country, gender, and age on shyness-related behaviors.

Source	Sum of Squares	*df*	Mean Square	F	*p*	Partial η^2
Within subjects						
Behaviors	24.357	3.66	6.654	7.325	<0.001	0.030
Behavior × Country	93.172	3.66	25.454	28.020	<0.001	0.106
Behavior × Gender	4.634	3.66	1.266	1.394	>0.05	0.006
Behavior × Country × Gender	9.476	3.66	2.589	2.850	0.027	0.012
Error (behaviors)	788.068	867.521	0.908			
Between subjects						
Country	9.834	1	9.834	8.731	0.003	0.036
Gender	0.069	1	0.069	0.061	0.805	0.000
Country × Gender	5.027	1	5.027	4.463	0.036	0.018
Age (Covariate)	0.461	1	0.461	0.409	0.523	0.002
Error	266.954	237	1.126			

3.2.1. Gaze Aversion

The results of the ANCOVA reveal that the main effect for country on gaze aversion is significant, $F(1, 243) = 42.04$, $p < 0.001$ (see Figure 1). As predicted, Chinese children ($M = 0.595$, $SE = 0.10$) displayed significantly more gaze aversion compared to Canadian children ($M = -0.245$, $SE = 0.07$). However, the main effect of gender on gaze aversion was not significant, $F(1, 243) = 2.13$, $p = 0.146$, indicating no significant difference in gaze aversion between boys ($M = 0.031$, $SE = 0.08$) and girls ($M = -0.058$, $SE = 0.09$). Moreover, the interaction effect between country and gender on gaze aversion was not significant, $F(1, 243) = 1.303$, $p = 0.255$.

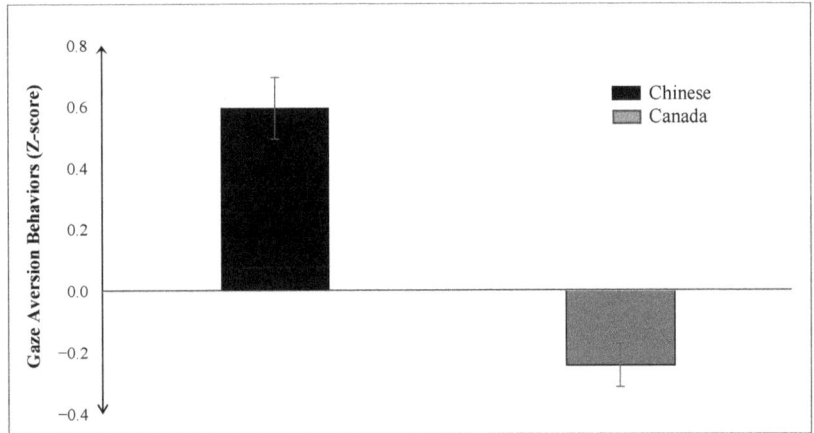

Figure 1. Main effect of country on gaze aversion behaviors. Error bars represent the standard error of the mean.

3.2.2. Time Spent Speaking

The results of the ANCOVA reveal that the main effect for country on time spent speaking is significant, $F(1, 243) = 21.09$, $p < 0.001$ (see Figure 2).

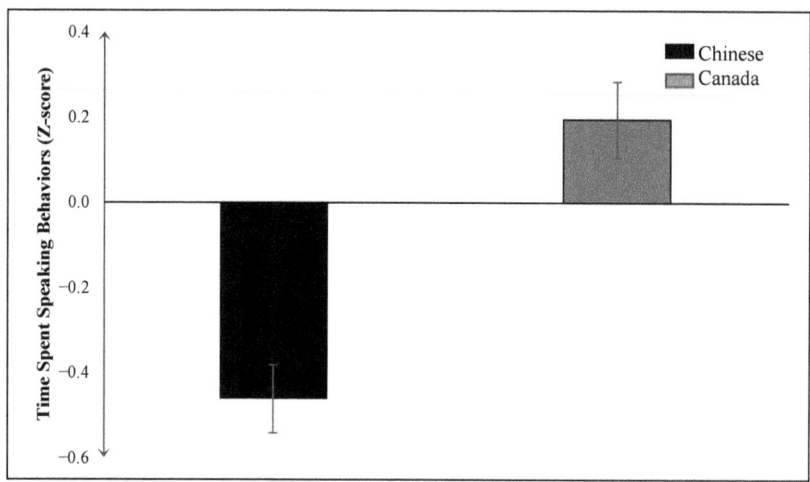

Figure 2. Main effect of country on time spent speaking behaviors. Error bars represent the standard error of the mean.

As predicted, Chinese children ($M = -0.46$, $SE = 0.09$) spent significantly less time speaking compared to Canadian children ($M = 0.19$, $SE = 0.07$). However, the main effect of gender was not statistically significant, $F(1, 243) = 0.11$, $p = 0.740$, indicating no significant difference in the time spent speaking between boys ($M = -0.053$, $SE = 0.08$) and girls ($M = 0.089$, $SE = 0.09$). Moreover, the interaction effect between country and gender on time spent speaking was not significant, $F(1, 243) = 0.794$, $p = 0.374$.

3.2.3. Fidgeting

The results of the ANCOVA reveal a significant interaction effect between country and gender on fidgeting, $F(1, 237) = 9.97$, $p = 0.002$ (see Figure 3). As shown in Figure 3, this interaction suggests that differences in fidgeting between boys and girls varied by country. Specifically, Canadian girls showed higher fidgeting scores ($M = 0.25$, $SE = 0.99$) compared to Chinese girls ($M = -0.78$, $SE = 1.10$), while Canadian boys had similar fidgeting scores ($M = -0.038$, $SE = 0.87$) compared to Chinese boys ($M = -0.14$, $SE = 1.02$).

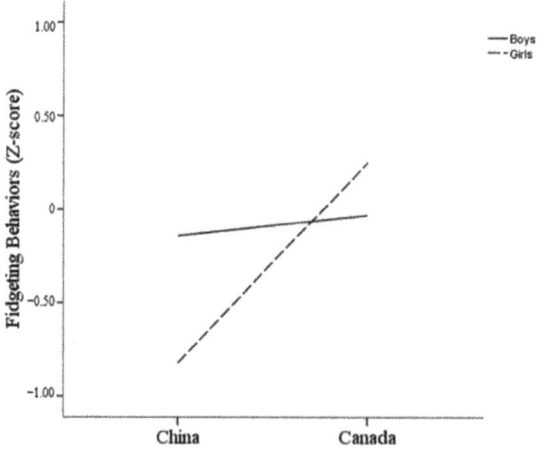

Figure 3. Interaction of country and gender on fidgeting.

3.2.4. Smiling Behaviors

The results of the ANCOVA reveal a significant interaction effect between country and gender on smiling, $F(1, 242) = 4.00$, $p = 0.047$ (see Figure 4). As shown in Figure 4, this interaction suggests that differences in smiling between boys and girls vary by country. Specifically, Canadian girls smiled more ($M = 0.31$, $SE = 0.09$) compared to Chinese girls ($M = -0.94$, $SE = 0.11$), while Canadian boys smiled more ($M = 0.19$, $SE = 0.10$) compared to Chinese boys ($M = -0.48$, $SE = 0.09$).

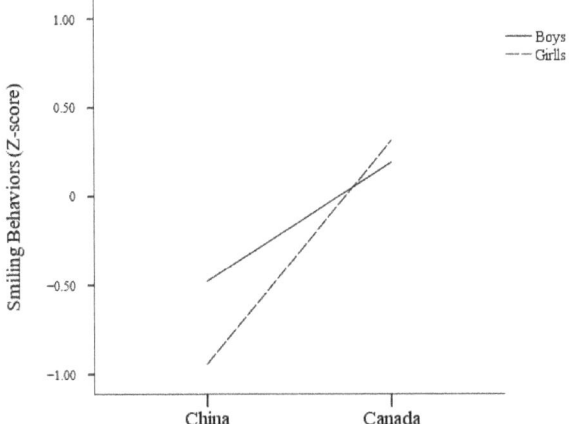

Figure 4. Interaction of country and gender on smiling.

3.2.5. Avoidance Behaviors

The country and gender interaction effect was not significant, $F(1,239) = 0.17$, $p = 0.683$), nor were the main effects for country, $F(1, 239) = 0.96$, $p = 0.329$ or gender, $F(1, 239) = 0.31$, $p = 0.577$ on avoidance behavior. There was no significant difference in avoidance behavior between Canadian ($M = -0.046$, $SE = 0.081$) and Chinese children ($M = 0.112$, $SE = 0.097$), as well as no significant differences between boys ($M = -0.042$, $SE = 0.088$) and girls ($M = 0.051$, $SE = 0.093$).

4. Discussion

In this study, we investigated whether Chinese and Canadian children differed in their observed expressions of shyness-related behaviors in response to a self-presentation task. As predicted, we found that Chinese children exhibited a higher frequency of gaze aversion, lower total time speaking, and a lower frequency of fidgeting and smiling compared with Canadian children during the speech task. Interestingly, the two countries did not differ in the avoidance measure. We also found that many of the observed measures during the speech task were not inter-related in either country, suggesting that the measures might affect different and unrelated behavioral aspects of shyness.

What do between-country and gender differences in children's observed shyness-related behaviors reflect? Previous studies have shown that Asian groups tend to exhibit more passive, deferential, unconfident, and anxious behaviors in social contexts, whereas Western groups are often characterized as more assertive [14,19]. Western cultures encourage lower levels of shyness, promoting peer acceptance and better well-being, and encouraging children to be more socially assertive [5,36]. In contrast, Eastern cultures emphasize self-restraint and non-assertiveness in interpersonal interactions, prioritizing social harmony [37,38]. Conforming to these social and cultural norms in both cultures is considered crucial for successful social development, even in young children [39]. Our findings support group differences in shyness-related behaviors in Chinese and Canadian children during a self-presentation task and suggest that culture may play a role in shaping these differences [18].

Eye contact can hold different cultural meanings regarding its directness [40]. In Western cultures, direct eye contact during communication is often encouraged, whereas in Eastern cultures, influenced by the etiquette values of Confucianism, direct eye contact is considered impolite and should be avoided when communicating [41]. Thus, this may be one explanation for the higher level of gaze aversion in the Chinese compared to the Canadian children. Researchers have posited that people who unknowingly attribute certain motives to eye avoidance (e.g., inattention, rudeness, shyness, and low intelligence) tend to be more biased [42].

Regarding the length of speech, previous research has supported the idea that children who are consistently shy and reticent are considered well-behaved in China [43]. Similarly, sensitive and silent children are considered *"guai"*, a common term used to praise children in China [43]. Therefore, Chinese children may be more likely to exhibit silent behavior due to Chinese acceptance than Canadian children.

The overall trend shows that fidgeting and smiling are relatively similar across cultures, with children from the same country exhibiting similar patterns. However, the differences in these behaviors between girls from China and Canada are more obvious than those observed between boys. This significant interaction between country and gender suggests that cultural expectations and norms play a critical role in shaping how boys and girls express discomfort or anxiety in social situations. In Canada, girls exhibited higher levels of fidgeting and smiling compared to their Chinese counterparts, while boys from both countries showed similar levels of fidgeting. Although Canadian boys smiled more frequently than Chinese boys, the difference was less obvious compared to that observed in girls. These patterns can be understood through the lens of cultural differences in the socialization of emotional expression.

In Chinese society, Confucianism plays an important role in influencing fidgeting behaviors, emphasizing the importance of considering others' views and evaluations [44,45]. As a result, Chinese children may be more susceptible to social threats in evaluative contexts, leading to fear-related behaviors, such as freezing or avoidance [46]. Therefore, Chinese children fidgeted less than Canadian children. Additionally, Chinese culture places greater social expectations on girls to behave delicately and quietly [28], which may explain why Chinese girls exhibit lower levels of fidgeting compared to boys.

Cultural differences in smiling behaviors can also be attributed to distinct norms and attributions regarding emotional expression. Researchers indicated that Canadian smile attributions may be based on internal emotional responses, while Chinese smile attributions may be based on modesty and assurance of the other person's face [47]. Therefore, these distinct cultural norms provide insights into why Chinese children may not smile as frequently in social settings. In Western cultures, smiling is often encouraged as a social behavior, especially for girls, who are typically socialized to be warm, friendly, and approachable [48]. This could explain why Canadian girls smile more compared to Chinese girls, who may be subject to cultural norms that emphasize modesty and emotional restraint [49–51]. For boys, while there is also the encouragement to smile in the Canadian culture, this expectation may not be as strongly enforced as it is for girls, leading to a smaller difference in smiling behavior between Canadian and Chinese boys. Therefore, although Chinese children generally exhibit lower levels of fidgeting and smiling compared to Canadian children, these differences are more pronounced among girls. This suggests that cultural norms place greater emphasis on behavioral expectations for girls, leading to more significant variations in how these behaviors are expressed across cultures.

Lastly, it is noteworthy that, although the mean level of avoidance behavior was higher in Chinese children than Canadian children, the two groups were not significantly different from one another regarding this behavioral measure. This may be due to the smaller sample size of Chinese children limiting the frequency of the behavior for this particular measure. Another possible explanation is that slight discrepancies in the positions of the experimenters and cameras between China and Canada resulted in deviations in the coding of avoidance behavior due to differences in the control of angles.

Strengths, Limitations, and Future Directions

The present study had several noteworthy strengths. These included (1) the collection of shyness-related behaviors from direct observations rather than a reliance on self-, teacher, and/or parent reports; (2) the developmental age studied, which coincides with the maturation and emergence of reliably measured social shyness; and (3) a direct comparison of children who were raised and residing in different countries, rather than comparing cultural differences among different cultural groups residing in the same country.

Despite these strengths, our study also had several limitations. First, unlike previous recent studies with self-report measures [52], we were unable to test for measurement invariance between the two countries to see if the coded measures were methodologically equivalent between China and Canada because of the relatively small sample sizes. Second, despite the advantages of observational methods, the micro-level behavioral variables chosen for coding in this study may not be equally sensitive to shyness, social anxiety, or social evaluation across ethnic groups [13]. Third, even though reliability among behavioral coders was established within and between countries, there may have been unmeasured variables and factors due to cultural differences in a setting that we did not control that may have adversely affected our observations. For example, the size of the observation room and the positioning of experimenters and cameras need to be considered. Fourth, the homogeneity of variance assumption was not met for smiling and avoidance behaviors, as indicated by Levene's test. This was likely due to cultural norms and individual coping strategies influencing these behaviors, leading to greater variability. Therefore, we need to exercise caution when interpreting the results for these two measures. Future research could use more robust statistical analyses to better understand cultural variances and may consider using alternative coding approaches and implementing more precise study designs to ensure consistency in behavioral observations. Future research should involve larger and more demographically diverse samples that incorporate multiple measurements of shyness in different contexts and establish measurement invariance for the measures to ensure trustworthiness between country comparisons. Future work should also consider examining psychophysiological measures between countries to extend and provide convergent evidence to the present findings. In terms of practical implications, it is important to consider how these findings can inform educational and social interventions, particularly for children transitioning between cultures. For example, when children from different cultures migrate or travel to new cultural contexts, understanding how cultural differences might condition the expression of shyness can be crucial for both educators and parents. Providing supportive environments that respect cultural differences in emotional expression may help children adapt more comfortably to new cultural settings and improve their social understanding.

5. Conclusions

To our knowledge, no previous studies have directly compared observed shyness-related behaviors in children in response to a self-presentation speech task at this age from Eastern and Western cultures. Our preliminary findings extend prior work examining cross-cultural differences in children's shyness using subjective measures of self-, teacher, and parent reports to measures obtained from direct observation. This study demonstrates the impact of culture on the expression of some shyness-related behaviors in children, highlighting the importance of cultural norms and individual behaviors. These findings also contribute to our understanding of how cultural context influences the manifestation of shyness-related behaviors in social contexts and also provide insights for educators, parents, and researchers interested in promoting the socioemotional development of children from diverse cultural backgrounds.

Behav. Sci. **2024**, *14*, 1147

Author Contributions: Conceptualization, X.K. and L.A.S.; methodology, X.K., T.L.M. and L.A.S.; validation, X.K. and L.A.S.; formal analysis, X.K.; investigation, X.K., S.W., Y.L. and L.A.S.; resources, T.L.M., Y.L. and L.A.S.; data curation, X.K., T.L.M., S.W., Y.L. and L.A.S.; writing—original draft preparation, X.K.; writing—review and editing, T.L.M., S.W., Y.L. and L.A.S.; supervision, Y.L. and L.A.S.; project administration, X.K., Y.L. and L.A.S.; funding acquisition, Y.L. and L.A.S. All authors have read and agreed to the published version of the manuscript.

Funding: This research was supported by the NSERC: 2017-05342 and STI 2030 Major Projects (Nos. 2022ZD0209000, 2022ZD0209001, 2022ZD0209002, 2022ZD0209003, 2022ZD0209004, 2022ZD0209005, and 2021ZD0200516).

Institutional Review Board Statement: The study was conducted in accordance with the Declaration of Helsinki, and approved by McMaster University (MREB# 2073, 8 July 2019) and the Institutional Review Board of Shanghai Normal University (No. 2021021, 28 October 2021).

Informed Consent Statement: Informed consent was obtained from all subjects involved in the study.

Data Availability Statement: The data presented in this study are available on request from the corresponding authors.

Conflicts of Interest: The authors declare no conflicts of interest.

References

1. Cheek, J.M.; Melchior, L.A. Shyness, Self-Esteem, and Self-Consciousness. In *Handbook of Social and Evaluation Anxiety*; Springer: Boston, MA, USA, 1990; pp. 47–82.
2. Coplan, R.J.; Weeks, M. Shy and Soft-Spoken: Shyness, Pragmatic Language, and Socio-Emotional Adjustment in Early Childhood. *Infant Child Dev.* **2010**, *19*, 238–254. [CrossRef]
3. Rubin, K.H.; Asendorpf, J.B. *Social Withdrawal, Inhibition, and Shyness in Childhood*; Erlbaum: Hillsdale, NJ, USA, 1993.
4. Schmidt, L.A.; Fox, N.A.; Rubin, K.H.; Hu, S.; Hamer, D.H. Molecular Genetics of Shyness and Aggression in Preschoolers. *Pers. Individ. Dif.* **2017**, *116*, 66–71. [CrossRef]
5. Chen, X.; Wang, L.; Wang, Z. Shyness-Sensitivity and Social, School, and Psychological Adjustment in Rural Migrant and Urban Children in China. *Child Dev.* **2009**, *80*, 1499–1513. [CrossRef] [PubMed]
6. Xu, Y.; Farver, J.M.; Zhang, Z.; Zeng, Q.; Yu, L.; Cai, B. Mainland Chinese Parenting Styles and Parent-Child Interaction. *Int. J. Behav. Dev.* **2007**, *31*, 210–217.
7. Chen, X. Culture and shyness in childhood and adolescence. *New Ideas Psychol.* **2019**, *53*, 58–66. [CrossRef]
8. Asendorpf, J.B. The Expression of Shyness and Embarrassment. In *Shyness and Embarrassment: Perspectives from Social Psychology*; Crozier, R., Ed.; Cambridge University Press: Cambridge, UK, 1990; pp. 87–118.
9. Colonnesi, C.; Napoleone, E.; Bögels, S.M. Positive and negative expressions of shyness in toddlers: Are they related to anxiety in the same way? *J. Pers. Soc. Psychol.* **2014**, *106*, 624–637. [CrossRef]
10. Kagan, J.; Snidman, N.; Arcus, D. Childhood derivatives of high and low reactivity in infancy. *Child Dev.* **1998**, *69*, 1483–1493. [CrossRef]
11. Poole, K.L.; Schmidt, L.A. Temperamental contributions to state expressions of shyness in children. *Pers. Individ. Dif.* **2022**, *186*, 111345. [CrossRef]
12. Rubin, K.H.; Coplan, R.J.; Bowker, J.C. Social withdrawal in childhood. *Annu. Rev. Psychol.* **2009**, *60*, 141–171. [CrossRef]
13. Okazaki, S.; Liu, J.F.; Longworth, S.L.; Minn, J.Y. Asian American-white American differences in expressions of social anxiety: A replication and extension. *Cult. Divers. Ethn. Minor. Psychol.* **2002**, *8*, 234–247. [CrossRef]
14. Chen, X.; French, D.C. Children's social competence in cultural context. *Annu. Rev. Psychol.* **2008**, *59*, 591–616. [CrossRef]
15. Coplan, R.J.; DeBow, A.; Schneider, B.H.; Graham, A.A. The social behaviours of inhibited children in and out of preschool. *Br. J. Dev. Psychol.* **2009**, *27*, 891–905. [CrossRef] [PubMed]
16. Rimm-Kaufman, S.E.; Kagan, J. Infant predictors of kindergarten behavior: The contribution of inhibited and uninhibited temperament types. *Behav. Brain Sci.* **2005**, *28*, 767–768. [CrossRef]
17. Gazelle, H.; Ladd, G.W. Anxious solitude and peer exclusion: A diathesis-stress model of internalizing trajectories in childhood. *Child Dev.* **2003**, *74*, 257–278. [CrossRef] [PubMed]
18. Rubin, K.H.; Hemphill, S.A.; Chen, X.; Hastings, P.; Sanson, A.; Coco, A.L.; Cui, L. A cross-cultural study of behavioral inhibition in toddlers: East–West–North–South. *Int. J. Behav. Dev.* **2006**, *30*, 219–226. [CrossRef]
19. Liu, M.; Wang, C.; Park, H. Cultural differences in shyness and modesty among Chinese and American children. *J. Cross-Cult. Psychol.* **2015**, *46*, 713–729.
20. Liu, J.; Chen, X.; Li, D. Shyness and Unsociability and Their Relations with Adjustment in Chinese and Canadian Children. *J. Cross-Cult. Psychol.* **2015**, *46*, 371–386. [CrossRef]

21. Chen, X. Shyness-Inhibition in Childhood and Adolescence: A cross-Cultural Perspective. In *The Development of Shyness and Social Withdrawal*; Rubin, K.H., Coplan, R.J., Eds.; The Guilford Press: New York, NY, USA, 2010; pp. 213–235.
22. Liu, J.; Bowker, J.C.; Coplan, R.J.; Yang, P.; Li, D.; Chen, X. Evaluating links among shyness, peer relations, and internalizing problems in Chinese young adolescents. *J. Res. Adolesc.* **2019**, *29*, 696–709. [CrossRef]
23. Kondratiuk, M. Phenomenon of self-consciousness and its development during infancy and childhood. In Proceedings of the E3S Web of Conferences, Virtual, 5 May 2020; EDP Sciences: Les Ulis, France; Volume 164, p. 12017.
24. Coplan, R.J.; Rubin, K.H.; Fox, N.A.; Calkins, S.D.; Stewart, S.L. Being alone, playing alone, and acting alone: Distinguishing among reticence and passive and active solitude in young children. *Child Dev.* **1994**, *65*, 129–137. [CrossRef]
25. Kagan, J.; Reznick, J.S.; Snidman, N. The physiology and psychology of behavioral inhibition in children. *Annu. Prog. Child Psychiatry Child Dev.* **1987**, *58*, 1459–1473. [CrossRef]
26. Mullen, M.; Snidman, N.; Kagan, J. Free-play behavior in inhibited and uninhibited children. *Infant Behav. Dev.* **1993**, *16*, 383–389. [CrossRef]
27. Liu, R.X.; Tein, J.Y.; Zhao, Z. Coping strategies and behavioral-emotional problems among Chinese adolescents. *Psychiatry Res.* **2004**, *126*, 275–285. [CrossRef]
28. Liu, F. Boys as only-children and girls as only-children—Parental gendered expectations of the only-child in the nuclear Chinese family in present-day China. *Gend. Educ.* **2006**, *18*, 491–505. [CrossRef]
29. Yu, C.; Zuo, X.; Lian, Q.; Zhong, X.; Fang, Y.; Lou, C.; Tu, X. Comparing the perceptions of gender norms among adolescents with different sibling contexts in Shanghai, China. *Children* **2022**, *9*, 1281. [CrossRef] [PubMed]
30. Pyke, K.D.; Johnson, D.L. Asian American Women and Racialized Femininities: "Doing" Gender across Cultural Worlds. *Gend. Soc.* **2003**, *17*, 33–53. [CrossRef]
31. Fox, N.A.; Rubin, K.H.; Calkins, S.D.; Marshall, T.R.; Coplan, R.J.; Porges, S.W.; Stewart, S. Frontal activation asymmetry and social competence at four years of age. *Child Dev.* **1995**, *66*, 1770–1784. [CrossRef]
32. MacGowan, T.L.; Colonnesi, C.; Nikolić, M.; Schmidt, L.A. Expressions of shyness and theory of mind in children: A psychophysiological study. *Cogn. Dev.* **2022**, *61*, 101138. [CrossRef]
33. Theall-Honey, L.A.; Schmidt, L.A. Do temperamentally shy children process emotion differently than nonshy children? Behavioral, psychophysiological, and gender differences in reticent preschoolers. *Dev. Psychobiol.* **2006**, *48*, 187–196. [CrossRef]
34. MacGowan, T.L.; Schmidt, L.A. Getting to the heart of childhood empathy: Relations with shyness and respiratory sinus arrhythmia. *Dev. Psychobiol.* **2021**, *63*, e22035. [CrossRef]
35. MacGowan, T.L.; Schmidt, L.A. Helping as prosocial practice: Longitudinal relations among children's shyness, helping behavior, and empathic response. *J. Exp. Child Psychol.* **2021**, *209*, 105154. [CrossRef]
36. Chen, X.; Tse, H.C.H. Social functioning and adjustment in Canadian-born children with Chinese and European backgrounds. *Dev. Psychol.* **2008**, *44*, 1184–1189. [CrossRef] [PubMed]
37. Chen, X.; Cen, G.; Li, D.; He, Y. Social functioning and adjustment in Chinese children: The imprint of historical time. *Child Dev.* **2005**, *76*, 182–195. [CrossRef] [PubMed]
38. Fukuyama, M.A.; Greenfield, T.K. Dimensions of assertiveness in an Asian-American student population. *J. Couns. Psychol.* **1983**, *30*, 429. [CrossRef]
39. Denham, S.A.; Bassett, H.H.; Brown, C.; Way, E.; Steed, J. "I know how you feel": Preschoolers' emotion knowledge contributes to early school success. *J. Early Child. Res.* **2015**, *13*, 252–262. [CrossRef]
40. McCarthy, A.; Lee, K.; Itakura, S.; Muir, D.W. Cultural display rules drive eye gaze during thinking. *J. Cross-Cult. Psychol.* **2006**, *37*, 717–722. [CrossRef]
41. Argyle, M.; Cook, M.; Cramer, D. Gaze and mutual gaze. *Br. J. Psychiatry* **1994**, *165*, 848–850. [CrossRef]
42. Sue, D.W.; Sue, D. Barriers to effective cross-cultural counseling. *J. Couns. Psychol.* **1977**, *24*, 420–429. [CrossRef]
43. Chen, X.; Rubin, K.H.; Sun, Y. Social reputation and peer relationships in Chinese and Canadian children: A cross-cultural study. *Child Dev.* **1992**, *63*, 1336–1343. [CrossRef]
44. Chen, X. Socioemotional Development in Chinese Children. In *Handbook of Chinese Psychology*; Bond, M.H., Ed.; Oxford University Press: Oxford, UK, 2010; pp. 37–52.
45. Henrich, C.C.; Blatt, S.J.; Kuperminc, G.P.; Zohar, A.; Leadbeater, B.J. Levels of interpersonal concerns and social functioning in early adolescent boys and girls. *J. Pers. Assess.* **2001**, *76*, 48–67. [CrossRef]
46. Broesch, T.; Callaghan, T.; Henrich, J.; Murphy, C.; Rochat, P. Cultural variations in children's mirror self-recognition. *J. Cross-Cult. Psychol.* **2011**, *42*, 1018–1029. [CrossRef]
47. Wiseman, R.L.; Pan, X. Smiling in the People's Republic of China and the United States: Status and situational influences on the social appropriateness of smiling. *Intercult. Commun. Stud.* **2004**, *13*, 1–18.
48. Hess, U.; Adams, R.B.; Kleck, R.E. The face is not an empty canvas: How facial expressions interact with facial appearance. *Philos. Trans. R. Soc. B Biol. Sci.* **2009**, *364*, 3497–3504. [CrossRef] [PubMed]
49. Buck, R.; Losow, J.I.; Murphy, M.M.; Costanzo, P. Social facilitation and inhibition of emotional expression and communication. *J. Pers. Soc. Psychol.* **1992**, *63*, 962–968. [CrossRef] [PubMed]
50. Gudykunst, W.B.; Ting-Toomey, S.; Chua, E. *Culture and Interpersonal Communication*; Sage Publications: Thousand Oaks, CA, USA, 1988.

51. Hofstede, G. *Culture's Consequences: International Differences in Work-Related Values*; Sage Publications: Beverly Hills, CA, USA, 1980.
52. Kong, X.; Brook, C.A.; Li, J.; Li, Y.; Schmidt, L.A. Shyness subtypes and associations with social anxiety: A comparison study of Canadian and Chinese children. *Dev. Sci.* **2024**, *27*, e13369. [CrossRef]

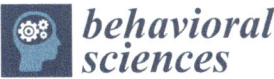

Article

Estimating the Heterogeneous Causal Effects of Parent–Child Relationships among Chinese Children with Oppositional Defiant Symptoms: A Machine Learning Approach

Haiyan Zhou [1,2,3,4], Fengkai Han [1,2,3,4], Ruoxi Chen [5,6], Jiajin Huang [1,2,3,4], Jianhui Chen [1,2,3,4] and Xiuyun Lin [5,6,*]

1   Faculty of Information Technology, Beijing University of Technology, Beijing 100124, China;
    zhouhaiyan@bjut.edu.cn (H.Z.); mochen12134@emails.bjut.edu.cn (F.H.); jhuang@bjut.edu.cn (J.H.);
    chenjianhui@bjut.edu.cn (J.C.)
2   Beijing International Collaboration Base on Brain Informatics and Wisdom Services, Beijing 100124, China
3   Engineering Research Center of Intelligent Perception and Autonomous Control, Ministry of Education,
    Beijing 100124, China
4   Engineering Research Center of Digital Community, Ministry of Education, Beijing 100124, China
5   Institute of Developmental Psychology, Faculty of Psychology, Beijing Normal University,
    Beijing 100875, China; chenruoxi@mail.bnu.edu.cn
6   Beijing Key Laboratory of Applied Experimental Psychology, National Demonstration Center for
    Experimental Psychology Education, Faculty of Psychology, Beijing Normal University, Beijing 100875, China
*   Correspondence: linxy@bnu.edu.cn

Abstract: Oppositional defiant symptoms are some of the most common developmental symptoms in children and adolescents with and without oppositional defiant disorder. Research has addressed the close association of the parent–child relationship (PCR) with oppositional defiant symptoms. However, it is necessary to further investigate the underlying mechanism for forming targeted intervention strategies. By using a machine learning-based causal forest (CF) model, we investigated the heterogeneous causal effects of the PCR on oppositional defiant symptoms in children in Chinese elementary schools. Based on the PCR improvement in two consecutive years, 423 children were divided into improved and control groups. The assessment of oppositional defiant symptoms (AODS) in the second year was set as the dependent variable. Additionally, several factors based on the multilevel family model and the baseline AODS in the first year were included as covariates. Consistent with expectations, the CF model showed a significant causal effect between the PCR and oppositional defiant symptoms in the samples. Moreover, the causality exhibited heterogeneity. The causal effect was greater in those children with higher baseline AODS, a worse family atmosphere, and lower emotion regulation abilities in themselves or their parents. Conversely, the parenting style played a positive role in causality. These findings enhance our understanding of how the PCR contributes to the development of oppositional defiant symptoms conditioned by factors from a multilevel family system. The heterogeneous causality in the observation data, established using the machine learning approach, could be helpful in forming personalized family-oriented intervention strategies for children with oppositional defiant symptoms.

Keywords: oppositional defiant symptoms; multilevel family model; parent–child relationship; causal forest model; causal effect; heterogeneity

1. Introduction

Oppositional defiant disorder includes a variety of emotional and behavioral problems characterized by a recurrent pattern of angry/irritable moods, argumentative/defiant behavior, and vindictiveness toward authority figures [1–3]. As one of the most prevalent mental health disorders among children, the average prevalence rate is approximately 3–4% [1]. In China, the prevalence rate is believed to be 2.3–8% [4–6]. Moreover, based on the rating of parents or teachers [3,7–9], oppositional defiant symptoms can be found in a larger group of children and adolescents not directly diagnosed as having oppositional defiant disorder by professional psychiatrists or authoritative organizations [9,10]. Previous studies have identified numerous factors associated with oppositional defiant symptoms, whereas family factors, such as weak and poor familial contextual conditions [7], bad parental psychopathology [3,8–10], poor disciplinary practices [7], frequent interpersonal conflicts [10], and low emotional regularity ability [7,10] are known to be significantly associated with the development of oppositional defiant symptoms in children. However, for forming more effective intervention strategies, research is needed to further clarify the underlying pathways linking these factors to oppositional defiant symptoms.

1.1. Multilevel Family Model and Oppositional Defiant Symptoms

The multilevel family model is proposed to explain the effects on the development and maintenance/exacerbation oppositional defiant symptoms in children across the entire family level, dyadic level, and individual level [9–11]. Factors at the entire family level include surface features (such as socioeconomic status) and deep features (such as family functions). Socioeconomic status is a comprehensive evaluation of a family's economic income and social status, and family monthly income is a representative indicator. Many studies have shown that poor economic conditions, such as low family income and unemployment [12,13], are closely related to oppositional defiant symptoms. Family function refers to the interaction of physical, emotional, and psychological activities among all family members and is composed of family cohesion and adaptability. Considering the family as a complete unit and system, factors at the entire family level have proven to be closely related to destructive behavior in children, including oppositional defiant symptoms. Specifically, excessive conflict and contradictions in the family will worsen the relationship between family members and lead to destructive behavior in children [14–17], while family cohesion is a protective factor for children in terms of them developing oppositional defiant symptoms [18]. Moreover, factors at the entire family level can not only impact oppositional defiant symptoms directly but also indirectly through factors at the dyadic level (e.g., the relationship between the parent and children) and the individual level (e.g., the child's emotion regulation abilities) [9].

The dyadic level, as a subsystem level, refers to the interactions between two or more family members, including a husband–wife subsystem and a parent–child subsystem. In the husband–wife subsystem, the marital relationship is one of the most impactful family risk factors in relation to children's disruptive behaviors. Lower marital quality, such as more marital conflict and violence between intimate partners, is associated with more oppositional defiant symptoms in children [19,20]. In the parent–child subsystem, a large number of research has emphasized the strong association with oppositional defiant symptoms. On the one hand, children with oppositional defiant symptoms have more conflicts with their parents in comparison with children without oppositional defiant symptoms [21], and children with oppositional defiant symptoms are associated more with subsequent depression and less happiness, which can be influenced by the parental attachment [4]. On the other hand, a maladaptive parenting style is very critical in increasing oppositional defiant symptoms [6,8,15]. Children with oppositional defiant symptoms are more likely to experience maltreatment, including physical and emotional abuse and emotional neglect [22,23]. It is also found that factors at the dyadic level can have direct effects on oppositional defiant symptoms and indirect effects through individual characteristics [9].

The individual level mainly focuses on the individual family members themselves, including both the parent's individual level and the child's individual level. With respect to individual parent factors, parental individual characteristics (e.g., parental depression, aggression, anxiety), cognitive factors (e.g., parental negative attribution style) and emotion factors (e.g., emotion regulation) are included [8,24–26]. One of the main contributing factors to the development of oppositional defiant symptoms in children is parental emotion regulation. Research shows that parental emotion dysregulation was significantly and positively related to child's oppositional defiant symptoms [22,27]. At the individual level of children, child emotion regulation has proven to be a consistently strong predictor of child emotional and behavioral problems [7,10]. The multilevel family model has proposed that factors at the individual level are the most proximal factors linked to oppositional defiant symptoms [9,11,22].

In summary, the multilevel family model respectively integrates the related family factors into the entire, dyadic and individual levels to increase understanding the development of oppositional defiant symptoms. Moreover, studies have demonstrated contributions from these factors to oppositional defiant symptoms. Many family factors could affect the development of oppositional defiant symptoms directly, but also, the factors highly interact and are associated with the oppositional defiant symptoms. It is still worthy of investigating the complicated linkages between these factors and oppositional defiant symptoms along with the family system perspective.

1.2. Parent–Child Relationship and Oppositional Defiant Symptoms

The parent–child relationship (PCR) is one of the most important factors at the dyadic level, and reflects the attention parents give to children and the attachment of children to parents [28]. Basically, a strong and secure PCR can provide a stable and supportive environment for children, which can mitigate the negative effects of family conflicts and be conducive to their healthy growth [29]. In contrast, a poor and impaired PCR can increase the risk of oppositional defiant symptoms. In a study with a large sample [7], the parents' support showed a direct association with the oppositional defiant symptoms in preschool children. It is also suggested that the PCR plays a pivotal role in the development and exacerbation of oppositional defiant symptoms in Chinese children [6,10]. Moreover, many intervention strategies are focused on the management of PCR [6,30], and have demonstrated the feasibility and effectiveness of improvements in PCR across different cultural contexts [31]. Behavioral problems in young children, including oppositional defiant symptoms, could be alleviated by improving PCRs with behavioral intervention strategies [32]. They can also enhance parents' parenting skills and sense of parenting efficacy [33]. However, despite the strong association, it is quite valuable to precisely predict the potential benefits of improvements in PCR in terms of oppositional defiant symptoms at the individual level or among different populations for providing personalized advice before implementing a targeted intervention strategy.

Additionally, as a two-way interpersonal relationship between parents and children, the impact of the PCR on oppositional defiant symptoms is quite complex. On the one hand, there are indirect associations the between the PCR and oppositional defiant symptoms mediated by other family factors. Firstly, the PCR could affect oppositional defiant symptoms through child emotional regulation [6,7]. Children with a poor PCR have more difficulties in regulating their emotions and behaviors, which leads to a greater risk of developing anxiety and other internalized problems [34]. Furthermore, the level of temperament-related negative affects and sensory regulation can further serve as mediators in the relationship between parent support and oppositional defiant symptoms [7]. Moreover, a longitudinal study further showed that the quality of the PCR in the first year could affect the risk of oppositional defiant symptoms in the third year through the level of parental depressive symptoms in the second year [5]. On the other hand, PCR can also serve as a mediator linking factors on the entire family level [4,11]. A family environment characterized by frequent conflicts and tense relationships may lead children to learn negative interpersonal patterns, including undesirable methods of emotional regulation and behavioral control, thereby increasing the risk of oppositional defiant symptoms [34]. Considering a specific dimension of the PCR, parental alienation plays a mediating role between family violence and oppositional defiant symptoms, which indicates that family violence increases children's feeling of alienation from parents and that higher parental alienation contributes to more oppositional defiant symptoms [35]. Hence, there is a need to more deeply understand the mechanisms of the PCR in the development of child oppositional defiant symptoms and explain the complex relationship between them by considering the family factors.

1.3. Causal Inference and Its Heterogeneity

Causal inference based on observational data has received attention from scholars in mathematics and machine learning, which can hierarchically consists of three layers with different causal concepts for reasoning: association, intervention, and counterfactuals [36–38]. Association deals with purely 'observational' and factual information, which is what machine learning usually achieves by recognizing what is happening. For example, regression models [38] are often used to assess the relationship between variables. In addition to this, the method of using the structural equation model (SEM) could establish correlations when considering multiple dependent variables simultaneously [39]. These methods have been widely used in human behavior and psychology studies.

The second layer of intervention is about the effect of the action, which encodes information about what would happen if a certain intervention is hypothesized. The typical question asked in child development is "What happens if we carry out the behavioral intervention strategy?". Finally, counterfactuals deal with information about what would have happened if a certain intervention had been carried out, from a counterfactual perspective. The typical question asked is "How would the outcome be different now if the behaviour had been different in the past?". A new data-driven approach, the causal forest (CF) model, has been proposed for explaining interventional causality as well as counterfactual causality with observational data [40–43].

The CF model comprises a number of causal trees consisting of a single root node and multiple child nodes with binary branches. First, the samples in the CF model are assigned into two groups according to the conditions of an independent variable. Then, every single causal tree is grown based on the principle of maximizing the variance in estimated causal effects in each node by comparing the outcomes or values of the dependent variable within the two groups in each node [43]. Meanwhile, all the covariates in each node are balanced between the two groups for controlling their effects on the causality estimation. Until the tree cannot be divided further, the causal effect estimated in the leaf nodes (the final nodes in the tree) serves as the individual-based causal effect or all the samples in both groups defined by independent variable. To decrease selection bias and increase robustness, the data samples and covariates are randomly selected to generate new trees and calculate new causal effects, iteratively forming the causal forest. Each sample may be allocated in a different node across the trees, and a weighted individual-based causal effect is obtained. Hence, based on the individual-based causal effects, the causal influence of an independent variable on the dependent variable is estimated without the traditional manipulation process of randomization. Thus, the CF model can explore interventional causality by estimating the individual-based causal effect between two groups as well as balancing the covariates in leaf nodes. Moreover, the CF model can further explore counterfactual causality via an estimation of the individual-based causal effect. Specifically, for the samples in both the groups defined by the independent variable, the counterfactual outcomes can be obtained by calculating the difference between the estimated individual-based causal effect and the factual outcomes. Actually, causal inference with observation data is a fundamental problem in a variety of domains, and the method of CF modeling has been widely used to evaluate causal effects, including policy evaluation [42], disease causality evaluation [44–46], and evaluations of the impact of psychological interventions on student achievement [41].

Moreover, the CF model divides samples into subgroups based on the differences in multiple covariates, which makes it possible to analyze the heterogeneity of causal effects. The heterogeneity of causal effects focuses on assessing different causal effects across individuals or subgroups. Individual-based causal inference in the CF model can predict the counterfactual results for each individual, e.g., what the treatment effect would be if the individuals in the control group received the treatment. This is very useful to guide personalized treatment strategies or the formation of public policies [46]. For instance, the causal effect of federal spending and its associated economic effects on decreasing crime was larger in below-median-income counties [47]. Preschool children in rural areas with less educated mothers benefited more from health insurance. The installation of cameras reduced the occurrence of traffic accidents in densely populated and poor areas more significantly.

1.4. Aims of the Study

In this study, to more deeply understand the underlying mechanism of the PCR in oppositional defiant symptoms and predict the potential benefits at the individual level or among different populations, we focused on the effect of the PCR on the development of oppositional defiant symptoms, to further infer the causal relationship and estimate the heterogeneity on observational data. To address the issue, we trained the CF model with follow-up ODD samples in China. The questions and hypotheses of interest are as follows: (1) Is there an "interventional" and "counterfactual" causality for the PCR in oppositional defiant symptoms with the machine learning-based approach of the CF model? Based on the strong association in previous research with the methods of SEM and intervention studies, we hypothesized that there would be a deeper causality between them via CF modeling. (2) Since many family factors were observed to link the PCR and oppositional defiant symptoms, what is the deeper mechanism of the PCR in the development of oppositional defiant symptoms and how can we explain the complex relationship between family factors? Guided by the multilevel family model and heterogeneous causality estimation in the CF model, we hypothesized that some related family factors from the entire, dyadic and individual family levels are involved in affecting causality, exhibiting the heterogeneity across individuals and subgroups. (3) Despite the strong association found in previous studies, testing it in these sample data as supplementary evidence is necessary. Therefore, the last goal is to further assess the "associational" level of causality and test the prediction of oppositional defiant symptoms for PCR. We hypothesized that improvements in the PCR could directly predict the development of oppositional defiant symptoms after controlling the related family factors with hierarchical multiple regression (HMR).

2. Materials and Methods

2.1. Participants

The samples came from a large-scale longitudinal research project on oppositional defiant disorder, and was taken from 14 elementary schools in northern (Beijing), eastern (Shandong Province) and southwestern (Yunnan Province) Mainland China during 2013 and 2014. First, invitation letters and informed consent forms were sent to the parents and children by school teachers to recruit the participants, then the parents and children with complete consent forms were involved in the subsequent investigation. The inclusion criteria were as follows: (1) Children were enrolled in the first grade to the six grade in the schools; (2) There was no obvious organic or neurological disease in the children. The children and parents who could not participate in the project during the follow-up period were excluded. The basic demographic information and assessments of oppositional defiant symptoms and other family factors of both children and parents were recorded and assessed in two consecutive years [4,10,11,14]. In total, there were 307 boys (62.1%) and 187 girls (37.8%) involved in this study. The children's ages ranged from 6 to 13 years old ($M = 9.37$, $SD = 1.59$), and the parents' ages ranged from 25 to 64 years old ($M_{mother} = 37.03$, $SD = 3.98$; $M_{father} = 39.23$, $SD = 4.91$).

Prior to conducting the study, the research protocol was reviewed and approved by the Ethics Committee of Beijing University of Technology (No. xxxb202404-2) and the Institutional Review Board of Beijing Normal University (No. 202003310034 and 202302280035), respectively. All procedures performed in the studies were in accordance with the ethical standards of the institutional research committee and with the 1964 Helsinki Declaration and its later amendments or comparable ethical standards.

2.2. Measures

2.2.1. Assessment of Oppositional Defiant Symptoms (AODS)

The children's parents assessed their oppositional defiant symptoms on an 8-item scale according to the Diagnostic and Statistical Manual of Mental Disorders (DSM-IV-TR) [48] both in the first year and second year, named baseline AODS and outcome AODS, respectively. The severity of oppositional defiant symptoms was evaluated by adding together the scores of items, with a higher total score indicating more oppositional defiant symptoms. Cronbach's α of the scale was 0.85 in this study.

2.2.2. PCR

The Chinese version of the Child-Parent Relationship Scale (CPRS) [49,50] was used to assess the PCR, which was calculated using the sum of two subscales: closeness and conflict. Closeness measured parents' feelings of affection and open communication with their children (10 items; e.g., I share an affectionate, warm relationship with my child). Conflict measured parents' conflict with their children (12 items; e.g., My child easily becomes angry at me). The higher the total summed score, the better and stronger the parent–child relationship. In this study, Cronbach's α of the scale was 0.82.

2.2.3. Monthly Income

A 5-point scale for monthly income was used to evaluate the entire family's economic level. A higher score suggested higher monthly income in a family.

2.2.4. Family Cohesion/Adaptability

The Family Adaptability and Cohesion Evaluation Scale (FACES-II) [51,52] was used to evaluate cohesion and adaptability in the family. The subscale of cohesion was used to evaluate the emotional connection between family members (16 items; e.g., At home, we do things together), and the subscale of adaptability examined the ability of a family to change in response to problems at different stages (14 items; e.g., Our family likes to try different ways to solve problems). The total score of the questionnaire was the sum of the two subscales scores. A higher score on the FACES suggested stronger adaptability and cohesion in the family. In this study, Cronbach's α for FACES-II was 0.84.

2.2.5. Marital Relationship

The Dyadic Adjustment Scale (DAS) [53] was a 32-item questionnaire used to measure the perception of the relationship with an intimate partner (e.g., Do you confide in your mate). A higher score of DAS indicated a higher-quality marriage. Cronbach's α for the DAS was 0.89 in this research.

2.2.6. Parenting Style

The Authoritative Parenting Index (API) [54] consisted of two subscales: responsiveness and demandingness. The responsiveness subscale (API-r) was reported by the parent and reflected the support of parents for their children (7 items; e.g., I listen patiently to my child). The higher the score, the higher the degree of support from parents. Cronbach's α for this subscale was 0.82. The demandingness subscale (API-d) reflected the control of parents over their children (9 items; e.g., I always tell my child what to do). The higher the score, the higher the degree of control from parents. In this research, Cronbach's α for this subscale was 0.81.

2.2.7. Parent Emotion Regulation

The self-reported Difficulties in Emotion Regulation Scale (DERS) [55,56] was used to assess parents' ability to engage in emotion regulation (36 items; e.g., When I am upset, I become angry with myself for feeling that way). A higher score on the DERS indicated greater difficulty in emotion regulation being experienced by the parents. Cronbach's α was found to be 0.84 in this study.

2.2.8. Child Emotion Regulation

The Emotion Regulation Checklist (ERC) [57] was a 24-item measure used to assess children's positive and negative emotion-related behaviors as reported by parents (e.g., Is easily frustrated). A higher score based on the ERC indicated poorer emotion regulation in children. In this study, Cronbach's α was 0.82.

2.3. CF Modeling

The procedure of CF modeling was implemented in R studio based on the GRF (Generalized Random Forests) package [58,59]. GRF is used as an R package that contains numerous models, such as causal forests, random forests, etc., which can provide corresponding methods and tools for the estimation of heterogeneous causal effects. For details on the package, please refer to its technical reference (https://github.com/grf-labs/grf accessed on 13 June 2022).

2.3.1. Data Preprocessing

As shown in Figure 1, the independent variable, X, dependent variable, Y and covariates, Cs, were first defined for CF modeling.

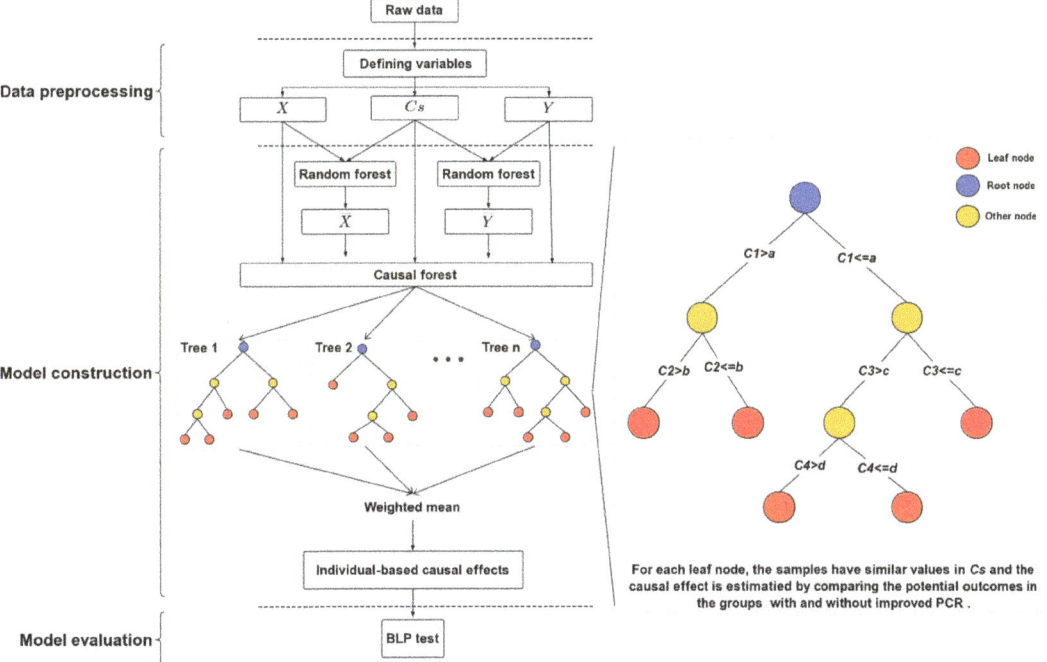

Figure 1. Overview of causal effect estimation with CF modeling.

The independent variable, X, is usually a binary value used to divide samples into two groups, and is further used to generate causal trees based on the principle of maximizing the variance in estimated causal effects in each node by comparing the values of the dependent variable within the two groups. To achieve this goal, we first defined the X values according to the difference in CPRS scores (range from -20 to 36) between the two consecutive years and divided the samples into an improved group and a control group. As shown in Figure 2, the differences in CPRS scores in the two consecutive years in most of the samples were within 10%. To balance the maximization of the difference between the improved PCR group and the control group as well as to ensure the inclusion of as many samples as possible, the samples with improvement in CPRS scores (10% change) were defined as the improved group, while those with relative stable scores (within 10% change) were defined as the control group. Therefore, in total, there were 423 qualified samples selected for CF modeling, with 155 children (37%) in the improved group and 268 children (63%) in the control group. In total, there were 274 boys (64.8%) and 149 girls (35.2%) involved. The children's ages ranged from 6 to 13 years old ($M = 9.35$, $SD = 1.58$), and the parents' ages ranged from 25 to 64 years old ($M_{mother} = 36.12$, $SD = 3.75$; $M_{father} = 38.26$, $SD = 4.63$).

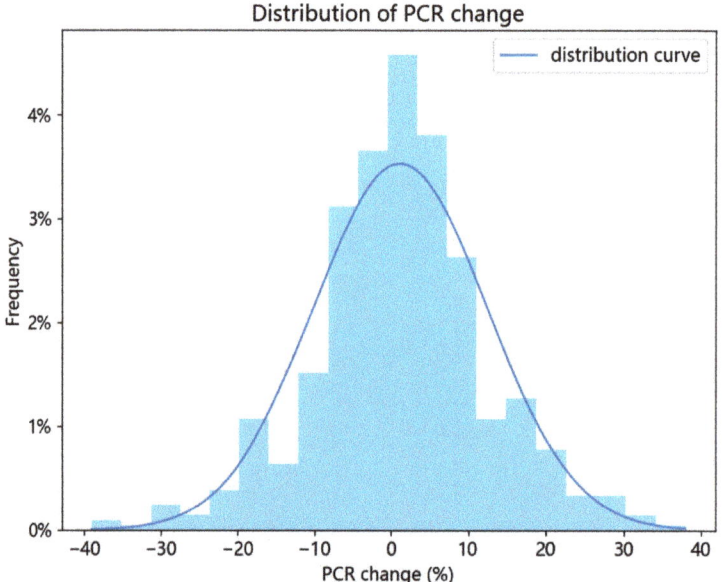

Figure 2. Histogram of the distribution of PCR changes in the two consecutive years.

For the outcome of oppositional defiant symptoms, the AODS score in the second year was defined as the dependent variable. The values of dependent variables were used to calculate the causal effects at the leaf nodes by comparing the differences between the improved PCR group and the control group.

The other measurements in the first year were used as Cs to evaluate their impacts on causality. The measurements at the entire family level (monthly income and FACES), dyadic level (DAS, API-r, and API-d measurements), and individual level (DERS and ERC) in the multilevel family model and the baseline AODS score in the first year were defined as Cs in the CF model.

The expectation–maximization (EM) method was employed to handle missing values. This statistical approach uses a probabilistic model and iteratively updates parameters until convergence is achieved for estimating missing values. SPSS 26.0 was utilized.

2.3.2. Model Construction

Because branch dividing in each node of the tree relies on the differences in covariates, the CF model may lead to over-sensitivity to heterogeneity. Hence, two regression forest models were first introduced to estimate the influences of the related family factors, Cs, on the causality of the PCR (X) and the outcome AODS (Y) (shown in Figure 1). Specifically, we put the previously defined Cs and Y into the random forest model to estimate the $\hat{Y}$. In the same way, we further put the Cs and X into the random forest model to estimate the

$\hat{X}$. Then, all the parameters (X, $\hat{X}$, Y, $\hat{Y}$, Cs) were put into the causal forest to adjust the influences of Cs on the estimation of causal effect.

Furthermore, the regular causal forests were used to estimate the causal effects and the differences across samples. As shown on the right in Figure 1, each causal tree was generated by fitting the data and characterized with binary branching in the root node, multiple leaf nodes, and other intermediate nodes. The trees were grown based on the principle of maximizing the variance in estimated causal effects in each node by considering Cs; therefore, the samples in the leaf nodes for each tree had similar values for Cs and the causal effect was estimated by comparing the outcome AODS (Y) in the groups with and without improved PCRs. Specifically, during the generation of causal trees, all the Cs were used for the division of the binary branch in each node. In this way, the influences of the covariates on the causality could be controlled to ensure a more rational estimation of the causal effect. Because each sample might have been assigned to different leaf nodes across trees, a weighted mean was calculated to obtain the individual-based causal effects for the samples during CF modeling. Hence, based on the individual-based causal effects, the causal influence of the PCR on the oppositional defiant symptoms in the second year was estimated without the traditional manipulation process of randomization. Furthermore, with the continuous branches being divided in the causal tree based on covariates, the heterogeneous causal effects of the PCR on oppositional defiant symptoms could be further estimated.

Moreover, the strategy of honest tree was adopted in the CF model to decrease overfitting. The training samples were divided into two sub-samples, with one used to generate the tree and the other used to estimate the causal effect within the leaf nodes. The optimal number of trees in the forest was adjusted to 300 to minimize the variance in causal effect. Other parameters were set to the package default.

2.3.3. Model Evaluation

The CF model serves as an estimator for quantifying causal effects, thereby obviating the necessity for cross-validation with the division of the training set and testing set, which is typically employed in predictive analytics in conventional machine learning. Nonetheless, it remains imperative to examine reliability when estimating causal effect and heterogeneity to ensure a comprehensive understanding of the variability across the subsets of samples in each tree. A test with the best linear predictor (BLP) was performed to assess the goodness of fit of the CF model to the longitudinal samples. Furthermore, it was also able to evaluate whether or not the heterogeneity of the causal effect had been well calibrated [60]. With the BLP test, the predicted dependent variable could be estimated as follows in Formulas (1) and (2):

$$Y = b_0(C)(X = 0) \tag{1}$$

$$Y = b_0(C) + \beta_1 \tau(C) + \beta_2 \Delta \tau(X = 1) \tag{2}$$

According to Formula (1) for the control group ($X = 0$), the output result was the baseline value, $b_0(C)$. On the other hand, according to Formula (2), for the improved group ($X = 1$), the output result included two more components. With the individual-based causal effects, the average causal effect, $\tau(C)$, reflected the overall difference between the improved and control groups. In addition, the heterogeneity ($\Delta \tau = \tau - \overline{\tau}$) reflected the fluctuations in the causal effect between individuals. Basically, a coefficient of 1 for β_1 reached the significant level, suggesting that the mean forest prediction was reasonable. Similarly, a coefficient of 1 for β_2 also reached the significant level, additionally suggesting that the heterogeneity across subgroups estimated from the forest was well calibrated.

2.3.4. Analysis of Causal Effect and Its Heterogeneity

Based on the CF modeling, the group-level causal effect could be further analyzed with the obtained individual-based causalities. The average causal effects (ACEs) for all samples, the improved group (ACI) and control group (ACC) and their 95% confidence intervals (CIs) were calculated. An independent two-sample *t*-test was used to compare the different causal effects between the improved group and control group.

The heterogeneity of the causal effect can typically be further analyzed in two ways. The first one is to compare the different causal effects between subgroups based on single *Cs*. Here, we divided the group into two subgroups according to the median value of each *C*, and then compared the differences between the high and low subgroups [14,42]. The second way is to analyze the heterogeneity based on a representative tree selected from the CF model, and was able to analyze the heterogeneous causal effects in several subgroups by considering the important *Cs* together [45].

2.4. Analysis of HMR

The selected samples in CF modeling were involved in HMR analysis with SPSS 26.0. Similarly, the critical independent variable was defined as the change in the PCR, which was calculated based on the difference of CPRS scores between the two consecutive years. The AODS score in the second year was defined as a dependent variable. Finally, the measurements at the entire family level (monthly income and FACES), dyadic level (DAS, API-r, and API-d measurements), and individual level (DERS and ERC) in the multilevel family model as well as the baseline AODS score in the first year were defined as covariates. Therefore, during the analysis, all the covariates were first entered as predictors into the regression model, and then the change in the PCR was entered as a predictor into the second regression model. The F-test was used to assess the fitting of the regression model, and the *t*-test was used to assess the contributions of the covariates and the independent variable.

3. Results

3.1. Descriptive Statistics

In the analysis of the *t*-test, there was no difference between the two groups for the baseline AODS, while the outcome of the AODS in the second year was different (t (421) = 2.571, $p < 0.001$) (Table 1), suggesting that oppositional defiant symptoms in the improved group had been alleviated more than they had been in the control group. The group difference was also observed in the API-d (t (421) = −1.131, $p < 0.05$) and ERC (t (421) = −2.843, $p < 0.001$).

Table 1. Summary in improved group and control group.

	Improved Mean/SD	Control Mean/SD	t	p
Outcome AODS	0.94/1.40	1.39/1.93	2.571	<0.001
Baseline AODS	2.12/2.29	1.62/2.23	−2.215	0.276
Income	2.87/0.87	3.07/1.05	1.970	0.066
FACES	121.97/14.18	124.94/15.69	1.941	0.734
DAS	134.63/15.08	135.13/17.70	0.294	0.755
API-r	18.96/3.75	17.71/3.63	−3.367	0.444
API-d	13.88/3.50	13.51/3.03	−1.131	<0.05
DERS	76.64/14.07	72.98/14.19	−2.564	0.639
ERC	56.94/11.35	52.41/17.88	−2.834	<0.001

3.2. Causal Effect of PCR on Oppositional Defiant Symptoms

The results of the BLP test are shown in Table 2. The estimated β_1 was 0.97 ($p < 0.001$), suggesting the causal effect was well estimated. The ACE for all samples was estimated as −0.727, and the negative value indicated significant improvements in oppositional defiant symptoms with PCR improvement. Moreover, as expected, there was a larger causal effect in the improved group (t (421) = 3.093, $p < 0.05$) (Table 3), which further indicated the causal effect of an improved PCR on oppositional defiant symptoms.

Table 2. BLP tests for causal effect and heterogeneity.

	Estimated	S.E.	*p*-Value
β_1	0.94	0.16	<0.001
β_2	1.37	0.36	<0.001

Note. S.E. standard error.

Table 3. Causal effect obtained from causal forest.

	Estimated	95% CI
ACE	−0.727	(−0.974, −0.480)
ACI	−0.854	(−0.881, −0.827)
ACC	−0.653	(−0.892, −0.414)

Note: ACE: average causal effect for the whole data; ACI: average causal effect in the improved group; ACC: average causal effect in the control group; CI, confidence interval.

3.3. Heterogeneous Causal Effects

3.3.1. General Analysis of Heterogeneity

The estimated value of β_2 was 1.37 ($p < 0.001$) (Table 2), indicating the reliable heterogeneity of the causality. Based on the weighted sum of how many times the *Cs* were split at each depth in the causal forest, we could analyze the contribution of the *Cs* to the heterogeneity prediction. The results are shown in Figure 3. The most important *Cs* were baseline ODD, on which the forest spent 37% of its split. Apart from that, the proportions of FACES, API-r, DERS, and ERC were higher than 10%.

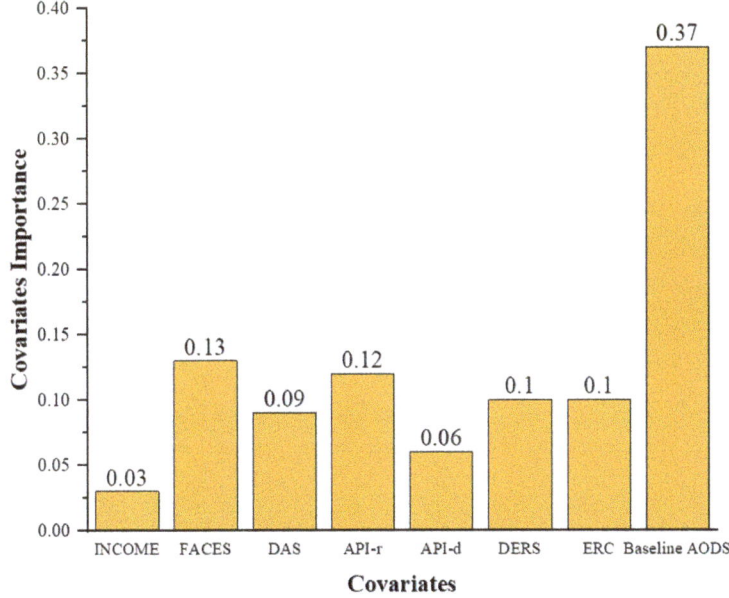

Figure 3. The ranking of importance of *Cs*.

3.3.2. Heterogeneity among *Cs*

As shown in Figure 4A, both the monthly income and FACES at the entire family level affected the causal effects, which suggested that children in families with a low income, or those from families with poor cohesion and adaptability, saw stronger benefits from PCR improvement (both $p < 0.05$).

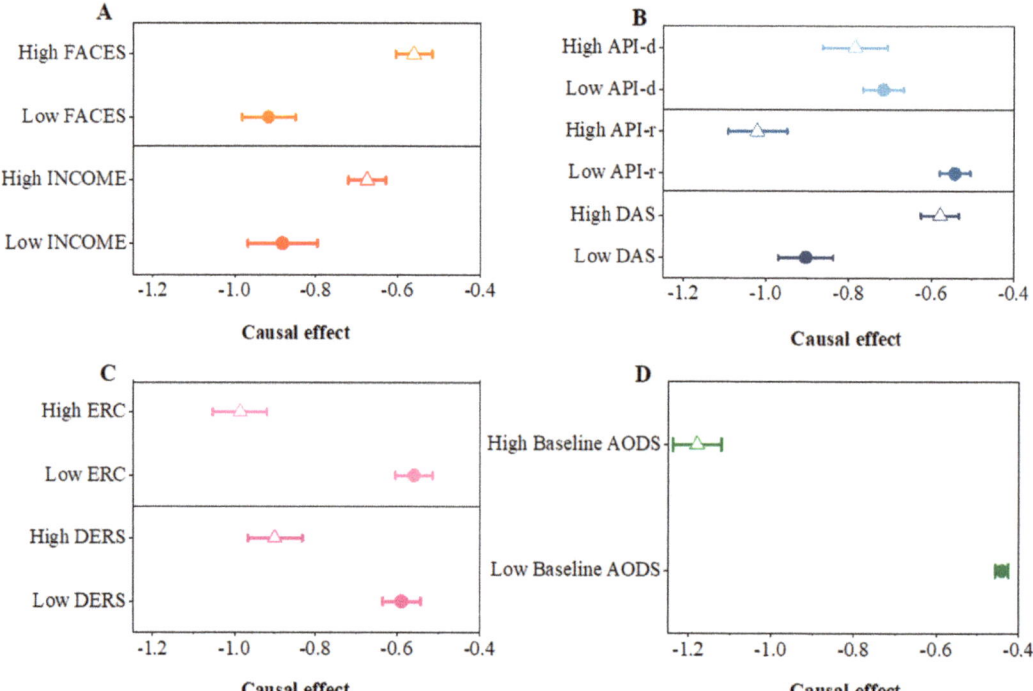

Figure 4. Heterogeneity along single covariates. The influence on the causality of PCR on the oppositional defiant symptoms from the factors in the entire family level (**A**), dyadic level (**B**), individual level (**C**) and the baseline AODS (**D**), respectively. The empty triangels represent the groups with higher values of the scales and the solid circles represent the groups with lower values.

As for the dyadic level (Figure 4B), first the children in families with a lower DAS score had greater causal effects ($p < 0.05$). Then, based on the two subscales of the API, we observed a reverse pattern of heterogeneity. The children in families with high API-r or high API-d value showed greater causal effects (both $p < 0.05$), suggesting the parenting style played a positive role in the causal effect.

The emotional regulation abilities of parents and children were crucial factors at the individual level. When parents and children had poorer emotional regulation abilities, the causality was greater ($p < 0.001$) (Figure 4C).

Finally, we also observed the role of this in heterogeneous causality based on the baseline AODS. Based on the division of subgroups according to the median value of the baseline AODS, the causal effect in the high-baseline AODS group was greater than that in the low-baseline AODS group ($p < 0.001$) (Figure 4D). This result further suggested that the causal effect was strongly dependent on the severity of oppositional defiant symptoms.

3.3.3. Heterogeneity Based on Causal Tree

Based on the *Cs* ranking result, we selected trees including the following five variables: baseline AODS, FACES, API-r, DERS, and ERC. There were three trees matching the criteria. Then, we selected one tree with the greatest difference in causal effects on the root node. As shown in Figure 5, the tree divided the sample of children into two parts on the root node based on the baseline AODS, and the children in the right part had more severe oppositional defiant symptoms than those in the left part. Their causal effect was mainly influenced by the FACES score, and Subgroup 6 showed the greatest causality in the whole tree. The findings were consistent with the results based on the ranking of important *Cs* and the heterogeneity between single variables, indicating the key roles of the FACES score and the severity of oppositional defiant symptoms in the causal effect. Moreover, to further maximize the variance in the causal effect, the causal tree continued to be divided into two branches with selected covariates, and this process was repeated until the causal tree could not be further divided. There were more covariates involved in influencing the causal effects. The smallest causal effect was observed in Subgroup 3 in the whole tree, in which the children had relatively lower ERC, higher DERS and lower API-r scores, indicating that multiple *Cs* affected the causality jointly.

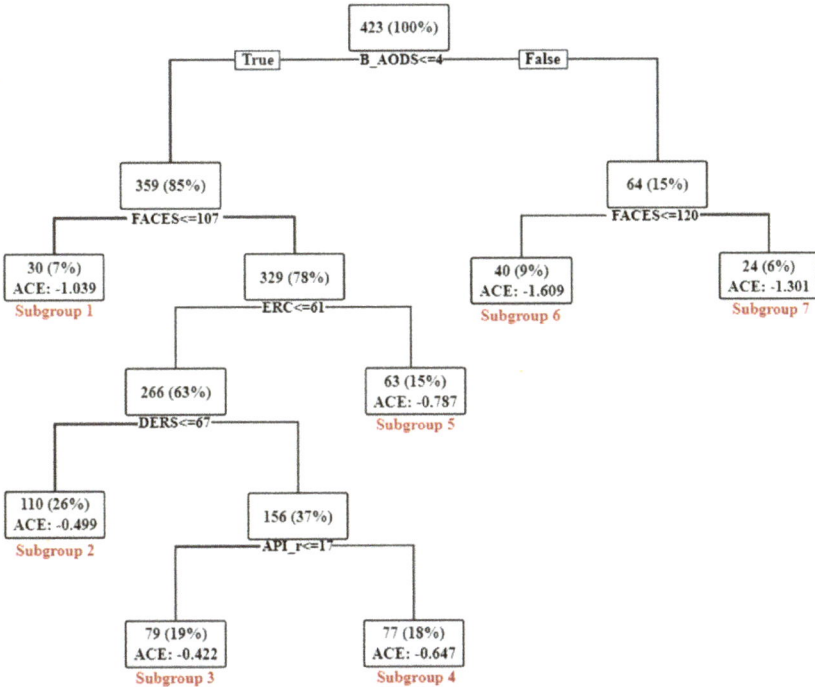

Figure 5. Subgroups identified by the representative causal tree. ACE: average causal effects.

3.4. Results of HMR Analysis

First, the VIF for all predictors included in the models ranged from 1.00 to 2.99, suggesting that the multicollinearity was not a concern in the study. Then, both the regression models significantly fit the data (both $p < 0.001$ with $F(8, 422) = 52.893$ in Model 1 and $F(9, 422) = 60.698$ in Model 2). Finally, the details of the regression models are listed in Table 4. After controlling the effects of other predictors, entering the change in the PCR significantly improved the explanation of the variance in Model 2 ($\Delta R^2 = 0.064$, $p < 0.001$), suggesting its unique contribution in predicting the oppositional defiant symptoms.

Table 4. Results of HMR analysis.

Predictors	Outcome AODS	
	ΔR^2	Beta
Model 1	0.505 ***	
Baseline AODS		0.609 ***
Income		−0.035
FACES		0.010
DAS		−0.244 ***
API-r		0.031
API-d		−0.116 **
DERS		−0.011
ERC		−0.048
Model 2	0.064 ***	
Baseline AODS		0.623 ***
Income		−0.042
FACES		−0.019
DAS		−0.193 ***
API-r		0.052
API-d		−0.094 **
DERS		0.002
ERC		0.002
Change in PCR		−0.266 ***

Note. level of significance: ** $p < 0.01$, *** $p < 0.001$.

4. Discussion

In this study, we aimed to train a data-driven CF model and elucidate the causal relationship and its heterogeneity between PCR and oppositional defiant symptoms under the framework of the multilevel family model. The CF model showed a significant causal effect of the PCR on oppositional defiant symptoms, which provides further evidence of causality estimation with observational and longitudinal data. Furthermore, we found that the causal effect was varied in individuals or subgroups based on the heterogeneity analysis, suggesting factors from multiple levels in a family play different roles in causality. These results contribute to a deeper understanding of the mechanism of the PCR on the development of oppositional defiant symptoms and enrich the theory of the multilevel family model [6,9,11]. From the perspective of prevention and intervention, the discovery of heterogeneous causality could be extremely helpful when forming more targeted strategies.

Based on previous research with the methods of SEM and intervention studies, there may be a potential causal link between the PCR and oppositional defiant symptoms [9,22,34, 61,62]. In the present study, we first observed a unique prediction of oppositional defiant symptoms from a PCR change with the method of HMR, which is consistent with the previous findings. Furthermore, a causal effect from the PCR on oppositional defiant symptoms was further clarified with the machine learning-based CF approach. During CF modeling, the causal trees were grown by maximizing the difference in causal effects between improved PCR group and control group in each node. At same time, the baseline AODS score and factors within the multilevel family model were accounted for to ensure comparability. Therefore, the approach of the CF model was very similar to the method of a randomized controlled trial (RCT), but the causality was estimated in naturally developing samples with no real intervention. To further eliminate the selection bias often found in intervention studies based on the RCT method, we repeated this process hundreds of times by randomly selecting samples and calculated individual-based causal effects with the weighted means in the CF model. Hence, by comparing it with SEM and HMR, the CF model was found to be able to uncover the causal relationships on the interventional and counterfactual levels rather than relying on association alone, and our results provide new evidence to demonstrate a deeper causal relationship between PCR and oppositional defiant symptoms in observational and longitudinal data.

Moreover, the prediction based on the CF model may be more practical in reality. Based on the methods with an associational causality reference, for a new sample, the development of oppositional defiant symptoms in the second year can be predicted using the difference in the PCR between the two consecutive years while controlling the influences from other related family factors in the first year, as observed from the results of the HMR. On the other hand, based on the interventional and counterfactual causality estimated with the CF model, just the PCR and other covariates in the first year are required to predict the oppositional defiant symptoms in the second year for a new sample, which provides the opportunity to make predictions in advance with time and cost savings. Hence, the findings with CF modeling may be very helpful in evaluating the potential benefits from the improvement in the PCR in terms of oppositional defiant symptoms at the individual level before implementing the targeted intervention strategy.

By considering the theoretical support for the multilevel family model, three factors are addressed. First, as many family factors contribute to the development of oppositional defiant symptoms [4–11], guided by the multilevel level family model, we can investigate the causal relationship between PCR and oppositional defiant symptoms by integrating all the factors from the entire, dyadic and individual family levels, along with the family system perspective of oppositional defiant symptoms. Second, consistent with the multilevel level family model [6,9–11], the findings for the direct association between PCR and oppositional defiant symptoms are further supported by the causal effect estimated via CF modeling and the prediction effect determined in the HMR analysis when family factors were taken as covariates in the present study. Finally, knowledge about the interactions between the family factors in the multilevel level family model is enriched in present study, which is mainly related to the heterogeneous effect of PCRs on oppositional defiant symptoms. The multilevel family model has illustrated the mediating role of the dyadic family level between the entire level and individual level in linking to oppositional defiant symptoms [4,7,9–11,35], whereas the present study exhibits the moderating roles of the family levels in the association of PCRs and oppositional defiant symptoms. FACES scores on the entire family level, API-r scores on the dyadic level, and the DERS and ERC scores on the individual family level were the most important factors contributing to the causal relationship between the PCR and oppositional defiant symptoms. Moreover, the heterogeneity can be further revealed by considering multiple family factors together with an illustration of a representative causal tree. The heterogeneous causal effects across individuals and subgroups indicate quite a complicated mechanism of the PCR in oppositional defiant symptoms, which can be divided into approximately three types.

The first one is related to the expectation of or support for oppositional defiant symptom alleviation. The baseline AODS and FACES scores were the most two important Cs and used as the root node and secondary node, respectively, in the representative tree. Notably, the effect of the baseline AODS score did not reflect the longitudinal change in the comparison between the baseline AODS and the outcome AODS scores as in intervention studies, while it was used as one covariate to estimate the influence of the causal effect during CF modeling. The multilevel family model proposes that factors at the entire family level play a basic supporting function in the family system [22], and are distal factors that affect oppositional defiant symptoms indirectly via more proximal factors, such as the PCR and child emotion regulation [16,22,62]. When children with oppositional defiant symptoms have more emotional and behavioral problems, there are more likely to be conflicts with their parents [4,9]. In such families, family members were less supported by each other [63]. Therefore, it might be more urgent for children with severe oppositional defiant symptoms and a less harmonious family atmosphere to alleviate oppositional defiant symptoms by improving the PCR.

The second type is related to the ethological or manipulable explanations for oppositional defiant symptoms. Children with lower emotion regulation abilities themselves or had parents with lower emotional regulation abilities could benefit more by reducing oppositional defiant symptoms via PCR improvement. The results advance the knowledge of the effects from individual family factors on the development of oppositional defiant symptoms. Research has emphasized that parents' negative emotional handling styles may easily impair children's emotional regulation skills, and subsequently lead to an increase in the risk of oppositional defiant symptoms [11,64]. Furthermore, a high-quality PCR could not only have a unilateral effect on a child's development but also can influence the parents' relationship and functioning [22]. Based on the multilevel family model, we further propose factors at the individual level might affect the causality of the PCR in oppositional defiant symptoms.

The last type of heterogeneity is related to the parenting style, particularly the factor API-r, which plays a compensatory role. The parenting style is one factor from the dyadic level of the parent–child subsystem. Generally, positive parenting styles play protective roles in the development of oppositional defiant symptoms [65]. It is suggested that factors at the dyadic level may directly or indirectly have an effect on oppositional defiant symptoms by mediating/linking the entire family-level factors and individual-level parent and children factors, so the interaction of family factors between levels exhibits a hierarchical connection [22]. However, the influence of factor interplay within the family levels in oppositional defiant symptoms is rarely considered in research. The observed compensatory role of parenting styles on the causality in this study provides preliminary knowledge about the mutual link in the parent–child subsystem at the dyadic level. Parenting style is highly related to the PCR, and emphasizes parents' leading role in behavior control and manipulation. To some extent, the PCR is a consequence of parenting style. A reasonable explanation for the larger causal effect in children with higher API-r scores is that parents can actively respond to their children's needs and, accordingly, the children's oppositional defiant symptoms can be alleviated significantly.

There are some limitations to this study that should be considered in the future. The first is related to the data samples. The samples used in this study were selected from an ordinary school population, and oppositional defiant symptoms were assessed by the parents of the children. Although this method is commonly used when investigating behavioral problems in children from a community [3,7–9,14], it is still very limited in terms of allowing us to generalize conclusions to the samples from clinical institutions. Moreover, the findings in this study need to be verified with larger sample sizes. The second limitation is related to the methodology. For some considerations, we set a criterion based on the difference between the two consecutive years for the binary group division, but it was still subjective and more validations are needed. Furthermore, in the CF model, the causal effect is estimated by comparing the group difference in each node with matching Cs. This group-based method may also still have selection bias. Currently, many "real" individual-based methods are being developed to predict counterfactual outcomes and are aimed at reducing the influence of the binary definition of the individual variable [66], so they could be introduced in future research. Finally, we mainly focused on the psychological factors under the framework of the multilevel family model to estimate the heterogeneous causality in this study, while research has found that the occurrence and development of oppositional defiant symptoms varies with the factors gender, age and social culture [2], so whether or not the causality effect would be different across the subgroups based on these factors is still not clear.

Despite these limitations, the following section briefly outlines some important implications for the prevention/intervention of oppositional defiant symptoms from both theoretical and practical perspectives. First, the findings from the current study highlight the importance of the management of the PCR in a family. Research has shown that there may be a reverse link, with severe oppositional defiant symptoms leading a to bad PCR [9], though we did not evaluate the causality in this direction. This is because based on a consideration of the practice, the effects of improvements in the PCR on alleviating oppositional defiant symptoms are of more interest. Second, the application of a machine learning-based CF model offers a novel research technique in investigating the causal relationship between PCR and oppositional defiant symptoms in observation data. Meanwhile, this approach can quantitatively represent the variability in this causal effect between different individuals or groups in detail, which may help in evaluating the intervention strategies aimed at more rational PCR management.

5. Conclusions

A machine learning-based CF model was introduced to investigate the causal relationship between PCR and oppositional defiant symptoms with observational and longitudinal data. The causality and heterogeneity across individuals and subgroups could be helpful in more deeply understanding the mechanism of PCR on the development of oppositional defiant symptoms as well as in forming precision- and personalization-based prevention/intervention strategies.

Author Contributions: H.Z.: conceptualization, methodology, and writing—reviewing and editing. F.H.: software, investigation, methodology, and writing—original draft. R.C.: investigation and conceptualization. J.H.: investigation and methodology. J.C.: methodology. X.L.: supervision and writing—reviewing and editing. All authors have read and agreed to the published version of the manuscript.

Funding: The present research is partially supported by the National Nature Science Foundation of China (Nos. 32071072 and 32371115) for X.L. and Beijing Natural Science Foundation (No. 4222022) for J.C. The content is solely the responsibility of the authors and does not necessarily represent the official views of the National Nature Science Foundation or Beijing Natural Science Foundation.

Institutional Review Board Statement: The research protocol was reviewed and approved by the Ethics Committee of Beijing University of Technology (No. xxxb202404-2 approved on 21 May 2024) and the Institutional Review Board of Beijing Normal University (No. 202003310034 approved on 31 March 2020 and 202302280035 approved on 1 March 2023), respectively. All procedures performed in studies were in accordance with the ethical standards of the institutional research committee and with the 1964 Helsinki Declaration and its later amendments or comparable ethical standards.

Informed Consent Statement: Invitation letters and informed consent forms were sent to the parents and children in the study, and those with completed consent forms were involved in the investigation.

Data Availability Statement: The datasets generated during and/or analyzed during the current study are available from the corresponding author on reasonable request.

Conflicts of Interest: The authors declare no conflicts of interest.

References

1. American Psychiatric Association. *DSM-5 Task Force. Diagnostic and Statistical Manual of Mental Disorders: DSM-5*^{TM}, 5th ed.; American Psychiatric Publishing, Inc.: Washington, DC, USA, 2013. [CrossRef]
2. Carter, M.J. Diagnostic and statistical manual of mental disorders. *Ther. Recreat. J.* **2014**, *48*, 275.
3. Ayano, G.; Lin, A.; Betts, K.; Tait, R.; Dachew, B.A.; Alati, R. Risk of conduct and oppositional defiant disorder symptoms in offspring of parents with mental health problems: Findings from the Raine Study. *J. Psychiatr. Res.* **2021**, *138*, 53–59. [CrossRef] [PubMed]
4. Ding, W.; Meza, J.; Lin, X.; He, T.; Chen, H.; Wang, Y.; Qin, S. Oppositional defiant disorder symptoms and children's feelings of happiness and depression: Mediating roles of interpersonal relationships. *Child Indic. Res.* **2020**, *13*, 215–235. [CrossRef]
5. He, T.; Su, J.; Jiang, Y.; Qin, S.; Chi, P.; Lin, X. Parenting Stress and Depressive Symptoms among Chinese Parents of Children with and without Oppositional Defiant Disorder: A Three-Wave Longitudinal Study. *Child Psychiatry Hum. Dev.* **2020**, *51*, 855–867. [CrossRef]
6. Lin, X.; Li, W.; Li, Y.; Zhao, Y.; Shen, J.; Fang, X. The family factors and family intervention program for child who have oppositional defiant disorder. *Adv. Psychol. Sci.* **2013**, *21*, 1983. [CrossRef]
7. Lavigne, J.V.; Gouze, K.R.; Hopkins, J.; Bryant, F.B.; LeBailly, S.A. A multi-domain model of risk factors for oppositional defiant symptoms in a community sample of 4-year-olds. *J. Abnorm. Child Psychol.* **2012**, *40*, 741–757. [CrossRef] [PubMed]
8. Antúnez, Z.; de la Osa, N.; Granero, R.; Ezpeleta, L. Parental psychopathology levels as a moderator of temperament and oppositional defiant disorder symptoms in preschoolers. *J. Child Fam. Stud.* **2016**, *25*, 3124–3135. [CrossRef]
9. Lin, X.; Li, L.; Heath, M.A.; Chi, P.; Xu, S.; Fang, X. Multiple levels of family factors and oppositional defiant disorder symptoms among Chinese children. *Fam. Process* **2018**, *57*, 195–210. [CrossRef] [PubMed]
10. Tang, Y.; Lin, X.; Chi, P.; Zhou, Q.; Hou, X. Multi-level family factors and affective and behavioral symptoms of oppositional defiant disorder in Chinese children. *Front. Psychol.* **2017**, *8*, 1123. [CrossRef]

11. Lin, X.; He, T.; Heath, M.; Chi, P.; Hinshaw, S. A Systematic Review of Multiple Family Factors Associated with Oppositional Defiant Disorder. *Int. J. Environ. Res. Public Health* **2022**, *19*, 10866. [CrossRef]
12. Burke, J.D.; Hipwell, A.E.; Loeber, R. Dimensions of oppositional defiant disorder as predictors of depression and conduct disorder in preadolescent girls. *J. Am. Acad. Child Adolesc. Psychiatry* **2010**, *49*, 484–492. [CrossRef]
13. Harvey, E.A.; Metcalfe, L.A.; Herbert, S.D.; Fanton, J.H. The role of family experiences and ADHD in the early development of oppositional defiant disorder. *J. Consult. Clin. Psychol.* **2011**, *79*, 784–795. [CrossRef]
14. Chen, H.; Lin, X.; Heath, M.A.; Ding, W. Family violence and oppositional defiant disorder symptoms in Chinese children: The role of parental alienation and child emotion regulation. *Child Fam. Soc. Work* **2020**, *25*, 964–972. [CrossRef]
15. Forssman, L.; Eninger, L.; Tillman, C.M.; Rodriguez, A.; Bohlin, G. Cognitive functioning and family risk factors in relation to symptom behaviors of ADHD and ODD in adolescents. *J. Atten. Disord.* **2012**, *16*, 284–294. [CrossRef]
16. Lavigne, J.V.; Gouze, K.R.; Hopkins, J.; Bryant, F.B. A multidomain cascade model of early childhood risk factors associated with oppositional defiant disorder symptoms in a community sample of 6-year-olds. *Dev. Psychopathol.* **2016**, *28*, 1547–1562. [CrossRef]
17. Raudino, A.; Fergusson, D.M.; Horwood, L.J. The quality of parent/child relationships in adolescence is associated with poor adult psychosocial adjustment. *J. Adolesc.* **2013**, *36*, 331–340. [CrossRef]
18. Lucia, V.; Breslau, N. Family cohesion and children's behavior problems: A longitudinal investigation. *Psychiatry Res.* **2006**, *141*, 141–149. [CrossRef]
19. Bornovalova, M.A.; Cummings, J.R.; Hunt, E.; Blazei, R.; Malone, S.; Iacono, W.G. Understanding the relative contributions of direct environmental effects and passive genotype–environment correlations in the association between familial risk factors and child disruptive behavior disorders. *Psychol. Med.* **2014**, *44*, 831–844. [CrossRef]
20. Braithwaite, S.R.; Steele, E.; Spjut, K.; Dowdle, K.K.; Harper, J. Parent–child connectedness mediates the association between marital conflict and children's internalizing/externalizing outcomes. *J. Child Fam. Stud.* **2015**, *24*, 3690–3699. [CrossRef]
21. Munkvold, L.H.; Lundervold, A.J.; Manger, T. Oppositional defiant disorder—Gender differences in co-occurring symptoms of mental health problems in a general population of children. *J. Abnorm. Child Psychol.* **2011**, *39*, 577–587. [CrossRef]
22. Lin, X.; Li, L.; Chi, P.; Wang, Z.; Heath, M.A.; Du, H.; Fang, X. Child maltreatment and interpersonal relationship among Chinese children with oppositional defiant disorder. *Child Abus. Negl.* **2016**, *51*, 192–202. [CrossRef]
23. Tseng, W.L.; Kawabata, Y.; Gau, S.S.F. Social adjustment among Taiwanese children with symptoms of ADHD, ODD, and ADHD comorbid with ODD. *Child Psychiatry Hum. Dev.* **2011**, *42*, 134–151. [CrossRef]
24. Duncombe, M.E.; Havighurst, S.S.; Holland, K.A.; Frankling, E.J. The contribution of parenting practices and parent emotion factors in children at risk for disruptive behavior disorders. *Child Psychiatry Hum. Dev.* **2012**, *43*, 715–733. [CrossRef]
25. Eisenberg, N.; Fabes, R.A. Emotion regulation and children's socioemotional competence. In *Child Psychology: A Handbook of Contemporary Issues*; Balter, L., Tamis-LeMonda, C., Eds.; Psychology Press: New York, NY, USA, 2006; pp. 357–381.
26. Wang, M.; Wang, J. Negative parental attribution and emotional dysregulation in Chinese early adolescents: Harsh fathering and harsh mothering as potential mediators. *Child Abus. Negl.* **2018**, *81*, 12–20. [CrossRef]
27. Muhtadie, L.; Zhou, Q.; Eisenberg, N.; Wang, Y. Predicting internalizing problems in Chinese children: The unique and interactive effects of parenting and child temperament. *Dev. Psychopathol.* **2013**, *25*, 653–667. [CrossRef]
28. Gong, J.; Zhou, Y.; Wang, Y.; Liang, Z.; Hao, J.; Su, L.; Wang, T.; Du, X.; Zhou, Y.; Wang, Y. How parental smartphone addiction affects adolescent smartphone addiction: The effect of the parent-child relationship and parental bonding. *J. Affect. Disord.* **2022**, *307*, 271–277. [CrossRef]
29. Brown, C.A.; Granero, R.; Ezpeleta, L. The Reciprocal Influence of Callous-Unemotional Traits, Oppositional Defiant Disorder and Parenting Practices in Preschoolers. *Child Psychiatry Hum. Dev.* **2017**, *48*, 298–307. [CrossRef]
30. Villodas, M.T.; Moses, J.O.; Cromer, K.D.; Mendez, L.; Magariño, L.S.; Villodas, F.M.; Bagner, D.M. Feasibility and promise of community providers implementing home-based parent-child interaction therapy for families investigated for child abuse: A pilot randomized controlled trial. *Child Abus. Negl.* **2021**, *117*, 105063. [CrossRef]
31. Parent, J.; Anton, M.T.; Loiselle, R.; Highlander, A.; Breslend, N.; Forehand, R.; Hare, M.; Youngstrom, J.K.; Jones, D.J. A randomized controlled trial of technology-enhanced behavioral parent training: Sustained parent skill use and child outcomes at follow-up. *J. Child Psychol. Psychiatry* **2022**, *63*, 992–1001. [CrossRef]
32. Scudder, A.; Wong, C.; Ober, N.; Hoffman, M.; Toscolani, J.; Handen, B.L. Parent–child interaction therapy (PCIT) in young children with autism spectrum disorder. *Child Fam. Behav. Ther.* **2019**, *41*, 201–220. [CrossRef]
33. Bjørseth, Å.; Wichstrøm, L. Effectiveness of parent-child interaction therapy (PCIT) in the treatment of young children's behavior problems. A randomized controlled study. *PLoS ONE* **2016**, *11*, e0159845. [CrossRef]
34. Brumariu, L.E.; Kerns, K.A. Pathways to Anxiety: Contributions of Attachment History, Temperament, Peer Competence, and Ability to Manage Intense Emotions. *Child Psychiatry Hum. Dev.* **2013**, *44*, 504–515. [CrossRef]
35. Chen, H.; Xing, J.; Yang, X.; Zhan, K. Heterogeneous Effects of Health Insurance on Rural Children's Health in China: A Causal Machine Learning Approach. *Int. J. Environ. Res. Public Health* **2021**, *18*, 9616. [CrossRef]
36. Bareinboim, E.; Correa, J.D.; Ibeling, D.; Icard, T. On Pearl's hierarchy and the foundations of causal inference. In *Probabilistic and Causal Inference: The Works of Judea Pearl*; ACM: New York, NY, USA, 2022; pp. 507–556.

37. Pearl, J.; Mackenzie, D. *The Book of Why: The New Science of Cause and Effect*; Basic Books: New York, NY, USA, 2018.
38. Montgomery, D.C.; Peck, E.A.; Vining, G.G. *Introduction to Linear Regression Analysis*; John Wiley & Sons: Hoboken, NJ, USA, 2021.
39. Wang, Y.; Wen, Z.; Li, W.; Fang, J. Methodological research and model development on structural equation models in China's mainland from 2001 to 2020. *Adv. Psychol. Sci.* **2022**, *30*, 1715–1733. [CrossRef]
40. Athey, S.; Imbens, G. Recursive partitioning for heterogeneous causal effects. *Proc. Natl. Acad. Sci. USA* **2016**, *113*, 7353–7360. [CrossRef]
41. Athey, S.; Wager, S. Estimating treatment effects with causal forests: An application. *Obs. Stud.* **2019**, *5*, 37–51. [CrossRef]
42. Zhang, Y.; Li, H.; Ren, G. Estimating heterogeneous treatment effects in road safety analysis using generalized random forests. *Accid. Anal. Prev.* **2022**, *165*, 106507. [CrossRef]
43. Knittel, C.R.; Stolper, S. *Using Machine Learning to Target Treatment: The Case of Household Energy Use (No. w26531)*; National Bureau of Economic Research: Cambridge, MA, USA, 2019. [CrossRef]
44. Yoon, J.; Jordon, J.; Van Der Schaar, M. GANITE: Estimation of individualized treatment effects using generative adversarial nets. In Proceedings of the International Conference on Learning Representations, Vancouver, BC, Canada, 30 April–3 May 2018.
45. Baum, A.; Scarpa, J.; Bruzelius, E.; Tamler, R.; Basu, S.; Faghmous, J. Targeting weight loss interventions to reduce cardiovascular complications of type 2 diabetes: A machine learning-based post-hoc analysis of heterogeneous treatment effects in the Look AHEAD trial. *Lancet Diabetes Endocrinol.* **2017**, *5*, 808–815. [CrossRef]
46. Gong, X.; Hu, M.; Basu, M.; Zhao, L. Heterogeneous treatment effect analysis based on machine-learning methodology. *CPT Pharmacomet. Syst. Pharmacol.* **2021**, *10*, 1433–1443. [CrossRef] [PubMed]
47. Hoffman, I.; Mast, E. Heterogeneity in the effect of federal spending on local crime: Evidence from causal forests. *Reg. Sci. Urban Econ.* **2019**, *78*, 103463. [CrossRef]
48. American Psychiatric Association. *Diagnostic and Statistical Manual of Mental Disorders*, 4th ed.; Text Revision Edition; American Psychiatric Association: Washington, DC, USA, 2000.
49. Pianta, R.C. *Beyond the Parent: The Role of Other Adults in Children's Lives*; Jossey-Bass: San Francisco, CA, USA, 1992.
50. Zhang, X.; Chen, H.; Zhang, G.; Zhou, B.; Wu, W. A longitudinal study of parent–child relationships and problem behaviors in early childhood: Transactional model. *Acta Psychol. Sin.* **2008**, *40*, 571–582. (In Chinese) [CrossRef]
51. Olson, D.H. Circumplex model of marital and family systems. *J. Fam. Ther.* **2000**, *22*, 144–167. [CrossRef]
52. Phillips, M.R.; West, C.L.; Shen, Q.; Zheng, Y. Comparison of schizophrenic patients' families and normal families in China, using Chinese versions of FACES-II and the family environment scales. *Fam. Process* **1998**, *37*, 95–106. [CrossRef]
53. Spanier, G.B. Measuring dyadic adjustment: New scales for assessing the quality of marriage and similar dyads. *J. Marriage Fam.* **1976**, *38*, 15–28. [CrossRef]
54. Weaver, S.R.; Prelow, H.M. A mediated-moderation model of maternal parenting style, association with deviant peers, and problem behaviors in urban African American and European American adolescents. *J. Child Fam. Stud.* **2005**, *14*, 343–356. [CrossRef]
55. Gratz, K.L.; Roemer, L. Multidimensional assessment of emotion regulation and dysregulation: Development, factor structure, and initial validation of the difficulties in emotion regulation scale. *J. Psychopathol. Behav. Assess.* **2004**, *26*, 41–54. [CrossRef]
56. Han, Z.R.; Lei, X.; Qian, J.; Li, P.; Wang, H.; Zhang, X. Parent and child psychopathological symptoms: The mediating role of parental emotion dysregulation. *Child Adolesc. Ment. Health* **2016**, *21*, 161–168. [CrossRef]
57. Shields, A.; Cicchetti, D. Emotion regulation among school-age children: The development and validation of a new criterion Q-sort scale. *Dev. Psychol.* **1997**, *33*, 906. [CrossRef]
58. Athey, S.; Tibshirani, J.; Wager, S. Generalized random forests. *Ann. Stat.* **2019**, *47*, 1148–1178. [CrossRef]
59. Chernozhukov, V.; Demirer, M.; Duflo, E.; Fernandez-Val, I. *Generic Machine Learning Inference on Heterogeneous Treatment Effects in Randomized Experiments, with an Application to Immunization in India (No. w24678)*; National Bureau of Economic Research: Cambridge, MA, USA, 2018. [CrossRef]
60. Hwang, W.J.; Park, E.H. Developing a structural equation model from Grandey's emotional regulation model to measure nurses' emotional labor, job satisfaction, and job performance. *Appl. Nurs. Res.* **2022**, *64*, 151557. [CrossRef]
61. Kong, J.; Lim, J.; Lindsey, D. The longitudinal influence of parent–child relationships and depression on cyber delinquency in South Korean adolescents: A latent growth curve model. *Child. Youth Serv. Rev.* **2012**, *34*, 908–913. [CrossRef]
62. Grant, K.E.; Compas, B.E.; Thurm, A.E.; McMahon, S.D.; Gipson, P.Y.; Campbell, A.J.; Krochock, K.; Westerholm, R.I. Stressors and child and adolescent psychopathology: Evidence of moderating and mediating effects. *Clin. Psychol. Rev.* **2006**, *26*, 257–283. [CrossRef]
63. Hopkins, J.; Lavigne, J.V.; Gouze, K.R.; LeBailly, S.A.; Bryant, F.B. Multi-domain models of risk factors for depression and anxiety symptoms in preschoolers: Evidence for common and specific factors. *J. Abnorm. Child Psychol.* **2013**, *41*, 705–722. [CrossRef]
64. Morris, A.S.; Criss, M.M.; Silk, J.S.; Houltberg, B.J. The impact of parenting on emotion regulation during childhood and adolescence. *Child Dev. Perspect.* **2017**, *11*, 233–238. [CrossRef]

65. Cruz-Alaniz, Y.; Martin, A.B.; Ballabriga, M. Parents' executive functions, parenting styles, and oppositional defiant disorder symptoms: A relational model. *Univ. Psychol.* **2018**, *17*, 39–48.
66. Ma, J.; Wan, M.; Yang, L.; Li, J.; Hecht, B.; Teevan, J. Learning causal effects on hypergraphs. In Proceedings of the 28th ACM SIGKDD Conference on Knowledge Discovery and Data Mining, Washington, DC, USA, 14–18 August 2022; pp. 1202–1212.

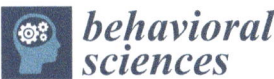

Article

Reciprocal Relations between Cognitive Empathy and Post-Traumatic Growth in School Bullying Victims

Fang Liu [1], Bo Chen [1], Xinrong Liu [1], Yifan Zheng [1], Xiao Zhou [2] and Rui Zhen [1,3,*]

[1] Jing Hengyi School of Education, Hangzhou Normal University, Hangzhou 311121, China
[2] Department of Psychology and Behavioral Sciences, Zhejiang University, Hangzhou 310058, China
[3] Zhejiang Philosophy and Social Science Laboratory for Research in Early Development and Childcare, Hangzhou Normal University, Hangzhou 310030, China
* Correspondence: zhenrui1206@126.com

Abstract: The association between post-traumatic growth (PTG) and cognitive empathy is well documented; however, few studies have tested the causal pathways explaining this association in school bullying victims' later recovery and growth in the long term. This study used a longitudinal design to examine the reciprocal relations between cognitive empathy and post-traumatic growth (PTG) in school bullying victims. We screened 725 adolescents who had experienced school bullying as our final subjects out of the 2173 adolescents we surveyed over three periods (November 2019, 2020, and 2021). Controlling for gender, cross-lagged analysis revealed that both cognitive empathy at T1 and T2 predicted adolescents' later PTG at T2 ($\gamma = 0.096$, $p < 0.05$) and T3 ($\gamma = 0.085$, $p < 0.05$), respectively, but the predictive effect across time points from PTG to cognitive empathy was not significant. The results delineated a specific directionality in the relation between cognitive empathy and PTG and suggested an important role of cognitive empathy in fostering school bullying victims' later recovery and growth. These findings contribute to ongoing research into ways researchers and educators may help and support school bullying victims.

Keywords: school bullying victimization; adolescents; cognitive empathy; post-traumatic growth; temporal relations

1. Introduction

Individuals who frequently endure aggressive behavior intended to cause harm—whether physically, psychologically, or socially—are identified as victims of bullying [1]. Research by Einarsen and his colleagues [2,3] presented the perspective that bullying can be equated to experiencing a traumatic event. A synthesis of numerous studies, both domestic and international, indicated that the prevalence of school bullying falls within a range of 20% to 33% [4]. Currently, school bullying has emerged as a chronic social issue, profoundly impacting the well-being and mental health of young individuals. This has led to heightened awareness and concern among nations globally [5].

Bullying victimization is increasingly recognized as a form of interpersonal violence that can be akin to a traumatic event [6]. Victims of bullying are susceptible to a spectrum of adverse outcomes, affecting them in both the short term and in the long term [7]. Nonetheless, a hopeful phenomenon was observed where, through personal resilience and external support [8], some individuals underwent a form of positive psychological transformation referred to as post-traumatic growth (PTG). This concept, introduced by Tedeschi and Calhoun [9], describes the beneficial psychological changes individuals experience as they navigate and overcome significant life crises. PTG encompasses three primary dimensions: transformations in self-perception, shifts in the nature of interpersonal relationships, and a re-evaluation of life's priorities [10]. The journey toward PTG is rich in cognitive and emotional processing. Recent research endeavors have embarked on

Behav. Sci. **2024**, *14*, 435. https://doi.org/10.3390/bs14060435

https://www.mdpi.com/journal/behavsci

unraveling the intricate interplay between post-traumatic growth and empathy, hinting at a potential interconnectedness between these constructs [11,12].

Cognitive empathy is the capability to grasp the emotional state of another individual [13]. As outlined by Davis [14,15], cognitive empathy sits at the heart of empathetic understanding, focusing on the cognitive aspect of stepping into someone else's shoes to view the world from their perspective. This form of empathy involves interpreting others' experiences in a manner that facilitates effective social negotiation and interaction [16]. It plays a critical role in fostering healthy interpersonal connections and securing a more robust network of social support. Recognized as a valuable socio-emotional skill, cognitive empathy involves top–down processing [15,17,18]. It is mirrored in the ability to identify and comprehend the emotions and viewpoints of others, a competency crucial for navigating and adapting to the ever-evolving social landscape [19].

Post-traumatic growth (PTG) and cognitive empathy are increasingly recognized as vital components of positive psychology. A substantial body of research has explored the linkage between these two factors, identifying post-traumatic growth as a phenomenon deeply intertwined with extensive cognitive and emotional processing [8]. Further investigations have uncovered a significant positive correlation between empathy and post-traumatic growth. For instance, Wang's research indicated a close connection between the level of PTG in individuals who have experienced trauma and their capacity for empathy [20]. However, it is noteworthy that the cognitive aspect of empathy has often been overlooked in research focusing on the dynamics between empathy and trauma derived from bullying [21].

According to de Waal and Preston's [22] Russian-doll model, empathy is structured in hierarchies, layering from the inside out, with cognitive empathy positioned at the outermost layer and emotional resonance at its core. Research by Shamay-Tsoory et al. [23] found that emotional empathy and cognitive empathy exhibited a dual separation, both behaviorally and anatomically. Moreover, cognitive empathy typically emerges during childhood and adolescence, a developmental stage when individuals begin to adeptly assume the perspectives of others [24–27]. This development highlights that, particularly for adolescents, the advancement of cognitive empathy takes precedence over emotional empathy in importance [28]. Given these insights, our study opts to disentangle cognitive empathy from its emotional counterpart, investigating it as an independent variable.

Post-traumatic growth (PTG) and cognitive empathy share a complex, bidirectional relations. On the one hand, post-traumatic growth appears to unlock an individual's latent cognitive empathy [11], while on the other, cognitive empathy may act as a catalyst for an individual's post-traumatic growth [12].

Evidence suggests that cognitive empathy serves as a predictor for post-traumatic growth. Zhou et al. [12] demonstrated that the activation of cognitive empathy enabled individuals to adopt broader perspectives, facilitating the re-evaluation of trauma-related events and fostering personal growth. Similarly, An et al. [29] found that empathetic individuals, being more open to external influences, underwent stress and negative emotions that prompted reflection on traumatic events, thus aiding in post-traumatic growth. Calhoun and Tedeschi [30] highlighted the significance of empathy among people as a potential source of post-traumatic growth for individuals experiencing trauma. The longitudinal study conducted by Wang and Wu [20] further confirmed that empathy can significantly enhance subsequent post-traumatic growth. Notably, cognitive empathy, a crucial element as outlined by Shamay-Tsoory et al. [23], played a pivotal and indispensable role in this process. Moreover, secondary post-traumatic growth studies hinted that cognitive empathy may be more conducive to individual growth than affective empathy [31,32]. Furthermore, pertinent theories endorse the contention that cognitive empathy serves as a contributor to post-traumatic growth. Drawing from the interpersonal model of stress and coping, when stressful occurrences endanger the well-being of a group, effective coping mechanisms encompass not merely problem-solving and the regulation of stress-induced negative emotions, but also the preservation of harmonious interpersonal relationships. Empathy emerges as a prototypical interpersonal-oriented coping strategy [33], with cognitive empathy occupying a pivotal role in interpersonal exchanges [34]. Additionally, the cognitive processing theory of trauma posits that cognitive factors are crucial for post-traumatic growth [35], suggesting a significant impact of cognitive empathy on positive growth outcomes. Together, these research findings imply the important role of cognitive empathy for post-traumatic growth.

Conversely, research also indicates that post-traumatic growth could predict cognitive empathy. Growth stemming from one's connection to vulnerability may enhance latent empathy, subsequently stimulating cognitive empathy [11]. Earlier studies suggested potential pathways where growth may lead to an enhancement in cognitive empathy [36–38]. The theory of suffering-based altruism [37] posits cognitive empathy as a potential outcome of growth, with psychological changes from trauma recovery enhancing cognitive empathy. Lifelong developmental models of empathy [39,40] and recent meta-analyses [28] further underscore the developmental trajectory of empathy, emphasizing that cognitive empathy, which evolves and strengthens over time, may be fostered by post-traumatic growth.

Yet, some research, such as that of Elam and Taku [41], pointed towards a non-significant relations between PTG and empathy, although it did not specifically dissect the relations between cognitive empathy and PTG. The relations between cognitive empathy and post-traumatic growth remains intricate, likely influenced by variables such as study populations, traumatic experiences, measurement timelines, and tools. Additionally, past relevant research paid less attention to adolescent victims of bullying [42]. Furthermore, a notable limitation in the existing literature is the reliance on cross-sectional designs, which hampers identifying definitive relationships and exploring causality.

This study, grounded in the interpersonal model of stress and coping and theories of suffering altruism, employs a longitudinal design with a cross-lagged approach. Our aim is to elucidate the relations and directionality between post-traumatic growth and cognitive empathy in the context of school bullying trauma, contributing valuable insights to empirical research in this domain.

2. Materials and Methods

2.1. Participants

In this investigation, we surveyed 2173 adolescents across Zhejiang Province, comprising 1384 junior high school students and 789 high school students. Following the guidelines proposed by Xie et al. [43], a participant was considered to have experienced bullying if they reported encountering such incidents "once or twice a month" or more often on any item of the Delaware Bullying Victimization Scale (student version). This criterion implicates that the individual has undergone bullying within the specific domain addressed by the question, thereby marking them as a victim of bullying. Applying this definition, we identified 802 out of the 2173 adolescents as having been bullied at the first time point. For this research, the focus was placed on these 802 adolescents who had encountered bullying. They were tracked and assessed at three distinct intervals: November 2019 (T1), November 2020 (T2), and November 2021 (T3). Due to various reasons such as school transfers and illnesses, some participants were unable to complete all three surveys. To ensure the reliability of the results, we retained subjects who had participated in at least two surveys, resulting in a sample size of 725 participants at the first time point. Within this group, there were 430 (59.3%) male students, 294 (40.6%) female students, and 1 individual who did not specify their gender. The average age of the participants was 14.44 years (SD = 1.40) at the first time point, with ages ranging from 10 to 18 years.

2.2. Measures

2.2.1. Bullying Victimization

In this study, the Delaware Bullying Victimization Scale (student version) revised by Xie et al. [44] was used to assess adolescents' school bullying victimization. The scale has 17 question items divided into four dimensions: verbal, physical, social/relational, and cyberbullying victimization, with item 13 as a screening item not counted in the data analysis. The items on the scale are scored on a six-point Likert scale, where 0 means "never," 1 means "occasionally", 2 means "once or twice a month," 3 means "once a week", 4 means "many times a week", and 5 means "every day". Higher scores indicate more severe bullying. Cronbach's alpha coefficients for this scale in this study ranged from 0.902 to 0.961.

2.2.2. Post-Traumatic Growth

In this study, the Post-Traumatic Growth Questionnaire (PTGQ) developed by Tedeschi and Calhoun [10] and revised by Zhou [45] was used. The questionnaire was designed to assess in what ways individuals changed significantly after experiencing bullying in school. The revised questionnaire consists of 22 questions, including three dimensions: changes in self-awareness, changes in interpersonal experiences, and changes in life values. The corresponding item numbers are 9, 7, and 6, respectively. The questionnaire is assessed on a 6-point scale, where 0 means "no change" and 5 means "very big change". The higher the score on the scale, the stronger the PTG, i.e., the more growth. Cronbach's alpha coefficients for this scale in this study ranged from 0.969 to 0.987.

2.2.3. Cognitive Empathy

In this study, a five-item version of the perspective-taking dimension of the Interpersonal Reactivity Index [14,15] was used to measure cognitive empathy. The scale has 5 question items, and a sample item included, "When my friends are having a disagreement or an argument, I try to listen to everybody before I decide who is right." Each item is scored on a five-point Likert scale (1 = completely inconsistent, 5 = completely consistent). Cronbach's alpha coefficients for cognitive empathy in this study ranged from 0.841 to 0.914.

2.3. Procedure and Data Analysis

In this research study, several graduate students specializing in psychology were meticulously trained to serve as examiners. This comprehensive training covered the test's content, administration requirements, procedural details, and essential precautions to be observed. Prior to test administration, the schools and teachers facilitated introductory sessions for parents and students to ensure a thorough understanding of the test's objectives and methodology. The testing was uniformly conducted across all classes, with students completing the questionnaires under the supervision of an invigilator who subsequently collected them immediately. This protocol was consistently applied across all three testing sessions. At the end of the survey, all participants were informed that psychological/counseling services were available from school psychologists or teachers if needed.

Data analysis was performed using SPSS 26.0, employing techniques for descriptive statistics, correlation analysis, and testing for common method bias. Furthermore, Mplus 8.3 software was utilized to develop a structural equation model for cross-lagged analysis. Model estimation was carried out using robust maximum likelihood estimation (MLR), while the full information maximum likelihood estimation (FIML) approach was adopted to handle missing data, following the methodology proposed by Muthén and Muthén [46].

2.4. Testing for Common Method Bias

To address the potential for common method bias in this study, we applied the Harman single-factor test. This analysis revealed twelve factors with eigenvalues exceeding 1 across the three time-points of measurement. Specifically, the proportion of variance explained by the first factor, both before and after rotation, was 28.87% and 16.67%, respectively. These findings suggest that common method bias does not pose a significant concern in this study, allowing for a more confident interpretation of the results.

Subsequently, we employed descriptive statistics and correlation analyses to explore the relationships between levels of variables and the variables themselves. Furthermore, cross-lagged regression analyses were conducted to investigate the dynamic relations between cognitive empathy and post-traumatic growth among school bullying victims.

3. Results

3.1. Correlations between Post-Traumatic Growth and Cognitive Empathy

Table 1 displays the mean values, standard deviations, and Pearson correlation co-efficients for the scores of post-traumatic growth and cognitive empathy among school bullying victims over a three-year period. The analysis revealed a positive correlation between the post-traumatic growth scores and cognitive empathy scores of school bullying victims at each respective time point, with all correlations being significant (rs ranging from 0.316 to 0.376, ps < 0.001). Furthermore, a significant positive correlation persisted over the course of the three years for both post-traumatic growth (rs ranging from 0.26 to 0.40, ps < 0.001) and cognitive empathy (rs ranging from 0.22 to 0.41, ps < 0.001) among the victims. Gender showed a significant correlation with both post-traumatic growth and cognitive empathy in school bullying victims, but age did not. As such, gender was incorporated as a control variable in subsequent cross-lagged modeling analyses to further investigate these relationships.

Table 1. Correlation analysis.

	M	SD	Sex	age	T1PTG	T2PTG	T3PTG	T1CE	T2CE	T3CE
sex	—	—	1							
age	14.44	1.4	0.014	1						
T1PTG	54.6	30.8	−0.052	−0.012	1					
T2PTG	48.6	30.2	−0.115 *	−0.054	0.263 ***	1				
T3PTG	46.7	33.3	0.014	−0.078	0.266 ***	0.395 ***	1			
T1CE	17.4	4.9	0.008	0.03	0.334 ***	0.182 ***	0.077	1		
T2CE	17.2	4.4	0.106 *	−0.038	0.073 #	0.316 ***	0.134 *	0.270 ***	1	
T3CE	16.6	4.5	−0.039	−0.005	0.1 #	0.095	0.376 ***	0.126 *	0.308 ***	1

Note: *** denotes $p < 0.001$; * denotes $p < 0.05$; # denotes borderline significant; PTG = post-traumatic growth, CE = cognitive empathy; gender coded as male = 0, female = 1.

3.2. Cross-Lagged Analysis of Post-Traumatic Growth and Cognitive Empathy

To ascertain the dynamic interplay between post-traumatic growth and cognitive empathy among school bullying victims, we proceeded with cross-lagged analyses that necessitated verifying the measurement invariance of these constructs over the three assessment points. We established and examined models for configural invariance, weak invariance, and strong invariance for the measures of post-traumatic growth and cognitive empathy among school bullying victims, with model fits detailed in Table 2.

Table 2. Measurement invariance test.

		χ^2	df	CFI	TLI	SRMR	RMSEA (90%CI)	ΔCFI	ΔRMSEA
PTG	Configural invariance	4053.911	1943	0.924	0.916	0.038	0.039 [0.037, 0.040]	—	—
	Weak invariance	4133.524	1981	0.923	0.916	0.039	0.039 [0.037, 0.040]	−0.001	0
	Strong invariance	4217.308	2019	0.921	0.916	0.041	0.039 [0.037, 0.040]	−0.002	0
CE	Configural invariance	93.428	69	0.991	0.987	0.037	0.022 [0.008, 0.033]	—	—
	Weak invariance	103.641	77	0.99	0.987	0.043	0.022 [0.009, 0.032]	−0.001	0
	Strong invariance	110.135	85	0.991	0.989	0.043	0.020 [0.006, 0.030]	0.001	0.002

Note: PTG = post-traumatic growth, CE = cognitive empathy.

A comparison was made between the configural invariance model (serving as the baseline model) against the weak invariance and strong invariance models. Although the chi-square test results indicated significant differences between the models, it is essential to note that the chi-square value is susceptible to sample size, rendering it a somewhat unstable indicator for model evaluation. Recognizing this limitation, it is prudent to consider variations in other fit indices when comparing models. In line with Cheung and Rensvold's [47] recommendation, we employed the ΔCFI for model comparison, since it remains unaffected by model parameters and sample size. The criterion for accepting measurement invariance, as suggested by these authors, is a ΔCFI of 0.01 or less. By examining the discrepancies across multiple fit metrics, we determined that both post-traumatic growth and cognitive empathy among school bullying victims exhibited sufficient configural and weak invariance over time. This finding paved the way for conducting in-depth cross-lagged analyses to further explore the relations between these variables.

Structural equation modeling was employed to explore the cross-lagged relations between post-traumatic growth and cognitive empathy among school bullying victims. In this model, gender served as a control variable, influencing both post-traumatic growth and cognitive empathy across the three time points. The results of this model are depicted in Figure 1, showcasing satisfactory model fits: Satorra–Bentler Scaled Chi-square (SBχ^2) (8) = 13.507, $p > 0.05$; Comparative Fit Index (CFI) = 0.982; Tucker–Lewis Index (TLI) = 0.953; Root Mean Square Error of Approximation (RMSEA) = 0.031 (90% CI [0.000, 0.058]); Standardized Root Mean Square Residual (SRMR) = 0.039. To simplify model presentation, path coefficients for the control variable—gender—are not included in Figure 1.

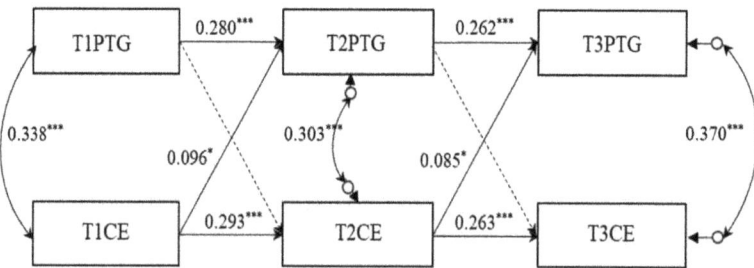

Figure 1. Cross-lagged analysis of post-traumatic growth and cognitive empathy. Note: *** denotes $p < 0.001$; * denotes $p < 0.05$; PTG = post-traumatic growth, CE = cognitive empathy. (In the model, solid lines indicate significant standardized path coefficients, while dashed lines represent non-significant path coefficients. For clarity, path coefficients related to control variables have been omitted from the visual representation).

As illustrated in Figure 1, both post-traumatic growth and cognitive empathy demonstrated moderate stability over the course of the three-year observation, with autoregressive path coefficients ranging from 0.26 to 0.29 (ps < 0.001). When controlling for autoregressive effects and within-time correlations between post-traumatic growth and cognitive empathy, cognitive empathy at the first time point (T1) was found to significantly and positively predict post-traumatic growth at the second time point (T2) ($\gamma = 0.096$, $p < 0.05$). Similarly, cognitive empathy measured at the second time point (T2) significantly and positively predicted post-traumatic growth at the third time point (T3) ($\gamma = 0.085$, $p < 0.05$). Contrarily, post-traumatic growth at T1 did not significantly predict cognitive empathy at T2 ($\gamma = -0.002$, $p = .0.948$), nor did post-traumatic growth at T2 significantly predict cognitive empathy at T3 ($\gamma = -0.002$, $p = 0.948$). This analysis therefore highlighted a temporal association where cognitive empathy precedes and positively influences the development of post-traumatic growth in school bullying victims over time.

4. Discussion

This research study utilized a cross-lagged design across three time points to delve into the dynamic interplay between post-traumatic growth and cognitive empathy among adolescent victims of bullying. The outcomes indicate that pre-existing cognitive empathy in victims can positively influence subsequent levels of post-traumatic growth. However, the emergence of post-traumatic growth does not appear to reciprocally amplify cognitive empathy. These findings partially corroborate the interpersonal modeling theory of stress and coping, as well as the cognitive processing theory related to post-traumatic growth [35,48], aligning with the trajectories observed in longitudinal research [20].

4.1. The Role of Cognitive Empathy in Post-Traumatic Growth

This study uncovered that cognitive empathy in adolescents who have experienced bullying significantly fosters post-traumatic growth one year following the initial trauma. This finding broadens the longitudinal insight previously established by other researchers [49], offering a novel lens through which we can view the psychological recuperation of school bullying victims. This observation is supported by similar findings across various studies [12,20,50–52].

Cognitive empathy, or the capacity to understand the perspectives and emotions of others, is identified as a crucial socio-emotional skill [53], vital for sustaining healthy social relationships [54]. This skill enables individuals to recognize and respond to the needs of others effectively. Among victims of bullying, those with heightened cognitive empathy exhibit better interpersonal-focused coping mechanisms when confronted with trauma. These strategies facilitate their recovery and psychological development. This aligns with the anticipations made by the interpersonal modeling theory of stress and coping [48], which elucidates how people can more efficaciously manage stressful situations. Additionally, the cognitive processing theory of trauma [35] suggests that recovery from trauma necessitates the reintegration of disrupted beliefs and disconcerting information emanating from the traumatic event. The cognitive dimension of empathy allows individuals to transcend self-centered perspectives and objectively view and understand the event from others' viewpoints, fostering recovery and post-traumatic progression. For bullying victims, heightened cognitive empathy can also engender a more reconciliatory stance towards perpetrators [55], transitioning from animosity towards others to self-improvement, enhancing adaptation to their environment, and fostering post-traumatic growth.

In addition, individuals exhibiting cognitive empathy are likely to adopt others' perspectives on issues [56], which strengthens personal connections and facilitates receiving more support [57]. This not only aids in effectively mitigating the trauma's adverse impacts but also enables victims to experience positive changes in their interpersonal relationships, further encouraging post-traumatic growth.

In summary, this result highlighted the significant influence of cognitive empathy on the psychological recovery and growth journey of school bullying victims. Enhancing cognitive empathy could potentially arm victims with more effective tools for coping with their trauma and achieving psychological development. These insights contribute to a deeper understanding of the psychological evolution of school bullying victims post trauma, offering valuable guidance for psychologists and educators in recognizing potential psychological outcomes and formulating suitable support strategies for victims. Moreover, by exploring post-traumatic growth among school bullying victims, this research introduces fresh perspectives and insights into the field, emphasizing that post-traumatic growth extends beyond catastrophic events to include daily life challenges such as bullying.

4.2. The Role of Post-Traumatic Growth in Cognitive Empathy

Contrary to initial predictions, this study revealed that post-traumatic growth observed in adolescents who had experienced bullying did not serve as a predictor for cognitive empathy in the subsequent year. According to Tedeschi and Calhoun [10], post-traumatic growth represents a positive change across three domains—self-perception, interpersonal relationships, and life's perceived value—following a traumatic event. Such transformation is a gradual process, and Yan et al. [28] asserted that the period from mid-childhood to early adulthood is primarily characterized by the development of cognitive empathy. However, the three-year duration of our study may not have been adequate to capture post-traumatic growth's potential to enhance cognitive empathy.

Moreover, the development of cognitive empathy in victims of bullying could be influenced by various factors, including previous bullying encounters. While our research focused on individuals who have suffered bullying, it failed to distinguish among different forms of bullying victimization. A recent meta-analysis by Meng et al. [58] proposed that the nature of the traumatic experience mediated the relations between trauma and empathy. Furthermore, the experience of post-traumatic growth and its influence on cognitive empathy might vary among individuals. For instance, Yan et al. [59] observed that women exhibited significantly higher levels of empathy compared to men. This is consistent with the results of this study, which found that women had higher levels of cognitive empathy at the T2 time point compared to men. Consequently, gender could play a certain role in mediating the relations between post-traumatic growth and cognitive empathy. But gender differences were not the main purpose of this study and gender was shown to be associated with cognitive empathy and post-traumatic growth only at the T2 time point. Therefore, while this study controlled for gender, it did not break down study results by men and women. This might have hidden specific gender-related dynamics in the interplay between post-traumatic growth and cognitive empathy. In future research, a deliberate classification of subjects by gender for separate analyses could offer deeper insights.

5. Implications and Limitations

The present study revealed that the cognitive empathy of victims of school bullying could predict their subsequent post-traumatic growth. This finding suggests that victims with higher levels of cognitive empathy are more likely to achieve positive psychological transformation and growth after experiencing bullying. These findings will enable a more comprehensive exploration of the evolving interplay between post-traumatic growth and cognitive empathy among bullying victims. Such efforts are anticipated to foster an understanding of the dynamics governing the relation between post-traumatic growth and cognitive empathy among this demographic and to refine interventions for enhancing bullying victims' post-traumatic growth by improving their cognitive empathy levels. Cognitive empathy training can be added to the intervention program for the bullied person; for example, cognitive empathy can be enhanced through methods and tools such as role-playing, emotional transposition, and empathy training games [60–62].

The current study also has some limitations. Firstly, while employing a longitudinal study design, the reliance on questionnaires for all three data collection points may have introduced susceptibility to social desirability biases and potential common method biases. Future studies are encouraged to incorporate methods such as interviews and observations to enhance study validity. Secondly, the current study was conducted during the COVID-19 pandemic, so some psychological responses may have been influenced to some extent by pandemic exposure. Future studies should control for COVID-19 pandemic exposure as a covariate when assessing psychological responses in the context of school bullying. Thirdly, the examination of the link between post-traumatic growth and cognitive empathy among bullying victims was confined to middle school students, predominantly from a specific city in Zhejiang Province, China. This limitation restricts the broader applicability of this study's findings. Future research endeavors will aim to broaden the sampling scope, employ diverse methodologies, and integrate measurements at various intervals.

Author Contributions: Conceptualization, F.L., B.C. and X.L.; methodology, F.L. and Y.Z.; software, F.L.; validation, B.C., X.L. and F.L.; formal analysis, F.L.; investigation, F.L. and B.C.; resources, X.Z.; data curation, X.Z.; writing—original draft preparation, F.L.; writing—review and editing,

R.Z.; visualization, F.L.; supervision, R.Z.; project administration, X.Z.; funding acquisition, R.Z. All authors have read and agreed to the published version of the manuscript.

Funding: This research was funded by "Zhijiang Youth" Special Project of Philosophy and Social Science Planning of Zhejiang Province, grant number 24ZJQN066Y.

Institutional Review Board Statement: This study was approved by the Research Ethics Committee of Hangzhou Normal University, the local education department, and the participating school principals (approval code 2019-004) on 28 February 2019.

Informed Consent Statement: The voluntary nature of students' participation in the research was highlighted, and informed consent was obtained from all students and their guardians.

Data Availability Statement: The data that support the findings of this study are available from the corresponding author or the first author upon reasonable request.

Conflicts of Interest: The authors declare no competing interests.

References

1. Olweus, D. *Bullying at School: What We Know and What We Can Do*; Blackwell: Oxford, UK, 1993.
2. Mikkelsen, E.G.; Einarsen, S. Relationships between exposure to bullying at work and psychological and psychosomatic health complaints: The role of state negative affectivity and generalized self-efficacy. *Scand. J. Psychol.* **2002**, *43*, 397–405. [CrossRef]
3. Matthiesen, S.B.; Einarsen, S. Psychiatric distress and symptoms of PTSD among victims of bullying at work. *Br. J. Guid. Counsell.* **2004**, *32*, 335–356. [CrossRef]
4. Wang, Y. Formation mechanism and countermeasures of school bullying under the perspective of psychology. *J. Beijing Norm. Univ. (Soc. Sci. Ed.)* **2019**, *4*, 32–45.
5. Sun, J. Research on the influencing factors of school bullying in China. *Fujian Forum Humanit. Soc. Sci.* **2021**, *6*, 181–191.
6. Kaess, M. Bullying: Peer-to-peer maltreatment with severe consequences for child and adolescent mental health. *Eur. Child Adolesc. Psychiatry* **2018**, *27*, 945–947. [CrossRef] [PubMed]
7. Moore, L.; Britten, N.; Lydahl, D.; Naldemirci, Ö.; Elam, M.; Wolf, A. Barriers and facilitators to the implementation of person-centred care in different healthcare contexts. *Scand. J. Caring Sci.* **2016**, *31*, 662–673. [CrossRef]
8. Tedeschi, R.G.; Calhoun, L.G. Target article: "Posttraumatic growth: Conceptual foundations and empirical evidence". *Psychol. Inq.* **2004**, *15*, 1–18. [CrossRef]
9. Tedeschi, R.G.; Calhoun, L.G. *Trauma & Transformation: Growing in the Aftermath of Suffering*; Sage Publications: Thousand Oaks, CA, USA, 1995.
10. Tedeschi, R.G.; Calhoun, L.G. The posttraumatic growth inventory: Measuring the positive legacy of trauma. *J. Trauma Stress* **1996**, *9*, 455–471. [CrossRef]
11. Canevello, A.; Hall, J.; Walsh, J.I. Empathy-Mediated Altruism in Intergroup Contexts: The Roles of Posttraumatic Stress and Posttraumatic Growth. *Emotion* **2022**, *22*, 1699–1712. [CrossRef] [PubMed]
12. Zhou, L.; Wu, X.; Yang, X.; Wang, W.; Tian, Y. The relationship between empathy and posttraumatic growth in post-earthquake adolescents: The mediating role of emotional expression and cognitive reappraisal. *Psychol. Sci.* **2019**, *6*, 1325–1331.
13. Jolliffe, D.; Farrington, D.P. Empathy and offending: A systematic review and meta-analysis. *Aggress. Violent Behav.* **2004**, *9*, 441–476. [CrossRef]
14. Davis, M.H. A Multidimensional Approach to Individual Differences in Empathy. *JSAS Cat. Sel. Doc. Psychol.* **1980**, *10*, 85.
15. Davis, M.H. Measuring individual differences in empathy: Evidence for a multidimensional approach. *J. Pers. Soc. Psychol.* **1983**, *44*, 113–126. [CrossRef]
16. Galinsky, A.D.; Ku, G.; Wang, C.S. Perspective-taking and self-other overlap: Fostering social bonds and facilitating social coordination. *Group Process. Intergroup Relat.* **2005**, *8*, 109–124. [CrossRef]
17. Decety, J.; Meyer, M. From emotion resonance to empathic understanding: A Social Developmental Neuroscience Account. *Dev. Psychopathol.* **2008**, *20*, 1053–1080. [CrossRef]
18. Heyes, C.M. *Cognitive Gadgets: The Cultural Evolution of Thinking*; The Belknap Press of Harvard University Press: Cambridge, MA, USA, 2018.
19. Smith, A. Cognitive empathy and emotional empathy in human behavior and evolution. *Psychol. Rec.* **2006**, *56*, 3–21. [CrossRef]
20. Wang, W.; Wu, X. The effects of empathy on pro-social behavior of post-disaster adolescents: The mediating roles of gratitude, social support, and post-traumatic growth. *J. Psychol.* **2020**, *3*, 307–316.
21. van Noorden, T.H.; Haselager, G.J.; Cillessen, A.H.; Bukowski, W.M. Empathy and involvement in bullying in children and adolescents: A systematic review. *J. Youth Adolesc.* **2014**, *44*, 637–657. [CrossRef]
22. de Waal, F.B.; Preston, S.D. Mammalian empathy: Behavioural manifestations and neural basis. *Nat. Rev. Neurosci.* **2017**, *18*, 498–509. [CrossRef]
23. Shamay-Tsoory, S.G.; Aharon-Peretz, J.; Perry, D. Two systems for empathy: A double dissociation between emotional and cognitive empathy in inferior frontal gyrus versus ventromedial prefrontal lesions. *Brain* **2009**, *132*, 617–627. [CrossRef]

24. Hoffman, M.L. Sex differences in empathy and related behaviors. *Psychol. Bull.* **1977**, *84*, 712–722. [CrossRef]
25. Preston, S.D.; de Waal, F.B. Empathy: Its ultimate and proximate bases. *Behav. Brain Sci.* **2002**, *25*, 1–20. [CrossRef] [PubMed]
26. Gallese, V. The roots of empathy: The shared manifold hypothesis and the neural basis of intersubjectivity. *Psychopathology* **2003**, *36*, 171–180. [CrossRef]
27. Decety, J.; Jackson, P.L. The functional architecture of human empathy. *Behav. Cogn. Neurosci. Rev.* **2004**, *3*, 71–100. [CrossRef]
28. Yan, C.; Su, Y. Developmental differences between cognitive and emotional empathy: A meta-analytic exploration. *Psychol. Dev. Educ.* **2021**, *1*, 1–9.
29. An, Y.; Zang, W.; Wu, X.; Lin, C.; Zhou, J. The effects of trauma exposure on posttraumatic growth of middle school students-the moderating role of resilience. *J. Psychol. Sci.* **2011**, *34*, 727–732.
30. Calhoun, L.G.; Tedeschi, R.G. The Foundations of Posttraumatic Growth: An Expanded Framework. In *Handbook of Posttraumatic Growth: Research and Practice*; Lawrence Erlbaum Associates: Mahwah, NJ, USA, 2006; pp. 3–23.
31. Wagner, S.L.; Pasca, R.; Regehr, C. Firefighters and Empathy: Does It Hurt to Care Too Much? *J. Loss Trauma* **2019**, *24*, 238–250. [CrossRef]
32. Zenasni, F.; Boujut, E.; Woerner, A.; Sultan, S. Burnout and empathy in primary care: Three hypotheses. *Br. J. Gen. Pract.* **2012**, *62*, 346–347. [CrossRef]
33. O'Brien, T.B.; DeLongis, A.; Pomaki, G.; Puterman, E.; Zwicker, A. Couples coping with stress. *Eur. Psychol.* **2009**, *14*, 18–28. [CrossRef]
34. Schurz, M.; Radua, J.; Tholen, M.G.; Maliske, L.; Margulies, D.S.; Mars, R.B.; Sallet, J.; Kanske, P. Toward a hierarchical model of social cognition: A neuroimaging meta-analysis and integrative review of empathy and theory of mind. *Psychol. Bull.* **2021**, *147*, 293–327. [CrossRef] [PubMed]
35. Epstein, R. Extinction-induced resurgence: Preliminary investigations and possible applications. *Psychol. Rec.* **1985**, *35*, 143–153. [CrossRef]
36. Tedeschi, R.G.; Park, C.L.; Calhoun, L.G. (Eds.) *Posttraumatic Growth: Positive Changes in the Aftermath of Crisis*; Lawrence Erlbaum Associates Publishers: Mahwah, NJ, USA, 1998.
37. Staub, E.; Vollhardt, J. Altruism born of suffering: The roots of caring and helping after victimization and other trauma. *Am. J. Orthopsychiatry* **2008**, *78*, 267–280. [CrossRef]
38. Greenberg, D.M.; Warrier, V.; Allison, C.; Baron-Cohen, S. Testing the empathizing–systemizing theory of sex differences and the extreme male brain theory of autism in half a million people. *Proc. Natl. Acad. Sci. USA* **2018**, *115*, 12152–12157. [CrossRef] [PubMed]
39. Decety, J.; Svetlova, M. Putting together phylogenetic and ontogenetic perspectives on empathy. *Dev. Cogn. Neurosci.* **2012**, *2*, 1–24. [CrossRef] [PubMed]
40. Huang, Y.; Su, Y. Lifelong development of empathy: A dual-process perspective. *Psychol. Dev. Educ.* **2012**, *4*, 434–441.
41. Elam, T.; Taku, K. Differences between posttraumatic growth and resiliency: Their distinctive relationships with empathy and emotion recognition ability. *Front. Psychol.* **2022**, *13*, 825161. [CrossRef] [PubMed]
42. Zhen, R.; Zhou, X. The relationship between school bullying victimization and post-traumatic stress symptoms: The role of just-world beliefs and social support. *Chin. J. Clin. Psychol.* **2023**, *1*, 148–152, 193.
43. Xie, J.; Wei, Y.; Zhu, Z. Exploration of patterns of bullying victimization among contemporary Chinese adolescents: Based on latent profile analysis. *Psychol. Dev. Educ.* **2019**, *35*, 95–102.
44. Xie, J.; Qin, F.; Bear, G.; Fu, Y. Revision of the Chinese version of the Delaware Student Involvement Scale (Student Volume). *Chin. J. Clin. Psychol.* **2019**, *2*, 277–281.
45. Zhou, X.; Wu, X.; An, Y.; Chen, J. The impact of adolescent core belief challenges on posttraumatic growth: The role of rumination and social support. *J. Psychol.* **2014**, *46*, 1509–1520.
46. Muthén, L.; Muthén, B. *Mplus User's Guide*, 7th ed.; Muthén & Muthén: Los Angeles, CA, USA, 2012.
47. Cheung, G.W.; Rensvold, R.B. Evaluating Goodness-of-Fit Indexes for Testing Measurement Invariance. *Struct. Equ. Model.* **2002**, *9*, 233–255. [CrossRef]
48. DeLongis, A.; O'Brien, T. An interpersonal framework for stress and coping: An application to the families of Alzheimer's patients. In *Stress and Coping in Later-Life Families*; Stephens, M.A.P., Crowther, J.H., Hobfoll, S.E., Tennenbaum, D.L., Eds.; Hemisphere Publishing Corp.: New York, NY, USA, 1990; pp. 221–239.
49. Cofini, V.; Cecilia, M.R.; Petrarca, F.; Bernardi, R.; Mazza, M.; Orio, F.D. Factors Associated with Post-Traumatic Growth after the Loss of a Loved One. *Minerva Psichiatr.* **2014**, *55*, 207–214.
50. Dou, J.; Liu, C.; Xiong, R.; Zhou, H.; Lu, G.; Jia, L. Empathy and post-traumatic growth among Chinese community workers during the COVID-19 pandemic: Roles of self-disclosure and social support. *Int. J. Environ. Res. Public Health* **2022**, *19*, 15739. [CrossRef] [PubMed]
51. Berzenski, S.R.; Yates, T.M. The Development of Empathy in Child Maltreatment Contexts. *Child Abus. Negl.* **2022**, *133*, 105827. [CrossRef]
52. Zhai, W.; Luo, S.; Li, K.; Liu, L.; Lai, D. A study of the interactive effects of empathy and self-expression on post-traumatic growth in gynecologic cancer couples. *J. Nurs. Manage.* **2023**, *23*, 31–36.
53. Bernhardt, B.C.; Singer, T. The Neural Basis of Empathy. *Annu. Rev. Neurosci.* **2012**, *35*, 1–23. [CrossRef] [PubMed]

54. Saarni, C. Emotional competence: How emotions and relationships become integrated. In *Nebraska Symposium on Motivation, 1988: Socioemotional Development*; Thompson, R.A., Ed.; University of Nebraska Press: Lincoln, NB, USA, 1990; pp. 115–182.
55. Berndsen, M.; Wenzel, M.; Thomas, E.F.; Noske, B. I Feel You Feel What I Feel: Perceived Perspective-taking Promotes Victims' Conciliatory Attitudes Because of Inferred Emotions in the Offender. *Euro J. Soc. Psychol.* **2018**, *48*, O103–O120. [CrossRef]
56. Ruby, P.; Decety, J. How would you feel versus how do you think she would feel? A neuroimaging study of perspective-taking with social emotions. *J. Cogn. Neurosci.* **2004**, *16*, 988–999. [CrossRef] [PubMed]
57. Swickert, R.J.; Hittner, J.B.; Foster, A. A proposed mediated path between gender and posttraumatic growth: The roles of empathy and social support in a mixed-age sample. *Psychology* **2012**, *3*, 1142–1147. [CrossRef]
58. Meng, X.; Yu, D.; Chen, Y.; Zhang, L.; Fu, X. The relationship between childhood trauma and empathy: A three-level meta-analysis. *J. Psychol.* **2023**, *55*, 1285–1303.
59. Yan, C.; Su, Y. Gender differences in empathy: Evidence from a meta-analysis. *Psychol. Dev. Educ.* **2018**, *34*, 129–136.
60. Using Role Playing in Teaching Empathy. Available online: http://www.blatner.com/adam/pdntbk/tchempathy.htm (accessed on 12 April 2024).
61. Li, L. The relationship between adolescents' empathy and prosocial behavior. *J. Psychol.* **1990**, *1*, 72–79.
62. Feshbach, N.D.; Feshbach, S. Empathy Training and the Regulation of Aggression: Potentialities and Limitations. *Acad. Psychol. Bull.* **1982**, *4*, 399–413.

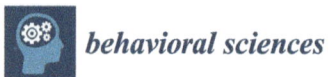 *behavioral sciences*

Article

Associations Between Emotional Resilience and Mental Health Among Chinese Adolescents in the School Context: The Mediating Role of Positive Emotions

Zhongmin Zhu [1,2], Biao Sang [1,2,*], Junsheng Liu [3], Yuyang Zhao [4] and Ying Liu [5]

1   Shanghai Academy of Educational Sciences, Shanghai 200032, China; zzmin@cnsaes.org.cn
2   Lab for Educational Big Data and Policymaking, Ministry of Education, P.R. China, Shanghai 200032, China
3   School of Psychology and Cognitive Science, East China Normal University, Shanghai 200062, China;
     jsliu@psy.ecnu.edu.cn
4   Department of Social Work, School of Sociology and Political Science, Shanghai University,
     Shanghai 200444, China; yuyang_zhao@yahoo.com
5   Wenbo College, East China University of Political Science and Law, Shanghai 200042, China;
     liuying3729@126.com
*   Correspondence: bsang@psy.ecnu.edu.cn

Abstract: Positive emotions play an essential role in adolescent resilience and mental healthy development, yet whether it affects emotional resilience, mental health, and the internal mechanism remains unknown. Therefore, the current study aims to, using a two-wave panel design, examine the relationship between emotional resilience and mental health, as well as the mediating role of positive emotion. We conducted this longitudinal study in two waves with a 6-month interval, surveyed 266 Chinese adolescents (54.9% boys, M_{age} = 14.11 years, SD = 1.77), and constructed a mediation model. The participants completed the measures of demographic information, positive emotions, emotional resilience, and mental health at two times. The results revealed that after controlling for gender and age, Time 2 positive emotions partially mediated the relationship between Time 1 emotional resilience and Time 2 mental health. In detail, emotional resilience is positively correlated with life satisfaction and self-esteem. It shows a negative correlation with symptoms of depression and anxiety, partly mediated by positive emotions. The findings highlighted the role of emotional resilience in mitigating psychological problems and enhancing mental health in Chinese adolescents. The implications and limitations were discussed.

Keywords: adolescents; emotional resilience; positive emotions; mental health

1. Introduction

Adolescence is a particularly crucial period for emotional development, as it presents opportunities for personal growth and the cultivation of lifelong well-being, as well as associated with a significant risk for mental health (Anderson & Priebe, 2021). During this period, episodes of mental health issues are common, with 10% to 20% of adolescents globally affected by mental health problems (Aguirre Velasco et al., 2020; Ma et al., 2021). It is crucial and urgent to comprehensively understand the factors and mechanisms that protect and harm adolescent mental health. Existing cross-sectional evidences demonstrated that emotional resilience as a type of resilience is recognized as an essential protective factor for adolescent mental health (i.e., Shapero et al., 2019; Wu et al., 2020).

Emotional resilience, stemming from the term "psychological resilience", is characterized by the ability of an individual to improve or maintain positive emotions and recover from negative emotions when faced with stress and adversity (Davidson, 2000). Previous documents have suggested that the emotional resilience linked with depression and anxiety symptoms (Davis, 2009; Mesman et al., 2021; Shi et al., 2022), well-being (Sterina et al., 2022), and self-efficacy (Rudolph et al., 2025). Moreover, existing findings have shown that emotional resilience is associated with positive emotion (Gloria & Steinhardt, 2016) and that positive emotion is crucial to mental health (Alexander et al., 2021). However, there is no research examining the positive emotion function as a mediational role of emotional resilience and mental health. Moreover, previous studies addressing the associations between emotional resilience and mental health are mostly cross-sectional designs, while data analysis methods focus on correlation and regression analysis rather than exploring causational relationships (i.e., Gatt et al., 2020; Li et al., 2020; Wu et al., 2020). To address abovementioned research gaps, the present study aimed to examine emotional resilience and positive emotion and explore potential mediating mechanisms for enhancing adolescent mental health through a two-wave panel design. The current study contributes to a deeper understanding of the positive emotional pathways that link emotional resilience and mental health, thereby broadening the existing body of research in this field. Furthermore, it provides valuable implications for the development of interventions aimed at promoting adolescent mental health.

1.1. Emotional Resilience and Mental Health

According to the Complete Mental Health Theory put forward by Keyes (2007), complete mental health implies not only the absence of disease but also a positive and flourishing mental state, which can lead to a high level of emotional and social adjustment (Arslan & Allen, 2022; Arslan & Renshaw, 2018). Given the theoretical points, complete mental health was supposed to contain two aspects: positive mental health and negative mental health (Mesman et al., 2021). Draper et al. (2022) identified depression and anxiety as indicators of negative mental health, while life satisfaction and self-esteem were also included in the indicators of positive mental health in previous studies (Moksnes & Espnes, 2013; Zhou & Cheng, 2022). Consequently, we chose positive mental health indicators (i.e., life satisfaction, self-esteem) and negative mental health indicators (i.e., depression, anxiety).

Previous research showed that there was a close and significant relationship between emotional resilience and negative mental health indicators such as depression and anxiety among adolescents (Chung et al., 2020; Ramos-Díaz et al., 2019). For example, Chung et al. (2020) found that adolescents who lived with single parents showed lower emotional resilience, which in turn was related to high levels of depression. Also, the results of a study conducted by Ramos-Díaz et al. (2019) highlighted that the importance of developing resilience improves life satisfaction among adolescents. High levels of emotional resilience trigger multiple and flexible coping strategies among adolescents as a result, which could generate high levels of self-esteem by solving problems easily (Chung et al., 2020). In spite of this, the possible mediated variable has not been examined. From the perspective of positive psychology, positive emotion is a vital variable that has received more attention in recent years.

1.2. Emotional Resilience and Positive Emotions

Positive emotions are featured by the pleasure feelings that arise when individuals' physical and mental needs are satisfied (Fredrickson, 2009). It is important to note that positive emotion and emotional resilience are both theoretically and functionally distinct constructs. Emotional resilience emphasizes a dynamic capacity to recover from adversity, rooted in stress-coping models that underscore cognitive–behavioral regulation (e.g., threat appraisal; Lazarus & Folkman, 1984; Ward et al., 2021). It prioritizes adaptive processes (e.g., restoring equilibrium) rather than transient affective states. In contrast, positive emotion emphasizes short-term hedonic experiences (e.g., joy) that enhance cognitive flexibility, as articulated in Fredrickson's (1998) broaden-and-build theory. While positive emotions may temporarily alleviate negative emotions states (Fredrickson et al., 2000), they lack the sustained self-regulatory mechanisms that are central to resilience. Crucially, emotional resilience involves actively confronting adversity (e.g., tolerating uncertainty), whereas positive emotions can arise independently of adversity (Tugade & Fredrickson, 2004). Thus, emotional resilience represents a capacity for recovery, while positive emotion constitutes an affective outcome that may coexist with, but is not essential to, resilient processes.

The broaden-and-build theory (BBT) supposed by Fredrickson (1998) of positive emotions highlights that if the relationship between emotional resilience and positive emotion is reciprocal, positive emotion can build emotional resilience, and the build of emotional resilience can generate more positive emotion (Fredrickson, 1998). It is worth noting that previous studies have focused more on the influence of positive emotion on emotional resilience (i.e., Gloria & Steinhardt, 2016; Zhu et al., 2023). However, an increasing amount of evidence regarding emotional resilience has shown strong associations with positive emotions recently (Gilchrist et al., 2023). For instance, a study involving adolescents demonstrated that those with low emotional resilience exhibited lower levels of emotional pleasure compared to their counterparts with high emotional resilience (Cohn et al., 2009). In another study involving 421 college students who reported their mood states, the results from implementing a structural equation model indicated that one dimension of emotional resilience, which is the capacity to generate positive emotions, could foster the emergence of positive emotions and contribute to the attenuation of negative emotions. Meanwhile, another dimension of emotional resilience, which is the ability to recover from negative emotions, also directly lessened negative emotions (Y. Wang et al., 2016). Overall, emotional resilience has been recognized as to be associated with positive emotions, whereas how emotional resilience predicts positive emotions needs to be further examined.

1.3. Positive Emotion and Mental Health

In the field of mental health, researchers have argued that positive emotions are crucial for complete mental health (Keyes, 2007). Recently, an increasing number of researchers have differentiated positive emotion and mental health as two distinct constructs through various operational definitions and different measurements (Fredrickson & Joiner, 2018; Z. Wang et al., 2011). Positive emotions as emotional states that are related to the satisfaction of personal needs and are usually accompanied by the subjective experience of pleasure, including both transient emotions (i.e., pleasure) and diffuse and persistent positive emotions (Z. Wang et al., 2011). Mental health is a functional component of an individual's overall psychological quality (L. Chen & Zhang, 2009). Therefore, the scope of mental health is larger and relatively stable than positive emotions and is generally used as an outcome variable in studies.

The undoing hypothesis proposed that positive emotions facilitate recovery from the autonomic arousal associated with negative emotions (Fredrickson & Levenson, 1998), indicating that positive emotions impact on negative indicators of mental health in a positive way. Furthermore, an individual with positive emotions in daily life or work experiences a high level of self-esteem (Nezlek & Kuppens, 2008), satisfies their own basic psychological and physical needs (Schutte & Malouff, 2021), and has access to complete mental health easily (Dong et al., 2012; Fredrickson & Joiner, 2018). Correspondingly, positive emotions helped individuals to relieve depression, fear, and anxiety (Santos et al., 2013). Cultivating positive emotions was an effective way to eliminate individual psychological barriers and promote healthy mental status (Gloria & Steinhardt, 2016). However, how to improve mental health through positive emotion remains to be addressed.

1.4. The Present Study

To address these gaps, the present study utilizes a two-wave panel design to investigate how emotional resilience predicts mental health outcomes among adolescents, and whether positive emotions serve as a key mediating mechanism in this relationship. By incorporating both positive and negative indicators of mental health, this study offers a more balanced and developmentally sensitive understanding of psychological well-being during adolescence. Given the existing evidence and the aims of the current study, the hypotheses were supposed as follows:

H1: *Emotional resilience significantly predicts mental health among Chinese adolescents.*

H2: *Positive emotions mediate the relationship between emotional resilience and mental health.*

H3: *T2 positive emotions mediate the relationship between T1 emotional resilience and T2 mental health.*

2. Methods

2.1. Participants

A longitudinal study was conducted involving three high school classes and five middle school classes. These medium-sized schools are located in urban areas of moderate socio-economic status. A total of 291 questionnaires were distributed, resulting in a final sample of 266 adolescents, comprising 146 boys (54.9%) and 120 girls (45.1%). The participants' ages ranged from 12 to 18 years, with a mean age of 14.11 years ($SD = 1.77$). Over 90% of the students were of Han nationality, the predominant ethnic group in China.

2.2. Measures

Emotional resilience was measured using the Adolescents' Emotional Resilience Questionnaire (AERQ) developed by Zhang and Lu (2010). The AERQ contains 11 items that yield two dimensions: the ability to generate positive emotions (GPE) (e.g., 'When I'm in a bad mood, I can think of happy things') and the ability to recover from negative emotions (RNE) (e.g., 'I can adjust my negative emotions in a short time'). Each item is rated on a 6-point scale (from 1 = completely disagree to 6 = completely agree). A higher score indicates a greater level of emotional resilience. During the T1 assessment, the overall scale demonstrated good reliability, with Cronbach's $\alpha = 0.91$. Furthermore, the reliabilities for the GPE and RNE dimensions were also very good at 0.90 and 0.85, respectively.

Positive emotion was measured using the positive affect items from the Positive Affect and Negative Affect Scale for Children (PANAS-C) (Pan et al., 2015), originally developed by Laurent et al. (1999). This measure consists of 15 items; each item describes a positive emotion, such as 'happy', among others. Participants rated their own emotional levels over recent weeks using a 5-point scale ranging from 1 (none) to 5 (very much). Higher total scores reflect higher levels of positive emotion. In this study, Cronbach's α for the Positive Emotion Questionnaire was found to be 0.92.

Life satisfaction was evaluated using the Satisfaction with Life Scale (SWLS), which includes five items and was developed by Diener et al. (1985). This scale has been widely utilized in China with established reliability and validity (Jiang et al., 2018). Participants rated their perceptions of life quality on a 7-point scale ranging from 1 (strongly disagree) to 7 (strongly agree), responding to statements such as 'I am satisfied with my life'. Higher total scores indicate greater life satisfaction; in this study, Cronbach's α for this measure was reported at 0.83.

Self-esteem was measured using the 10-item Self-Esteem Scale (Wu et al., 2017), which uses 5 scoring points ranging from 1 (complete non-conformity) to 5 (complete conformity).

A higher total score indicated a higher level of self-esteem (e.g., 'Overall, I am satisfied with myself'). Previous studies have shown that the scale has good reliability and validity (Wu et al., 2017; Xie et al., 2019). Cronbach's α in this study was 0.87.

Depression was assessed using the Center for Epidemic Studies Depression Scale (CES-D), which comprises 20 items (Radloff, 1977). This scale required participants to subjectively evaluate the frequency of depressive symptoms experienced over the past week (e.g., 'It's hard for me to concentrate'), and it has been previously validated in Chinese adolescents (Tang et al., 2019). The questionnaire employed a 4-point scale ranging from 0 to 3, where scores of 0, 1, 2, and 3 corresponded to occasional or none (less than one day per week), sometimes (1–2 days per week), frequently or about half the time (3–4 days per week), and most of the time or nearly every day (5–7 days per week). A higher total score indicated a greater level of depressive symptoms. In this study, Cronbach's α was found to be 0.91.

Anxiety was assessed using the 'Trait Anxiety Questionnaire', which consists of 20 items adapted from prior research (J. Chen et al., 2015; Shek, 1993). Participants were instructed to reflect on their own emotional experiences and provide ratings for four statements presented in the scale (e.g., 'I worry too much about things that don't really matter'), with a scoring system ranging from 1 (almost none) to 4 (almost always). A higher total score indicated a greater level of anxiety. Previous studies have demonstrated that the reliability and validity of this questionnaire fulfill psychometric standards (J. Chen et al., 2015; Shek, 1993). In this study, Cronbach's α was found to be 0.89.

2.3. Procedures

The current study received initial approval from the Institutional Review Board (IRB) of BLINDED University prior to data collection. Data for Time 1 (T1) were collected in April and May of 2021. Subsequently, all Time 2 (T2) data were gathered six months after T1, specifically in October and November of 2021. Participants included students aged 12 to 18, as well as their parents, who were informed about this study and asked to provide voluntary consent by signing an informed consent form. Students had the right to withdraw from this research at any time, even if they had previously signed the informed consent.

All data utilized in this study were obtained from students through a paper-based questionnaire. Trained investigators administered these questionnaires by providing face-to-face instructions to all participating students. Afterward, the investigators collected the completed questionnaires and securely stored them in a laboratory setting for further analysis.

2.4. Statistical Analysis

The analyses conducted in the current study utilized SPSS 22.0 and the SPSS Process Macro. First, we performed a test for common method bias to confirm that there was no significant effect of common method bias present. Second, we examined the correlations among the variables under investigation. Finally, we employed the SPSS Process Macro to assess the mediating role of positive emotions between emotional resilience and mental health, utilizing bias-corrected bootstrap tests with a 95% confidence interval to determine whether the indirect effects were statistically significant.

3. Results

3.1. The Control and Verification of Common Method Variance

Since all variables utilized in the current study were measured through students' self-reports, there is a potential for common method variance (CMV) effects. To assess this possibility, the Harman single-factor test was conducted to evaluate CMV (Podsakoff et al., 2003). All variables were subjected to exploratory factor analysis without rotation.

For the T1 assessment, results indicated that there were 13 factors with characteristic roots greater than 1, and the variance explained by the first factor was 31.88%, which falls below the critical threshold of 40%. In the T2 assessment, findings revealed that there were 15 factors with characteristic roots exceeding 1, and the variance accounted for by the first factor was 32.73%, also less than the critical value of 40%. Consequently, no significant CMV effects were identified in this study.

3.2. Descriptive Statistics

As presented in Table 1, the descriptive statistics and the interrelationships among T1 emotional resilience, T2 positive emotions, and T2 mental health indicators are reported. The findings revealed a robust positive correlation between T1 emotional resilience, T2 positive emotions, and the positive indicators of mental health at T2 (i.e., life satisfaction and self-esteem). In contrast, there exists a significant negative correlation between T1 emotional resilience, T2 positive emotions, and the negative indicators of mental health at T2 (i.e., depression and anxiety).

Table 1. Mean, standard deviation (SD), and correlation coefficient of emotional resilience, positive emotion, and mental health (n = 266).

Variables	*M*	*SD*	1	2	3	4	5	6
1. T1 Emotional resilience	41.62	12.90	-					
2. T2 Positive emotions	47.49	10.27	0.34 ***	-				
3. T2 Life satisfaction	22.92	5.94	0.44 ***	0.43 ***	-			
4. T2 Self-esteem	28.67	4.33	0.43 ***	0.43 ***	0.47 ***	-		
5. T2 Depression	16.19	8.79	−0.47 ***	−0.37 ***	−0.60 ***	−0.72 ***	-	
6. T2 Anxiety	43.80	7.18	−0.43 ***	−0.47 ***	−0.57 ***	−0.71 ***	0.78 ***	-

Note. *** $p < 0.001$.

3.3. The Mediating Effect of Positive Emotion on the Relationship Between Emotional Resilience and Mental Health

By using the SPSS Process Macro, the mediating effects of T2 positive emotions on the relationship between T1 emotional resilience and four T2 mental health indicators were tested. As shown in Table 2, after controlling for gender and age, the results suggested that T2 positive emotions partially mediated the relationship between T1 emotional resilience and T2 mental health. The Bootstrap test results showed that the 95% confidence interval did not include the number 0, and the mediating effect was significant. As can be seen from Figure 1, the total and direct effects of emotional resilience were also significant.

Table 2. Test of mediating effect of positive emotions on the relationship between emotional resilience and mental health (n = 266).

Dependent Variable		Gender	Age	T1 Emotional Resilience	T2 Positive Emotion	Indirect Effect (95% Confidence Interval)
T2 Positive emotion	B	−0.85	−1.46	0.33		
	t	−0.53	−3.49 **	5.51 ***		
	95%CI	[−4.03, 2.33]	[−2.28, −0.64]	[0.21, 0.45]		

Table 2. *Cont.*

Dependent Variable		Gender	Age	T1 Emotional Resilience	T2 Positive Emotion	Indirect Effect (95% Confidence Interval)
T2 Life satisfaction	B	0.71	0.17	0.20	0.17	
	t	0.82	0.74	5.66 ***	4.37 ***	0.06 [0.03, 0.10]
	95%CI	[−0.99, 2.41]	[−0.28, 0.63]	[0.13, 0.27]	[0.09, 0.25]	
T2 Self-esteem	B	−0.58	0.49	0.13	0.15	
	t	−0.93	2.96 **	5.22 ***	5.34***	0.05 [0.03, 0.08]
	95%CI	[−1.80, 0.65]	[0.16, 0.82]	[0.08, 0.18]	[0.09, 0.21]	
T2 Depression	B	0.13	0.23	−0.34	−0.16	
	t	0.10	0.68	−6.71 ***	−2.80 ***	−0.05 [−0.10, −0.02]
	95%CI	[−2.40, 2.67]	[−0.44, 0.91]	[−0.44, −0.24]	[−0.28, −0.05]	
T2 Anxiety	B	0.68	0.23	−0.21	−0.23	
	t	0.66	0.84	−4.95 ***	−4.86 ***	−0.08 [−0.13, −0.04]
	95%CI	[−1.36, 2.74]	[−0.32, 0.79]	[−0.29, −0.13]	[−0.32, −0.14]	

Note. ** $p < 0.01$, *** $p < 0.001$.

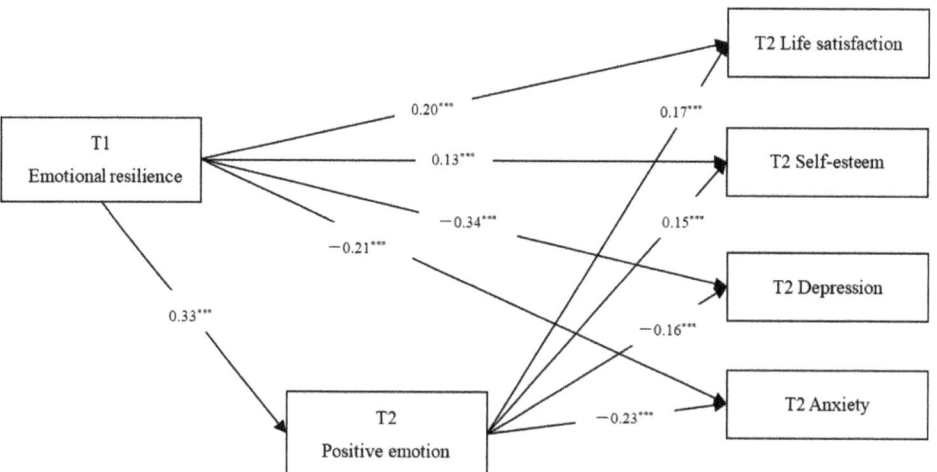

Figure 1. The mediating model of positive emotion on the relationship between emotional resilience and mental health. Note. *** $p < 0.001$.

4. Discussion

This study explored the impact of emotional resilience on adolescent mental health in a two-wave panel design, highlighting the mediating role of positive emotion. The findings indicated the critical role emotional resilience plays in both reducing mental health problems and promoting positive mental health outcomes. Specifically, the results demonstrate that emotional resilience positively influences life satisfaction and self-esteem while mitigating the effect of depression and anxiety. Moreover, positive emotions partially mediate these relationships, indicating that emotional resilience not only exerts direct effects on mental health but also facilitates improvements through the enhancement of positive emotional experiences.

Previous studies found that psychological resilience had a significant influence on mental health (Liu et al., 2019; Chung et al., 2020; Gloria & Steinhardt, 2016). The current study focused on a specific type of psychological resilience, emotional resilience, and found that it also had a significant effect on mental health, consistent with H1, which deepens the research on the relationship between psychological resilience and mental health. The integration of positive and negative mental health indicators into a single framework aligns with Keyes' theory of complete mental health (Keyes, 2007). This approach underscores the importance of addressing both the reduction of mental illnesses and the promotion of flourishing mental states. By focusing on a sample of adolescents, this study expands the literature beyond younger adults and seniors, offering valuable insights into a critical developmental period. Moreover, the broaden-and-build theory of positive emotions (Fredrickson, 1998) provides a theoretical basis for understanding the mechanisms through which emotional resilience fosters mental health. Positive emotions, as posited by this theory, not only broaden cognitive and behavioral repertoires but also build enduring psychological resources such as resilience and well-being. The current findings align with prior research, suggesting that positive emotions serve as a key driver in this dynamic process.

The significant mediating effect of positive emotions indicated that they played a significant role in promoting mental health, consistent with H2 and H3. Positive emotions have been a cornerstone of contemporary positive psychology, receiving considerable attention for their role in enhancing mental health. Seligman (2018) considered positive emotions as one of the three main concepts of positive psychology and built the PERMA model of positive psychology. Seligmans's PERMA model underscores the importance of positive emotions as one of five key pillars of well-being, alongside engagement, relationships, meaning, and achievement. Positive emotions not only initiate and sustain positive mental states but also counterbalance the human tendency to focus on negative experiences. Extensive research on positive emotions emerged during the beginning of the 20th century; more attention was given to the important role of positive emotions on mental health (Gruber & Purcell, 2015; Sang et al., 2014). Meanwhile, positive emotions are usually associated with positive feedback on individuals' behaviors. When individuals experience positive emotions while they are performing certain activities, they are more likely to show such behaviors, especially for healthy behavior. Positive emotions promote mental and physical health. People should cultivate positive emotions in their daily lives not only because they feel good in the moment but also because they help them to feel better and lead them to prosperity, health, and longevity. The BBT of positive emotions emphasized that positive emotions were the core factors in helping individuals reach their optimum functions and moving forward to a more psychologically healthy status (Fredrickson, 2009; Fredrickson & Joiner, 2018).

4.1. Educational Implications from the Current Investigation

Integrating the findings from previous research (focused on how positive emotions promote emotional resilience) and the current study (focused on how emotional resilience promotes positive emotions), this study highlights the potential of positive emotions to create a virtuous cycle in building psychological resources. Positive emotions foster emotional resilience, which, in turn, generates further positive emotions, leading to a dynamic upward spiral of mental health and well-being.

Positive emotions can be cultivated in daily life through accessible activities such as interacting with others, helping others, playing, and learning. These activities utilize abundant endogenous resources that remain largely untapped (Troy & Mauss, 2011). Positive emotions generated in such contexts can stimulate a process of spiral escalation: positive emotions build psychological resources, and these resources lead to more positive emotions, creating a self-reinforcing cycle (Fredrickson & Joiner, 2018). Psychological resilience, while often associated with positive emotions experienced during difficult situations, is not necessarily linked to a reduction in negative emotional arousal but contributes meaningfully to overall well-being.

These findings provide important implications for promoting mental health practices. Individuals can actively cultivate positive emotions through small, intentional actions, carving a pathway to improved health and well-being (LaBelle, 2023). Interventions should focus on embedding these practices into educational and community programs to foster resilience and mental health on a larger scale.

4.2. Limitations and Future Research

Even though this study provides significant insights into the interplay between emotional resilience and positive emotions, several implications and avenues for further research emerge. First, the findings rely primarily on self-reported data, which could introduce biases. While this study utilized longitudinal data, future research should incorporate mixed methods, including behavioral experiments and cognitive neuroscience approaches, to yield more convergent conclusions about the influence of emotional resilience on mental health.

Second, more nuanced studies are needed to explore the effects of emotional resilience on specific types of positive emotions. Research suggests that positive emotions can be categorized into high-approach emotions (e.g., enthusiasm, desire, excitement) and low-approach emotions (e.g., contentment, satisfaction, love, gratitude) (Gilbert, 2012). High-approach emotions are associated with reward-seeking behaviors and motivate actions, whereas low-approach emotions emphasize savoring the present moment without necessarily prompting action. Understanding whether emotional resilience exerts differential effects on these categories, and how each influences mental health, remains an important area for future research.

Third, while positive emotions generally enhance mental health, disturbances in positive emotional regulation may have adverse effects. Excessive positive emotions have been linked to clinical syndromes such as problematic drug and alcohol use, risky sexual behavior, bulimia, gambling, and mania (Gruber & Purcell, 2015). Individuals who fail to down-regulate overly heightened positive emotions are particularly susceptible to these risks. Future study could explore the boundaries of positive emotional experiences on different types of behaviors, as well as the strategies to regulated excessive positive emotions, which will provide theoretical evidence for psychological and educational interventions.

Lastly, the reliance on two-time-point data restricts the ability to model nonlinear trajectories, limiting insights into dynamic processes that may unfold over multiple intervals. Methodologically, while the SPSS Process Macro was selected for its accessibility and capacity to test mediation, future study might employee latent variable modeling or advanced longitudinal techniques (e.g., cross-lagged models) to replicate this study. Additionally, the absence of measurement invariance testing between time points might raise concerns about whether observed changes reflect true differences or measurement artifacts; the observational design and limited temporal resolution preclude definitive conclusions about causality. Future research should incorporate multi-wave designs, validate measures across time points, and employ robust longitudinal analyses to strengthen temporal and causal claims.

5. Conclusions

This study highlights the pivotal role of emotional resilience in promoting adolescent mental health, both directly and through the mediating influence of positive emotions using a two-wave panel design. Integrating the findings from prior research (focused on how positive emotions foster emotional resilience) and the current study (focused on how emotional resilience promotes positive emotions), the results suggest a self-reinforcing cycle between positive emotions and psychological resources. Positive emotions facilitate

Behav. Sci. **2025**, *15*, 567

the development of emotional resilience, which, in turn, fosters further positive emotional experiences, creating a dynamic upward spiral of well-being. Positive emotions can be cultivated in daily life through activities such as social interactions, acts of kindness, play, and learning. These easily accessible endogenous resources provide a foundation for improving health and well-being. By leveraging this positive cycle, individuals can enhance their mental health and achieve flourishing states.

Author Contributions: Conceptualization, Z.Z. and B.S.; Data curation, Z.Z., J.L., Y.Z. and Y.L.; Formal analysis, Z.Z. and J.L.; Investigation, Y.Z.; Methodology, Z.Z., B.S., J.L. and Y.L.; Project administration, B.S.; Resources, B.S.; Software, Z.Z. and J.L.; Validation, J.L.; Visualization, Y.Z.; Writing—original draft, Z.Z.; Writing—review and editing, Z.Z., B.S. and J.L. All authors have read and agreed to the published version of the manuscript.

Funding: This research received no external funding.

Institutional Review Board Statement: This study was conducted in accordance with the Declaration of Helsinki and approved by the Institutional Review Board of East China Normal University: IRB protocol HR 229-2019; 14 September 2019.

Informed Consent Statement: Informed consent was obtained from all subjects involved in this study.

Data Availability Statement: Data are unavailable due to privacy restrictions and ethical concerns.

Acknowledgments: We would like to thank all the participants of this study.

Conflicts of Interest: The authors declare no conflicts of interest.

References

Aguirre Velasco, A., Cruz, I. S. S., Billings, J., Jimenez, M., & Rowe, S. (2020). What are the barriers, facilitators and interventions targeting help-seeking behaviours for common mental health problems in adolescents? A systematic review. *BMC Psychiatry*, *20*, 1–22. [CrossRef] [PubMed]

Alexander, R., Aragón, O. R., Bookwala, J., Cherbuin, N., Gatt, J. M., Kahrilas, I. J., Kästner, N., Lawrence, A., Lowe, L., Morrison, R. G., Mueller, S. C., Nusslock, R., Papadelis, C., Polnaszek, K. L., Helene Richter, S., Silton, R. L., & Styliadis, C. (2021). The neuroscience of positive emotions and affect: Implications for cultivating happiness and wellbeing. *Neuroscience and Biobehavioral Reviews*, *121*, 220–249. [CrossRef] [PubMed]

Anderson, K., & Priebe, S. (2021). Concepts of resilience in adolescent mental health research. *Journal of Adolescent Health*, *69*(5), 689–695. [CrossRef] [PubMed]

Arslan, G., & Allen, K. A. (2022). Complete mental health in elementary school children: Understanding youth school functioning and adjustment. *Current Psychology*, *41*, 1174–1183. [CrossRef]

Arslan, G., & Renshaw, T. L. (2018). Student subjective wellbeing as a predictor of adolescent problem behaviors: A comparison of first-order and second-order factor effects. *Child Indicators Research*, *11*, 507–521. [CrossRef]

Chen, J., Yu, J., Li, X., & Zhang, J. (2015). Genetic and environmental contributions to anxiety among Chinese children and adolescents–a multi-informant twin study. *Journal of Child Psychology and Psychiatry*, *56*, 586–594. [CrossRef]

Chen, L., & Zhang, D. (2009). The progress and trend of adolescent mental health research in China in the past 20 years. *Higher Education Research*, *30*, 74–79.

Chung, J. O. K., Lam, K. K. W., Ho, K. Y., Cheung, A. T., Ho, L. L. K., Gibson, F., & Li, W. H. C. (2020). Relationships among resilience, self-esteem, and depressive symptoms in Chinese adolescents. *Journal of Health Psychology*, *25*, 2396–2405. [CrossRef]

Cohn, M. A., Fredrickson, B. L., Brown, S. L., Mikels, J. A., & Conway, A. M. (2009). Happiness unpacked: Positive emotions increase life satisfaction by building resilience. *Emotion*, *9*, 361–368. [CrossRef]

Davidson, R. J. (2000). Affective style, psychopathology, and resilience: Brain mechanisms and plasticity. *The American Psychologist*, *55*(11), 1196–1214. [CrossRef]

Davis, M. C. (2009). Building emotional resilience to promote health. *American Journal of Lifestyle Medicine*, *3*(Suppl. 1), 60–63. [CrossRef] [PubMed]

Diener, E., Emmons, R. A., Larsen, R. J., & Griffin, S. (1985). The satisfaction with life scale. *Journal of Personality Assessment*, *49*(1), 71–75. [CrossRef] [PubMed]

Dong, Y., Wang, Q., & Xing, C. (2012). Progress in the study on the relationship between positive emotion and physical and mental health. *Journal of Psychological Science*, *35*, 487–493.

Draper, C. E., Cook, C. J., Redinger, S., Rochat, T., Prioreschi, A., Rae, D. E., Ware, L. J., Lye, S. J., & Norris, S. A. (2022). Cross-sectional associations between mental health indicators and social vulnerability, with physical activity, sedentary behavior and sleep in urban African young women. *International Journal of Behavioral Nutrition and Physical Activity, 19*, 1–12. [CrossRef]

Fredrickson, B. L. (1998). What good are positive emotions? *Review of General Psychology, 2*(3), 300–319. [CrossRef]

Fredrickson, B. L. (2009). *Positivity: Groundbreaking research reveals how to embrace the hidden strength of positive emotions, overcome negativity, and thrive.* Crown Publishers.

Fredrickson, B. L., & Joiner, T. (2018). Reflections on positive emotions and upward spirals. *Perspectives on Psychological Science, 13*, 194–199. [CrossRef]

Fredrickson, B. L., & Levenson, R. W. (1998). Positive emotions speed recovery from the cardiovascular sequelae of negative emotions. *Cognition and Emotion, 12*(2), 191–220. [CrossRef]

Fredrickson, B. L., Mancuso, R. A., Branigan, C., & Tugade, M. M. (2000). The undoing effect of positive emotions. *Motivation and Emotion, 24*, 237–258. [CrossRef]

Gatt, J. M., Alexander, R., Emond, A., Foster, K., Hadfield, K., Mason-Jones, A., Reid, S., Theron, L., Ungar, M., Wouldes, T. A., & Wu, Q. (2020). Trauma, resilience, and mental health in migrant and non-migrant youth: An international cross-sectional study across six countries. *Frontiers in Psychiatry, 10*, 997. [CrossRef]

Gilbert, K. E. (2012). The neglected role of positive emotion in adolescent psychopathology. *Clinical Psychology Review, 32*, 467–481. [CrossRef]

Gilchrist, J. D., Gohari, M. R., Benson, L., Patte, K. A., & Leatherdale, S. T. (2023). Reciprocal associations between positive emotions and resilience predict flourishing among adolescents. *Health Promotion and Chronic Disease Prevention in Canada: Research, Policy and Practice, 43*(7), 313–320. [CrossRef]

Gloria, C. T., & Steinhardt, M. A. (2016). Relationships among positive emotions, coping, resilience and mental health. *Stress and Health, 32*(2), 145–156. [CrossRef]

Gruber, J., & Purcell, J. (2015). Positive Emotion Disturbance. In R. A. Scott, S. M. Kosslyn, & M. C. Buchmann (Eds.), *Emerging trends in the social and behavioral sciences: An interdisciplinary, searchable, and linkable resource* (pp. 1–12). John Wiley & Sons.

Jiang, X., Fang, L., Stith, B. R., Liu, R. D., & Huebner, E. S. (2018). A psychometric evaluation of the Chinese version of the student's life satisfaction scale. *Applied Research in Quality of Life, 13*, 1081–1095. [CrossRef]

Keyes, C. L. (2007). Promoting and protecting mental health as flourishing: A complementary strategy for improving national mental health. *The American Psychologist, 62*(2), 95–108. [CrossRef] [PubMed]

LaBelle, B. (2023). Positive outcomes of a social-emotional learning program to promote student resiliency and address mental health. *Contemporary School Psychology, 27*, 1–7. [CrossRef]

Laurent, J., Catanzaro, S. J., Joine, T. E., Jr., Rudolph, K. D., Potter, K. I., Lambert, S., Osborne, L., & Gathright, T. (1999). A measure of positive and negative affect for children: Scale development and preliminary validation. *Psychological Assessment, 11*, 326–338. [CrossRef]

Lazarus, R. S., & Folkman, S. (1984). *Stress, appraisal, and coping.* Springer.

Li, J., Chen, Y. P., Zhang, J., Lv, M. M., Välimäki, M., Li, Y. F., Yang, S. L., Tao, Y. X., Ye, B. Y., Tan, C. X., & Zhang, J. P. (2020). The mediating role of resilience and self-esteem between life events and coping styles among rural left-behind adolescents in China: A cross-sectional study. *Frontiers in Psychiatry, 11*, 560556. [CrossRef] [PubMed]

Liu, W., Yu, Z., & Lin, D. (2019). Meta-analysis of the relationship between psychological resilience and mental health in children and adolescents. *Psychology and Behavior, 17*, 31–37.

Ma, L., Mazidi, M., Li, K., Li, Y., Chen, S., Kirwan, R., Zhou, H., Yan, N., Rahman, A., Wang, W., & Wang, Y. (2021). Prevalence of mental health problems among children and adolescents during the COVID-19 pandemic: A systematic review and meta-analysis. *Journal of Affective Disorders, 293*, 78–89. [CrossRef]

Mesman, E., Vreeker, A., & Hillegers, M. (2021). Resilience and mental health in children and adolescents: An update of the recent literature and future directions. *Current Opinion in Psychiatry, 34*(6), 586–592. [CrossRef]

Moksnes, U. K., & Espnes, G. A. (2013). Self-esteem and life satisfaction in adolescents—Gender and age as potential moderators. *Quality of Life Research, 22*, 2921–2928. [CrossRef] [PubMed]

Nezlek, J. B., & Kuppens, P. (2008). Regulating positive and negative emotions in daily life. *Journal of Personality, 76*(3), 561–580. [CrossRef] [PubMed]

Pan, T., Ding, X., Sang, B., Liu, Y., Xie, S., & Feng, X. (2015). Reliability and validity of positive and negative affective scale for children (PANAS-C). *Chinese Journal of Clinical Psychology, 23*, 397–400.

Podsakoff, P. M., Mackenzie, S. B., Lee, J. Y., & Podsakoff, N. P. (2003). Common method biases in behavioral research: A critical review of the literature and recommended remedies. *Journal of Applied Psychology, 88*, 879–903. [CrossRef]

Radloff, L. S. (1977). The CES-D scale: A self-depression scale for research in the general population. *Journal of Applied Psychological Measurement, 1*, 384–401. [CrossRef]

Ramos-Díaz, E., Rodríguez-Fernández, A., Axpe, I., & Ferrara, M. (2019). Perceived emotional intelligence and life satisfaction among adolescent students: The mediating role of resilience. *Journal of Happiness Studies*, *20*, 2489–2506. [CrossRef]

Rudolph, K. D., Troop-Gordon, W., Skymba, H. V., Modi, H. H., Ye, Z., Clapham, R. B., Dodson, J., Finnegan, M., & Heller, W. (2025). Cultivating emotional resilience in adolescent girls: Effects of a growth emotion mindset lesson. *Child Development*, *96*(1), 389–406. [CrossRef]

Sang, B., Deng, X., & Luan, Z. (2014). Which emotional regulatory strategy makes Chinese adolescents happier? a longitudinal study. *International Journal of Psychology*, *49*, 513–518. [CrossRef]

Santos, V., Paes, F., Pereira, V., Arias-Carrión, O., Silva, A. C., Carta, M. G., Nardi, A. E., & Machado, S. (2013). The role of positive emotion and contributions of positive psychology in depression treatment: Systematic review. *Clinical Practice and Epidemiology in Mental Health*, *9*, 221–237. [CrossRef]

Schutte, N. S., & Malouff, J. M. (2021). Basic psychological need satisfaction, affect and mental health. *Current Psychology*, *40*, 1228–1233. [CrossRef]

Seligman, M. (2018). PERMA and the building blocks of well-being. *Journal of Positive Psychology*, *13*, 1–3. [CrossRef]

Shapero, B. G., Farabaugh, A., Terechina, O., DeCross, S., Cheung, J. C., Fava, M., & Holt, D. J. (2019). Understanding the effects of emotional reactivity on depression and suicidal thoughts and behaviors: Moderating effects of childhood adversity and resilience. *Journal of Affective Disorder*, *245*, 419–427. [CrossRef] [PubMed]

Shek, D. T. (1993). The Chinese version of the State-Trait Anxiety Inventory: Its relationship to different measures of psychological well-being. *Journal of Clinical Psychology*, *49*, 349–358. [CrossRef]

Shi, W., Zhao, L., Liu, M., Hong, B., Jiang, L., & Jia, P. (2022). Resilience and mental health: A longitudinal cohort study of Chinese adolescents before and during COVID-19. *Frontiers in Psychiatry*, *13*, 948036. [CrossRef]

Sterina, E., Hermida, A. P., Gerberi, D. J., & Lapid, M. I. (2022). Emotional resilience of older adults during COVID-19: A systematic review of studies of stress and well-being. *Clinical Gerontologist*, *45*(1), 4–19. [CrossRef]

Tang, X., Tang, S., Ren, Z., & Wong, D. F. K. (2019). Prevalence of depressive symptoms among adolescents in secondary school in mainland China: A systematic review and meta-analysis. *Journal of Affective Disorders*, *245*, 498–507. [CrossRef]

Troy, A. S., & Mauss, I. B. (2011). Resilience in the face of stress: Emotion regulation as a protective factor. *Resilience and Mental Health: Challenges Across the Lifespan*, *1*, 30–44.

Tugade, M. M., & Fredrickson, B. L. (2004). Resilient individuals use positive emotions to bounce back from negative emotional experiences. *Journal of Personality and Social Psychology*, *86*(2), 320. [CrossRef]

Wang, Y., Xu, W., & Luo, F. (2016). Emotional resilience mediates the relationship between mindfulness and emotion. *Psychological Reports*, *118*, 725–736. [CrossRef]

Wang, Z., Lu, W., Du, J., & Wang, K. (2011). The relationship between positive emotion and mental health of college students: The mediating effect of personal resources. *Chinese Journal of Mental Health*, *25*, 521–527.

Ward, R. N., Brady, A. J., Jazdzewski, R., & Yalch, M. M. (2021). Stress, resilience, and coping. In *Emotion, well-being, and resilience* (pp. 3–14). Apple Academic Press.

Wu, Y., Sang, Z., Zhang, X., & Margraf, J. (2020). The relationship between resilience and mental health in Chinese college students: A longitudinal cross-lagged analysis. *Frontiers in Psychology*, *11*, 108. [CrossRef] [PubMed]

Wu, Y., Zuo, B., Wen, F., & Yan, L. (2017). Rosenberg self-esteem scale: Method effects, factorial structure and scale invariance across migrant child and urban child populations in China. *Journal of Personality Assessment*, *99*, 83–93. [CrossRef] [PubMed]

Xie, F., Xin, Z., Chen, X., & Zhang, L. (2019). Gender difference of Chinese high school students' math anxiety: The effects of self-esteem, test anxiety and general anxiety. *Sex Roles*, *81*, 235–244. [CrossRef]

Zhang, M., & Lu, J. (2010). Research report on the emotional resilience questionnaire for adolescents. *Journal of Psychological Science*, *33*, 24–27.

Zhou, Z., & Cheng, Q. (2022). Relationship between online social support and adolescents' mental health: A systematic review and meta-analysis. *Journal of Adolescence*, *94*, 281–292. [CrossRef]

Zhu, Y., Zhang, G., & Anme, T. (2023). Adverse childhood experiences, resilience, and emotional problems in young chinese children. *International Journal of Environmental Research and Public Health*, *20*(4), 3028. [CrossRef]

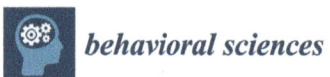

Article

The Relationship Between Mental Health Literacy and Social Well-Being: A Longitudinal Study in China

Jiali Pan [1,†], Tianyu Xu [2,†] and Dan Li [2,*]

[1] Mental Health Education and Counseling Center, Shanghai Business School, Shanghai 201400, China; panjl@sbs.edu.cn
[2] School of Psychology, Shanghai Normal University, Shanghai 200234, China; xuty_psy@163.com
* Correspondence: lidan@shnu.edu.cn
† These authors contributed equally to this work.

Abstract: In this study, 793 college students were examined through the utilization of the socioeconomic status scale, mental health literacy scale, and social well-being questionnaire at T1 and T2, respectively, with the aim of exploring the relationship between mental health literacy and social well-being and the relative static and dynamic development of the two. The results indicated that mental health literacy was significantly and positively correlated with social well-being to a moderate extent (T1: $r = 0.31$; T2: $r = 0.35$). Furthermore, the across-lagged model was employed to determine the relationship between mental health literacy and social well-being over time, revealing that mental health literacy and social well-being merely have a unidirectional predictive relationship; social well-being at T1 can significantly and positively predict mental health literacy at T2, but mental health literacy at T1 cannot predict social well-being at T2. We carried out the latent change score model and discovered that a higher level of T1 social well-being can facilitate the enhancement of mental health literacy subsequently.

Keywords: mental health literacy; social well-being; late adolescent; cross-lagged model; latent change score model

1. Introduction

Mental health literacy (MHL) is a multifaceted and evolving concept characterized by various definitions (Jorm, 2015; Jorm et al., 1997; Wei et al., 2015). Jorm and his colleagues, who were the pioneers in introducing the notion of MHL, defined it as "knowledge and beliefs about mental disorders which aid their recognition, management or prevention" (Jorm et al., 1997). For an extended period, researchers have mainly concentrated on the prevention and intervention of mental disorders rather than on promoting well-being and personal development (Jorm, 2000; Jorm, 2012). There is an increasing consensus among scholars that mental health literacy encompasses individuals' knowledge, beliefs, and behaviors related to mental disorders, including an understanding of how to achieve and maintain positive mental health, a comprehensive awareness of mental disorders and their treatments, efforts to reduce the stigma associated with these conditions, as well as strategies for enhancing self-help and supporting others (Bjornsen et al., 2017; Kutcher et al., 2015, 2016). Most of the existing MHL measures adopt self-reported evaluations of a single dimension, such as a person's beliefs or knowledge regarding depression (Gabriel & Violato, 2010; Wang et al., 2013). Spiker and Hammer (2019) contend that MHL ought to be multiconstruct rather than single-dimensional. This contention is upheld by Jiang's team, which not only incorporates mental illness and health promotion but also considers two dimensions of self-seeking

https://doi.org/10.3390/bs15010029

help and assisting others, and can enhance individuals' mental health literacy from three aspects: knowledge, attitude, and behavior (Jiang et al., 2020).

As a critical component of health literacy, it is essential for enhancing both individual and population health outcomes (Kajawu et al., 2016; Zhong et al., 2024). Previous investigations have demonstrated that low mental health literacy is correlated with adverse mental health conditions, such as depression and anxiety (Jacka et al., 2017; Tambling et al., 2023), stress (Tambling et al., 2023), internalized stigma (Tambling et al., 2023), suboptimal sleep quality (Jacka et al., 2017), and unhealthy lifestyles (Tambling et al., 2023). However, there are also studies indicating that individuals diagnosed with specific mental health disorders exhibit higher levels of MHL (BinDhim et al., 2023; O'Connor & Casey, 2015; Zeng et al., 2023). This might imply that people with mental illnesses are more prone to seek information on the subject, which promotes positive health behaviors and subsequently leads to enhancements in MHL. Brijnath et al. (2016) carried out a meta-analysis of 14 intervention investigations concerning MHL from 2000 to 2015 and discovered that enhancing MHL ameliorates mental health outcomes. For major mental illnesses, it is widely acknowledged that increasing public awareness of preventive measures, early intervention strategies, and treatment options can significantly benefit individuals (Jafari et al., 2021; Ming & Chen, 2020). Elevated levels of mental health literacy empower individuals to recognize mental illness at an early stage, reduce the stigma surrounding mental disorders, and facilitate access to timely and effective support and treatment, thereby enhancing their overall mental health and quality of life (Jafari et al., 2021; Ming & Chen, 2020; Morales-Torres et al., 2023; Tang et al., 2024). It is evident that mental health literacy is closely associated with mental health.

As one of the indicators closely related to mental health, well-being has garnered the attention of numerous researchers. Concurrent with the progress of well-being theory and empirical research, the conceptual orientation of well-being manifests two principal viewpoints. The prevailing perspective on hedonism suggests that well-being encompasses the pursuit of pleasure or the acknowledgment of distressing encounters (Kahneman et al., 1999); eudaimonism reflects the perspective that well-being encompasses not only being happy but also realizing human potential (Waterman, 1993). Thus, from the eudaimonic perspective, subjective well-being cannot be equated with well-being (Diener, 2009; Ryan & Deci, 2001). Prior research on well-being has predominantly concentrated on individual-level factors, such as subjective well-being and physical health, while neglecting social-level determinants, including social adjustment and social support (Larson, 1993). Mental well-being is increasingly regarded as comprising happiness, contentment, subjective well-being, self-realization, and positive functioning (Ryan & Deci, 2001). In fact, well-being is not merely manifested in terms of satisfaction with relationships, family life, employment, health, and finances, but also in terms of the connections with various aspects of the environment (Moser, 2009). In 1947, the World Health Organization established a conceptual link between mental health and social health, and defined health as a state of complete physical, mental, and social well-being. Since then, a growing body of research has focused on social well-being, with most scholars believing that social health and social well-being are synonymous (Diener, 2009). Keyes (1998) defined social well-being as individuals' appraisal of their present social circumstances and their social functions, which reflects the significance or value of the realization of personal skills for others or society, as well as whether social skills are in a propitious state. According to Keyes, social well-being includes five aspects: social integration, social actualization, social contribution, social acceptance, and social coherence (Keyes, 1998). Keyes further maintains that well-being represents a comprehensive state of individual psychological experience and the integration of emotional well-being, psychological well-being, and social well-being, which are interrelated yet independent (Keyes, 2005, 2007; Ryff & Keyes, 1995). These three types of indicators of mental health, respectively, mirror the individual's evaluation of their own quality of life in three aspects, namely, their sense of a good life, proper self-functioning, and sound social functioning (Keyes, 2003, 2007). Through confirmatory factor analysis, it is revealed that the goodness of fit of the three-factor model of emotional well-being, psychological well-being, and social well-being is significantly higher than that of the single-factor and two-factor models (Gallagher et al., 2009). To sum up, well-being encompasses three dimensions that possess certain correlation and independence: emotional well-being, psychological well-being, and social well-being. A considerable number of studies contend that positive mental health literacy is positively associated with subjective well-being, and positive mental health literacy can positively predict subjective well-being (Bjornsen et al., 2019; Mahmoodi et al., 2023; Nalipay et al., 2024). Previous research has mostly approached the relationship between mental health literacy and well-being from an individual perspective. However, as members of social groups, individuals are influenced by interactions with others and the social environment, which in turn affects their self-assessment of their environment and social functions. This well-being, which places emphasis on sociality, is equally important for individual development. However, limited knowledge is available regarding the associations between mental health literacy and social well-being (de Carvalho et al., 2022). The relationship between mental health literacy and social well-being is still unclear.

Some researchers assert at the theoretical level that mental health literacy could be one of the significant related factors influencing social well-being. Firstly, the ecological systems theory elucidates the promotional impact of mental health literacy on social well-being (Bronfenbrenner, 1979). This theory highlights the dynamic interaction between individuals and the environment, and posits that people's psychology and behavior are the outcomes of the interaction with their environmental system. This environmental system encompasses multiple levels, ranging from the micro individual environment to the macro social and cultural environment, which jointly affect individual psychological development and well-being. Individuals with higher mental health literacy are capable of coping more effectively with challenges and pressures in life (Winding et al., 2023), maintaining a positive attitude and emotional state, making better utilization of social support resources, establishing positive interpersonal relationships, enhancing their social competence, and having positive social ties, thereby augmenting social well-being. Secondly, the theory of positive psychology (Seligman & Csikszentmihalyi, 2000) also discloses the facilitating effect of mental health literacy on social well-being. This theory emphasizes the significance of positive emotions and coping styles for individual mental health and well-being. Individuals with high mental health literacy are better equipped to identify, express, and regulate their emotions, and adopt positive behavioral strategies, such as seeking social support and participating in community activities (Cicognani et al., 2008; Son & Wilson, 2012). Individuals experience more positive emotions in daily life, which enhances the connections and activities between individuals and others and the community, thus enhancing social well-being. Based on the foregoing theories, we hypothesize that mental health literacy exerts a positive predictive effect on social well-being.

On the other hand, social well-being may also be predictive of mental health literacy. The cognitive behavioral theory contends that an individual's emotions, behaviors, and responses are shaped by their cognitive processes, such as thinking, beliefs, and assumptions. When individuals experience a higher level of social well-being, they are more inclined to hold positive cognitive appraisals of the social environment (e.g., the society is improving, I have made my own contribution to the development of the society, people are willing to assist others, etc.), establish healthier thinking patterns and behavioral habits, and thereby fulfill interpersonal functions optimistically and confidently (Baldwin et al., 2020). This positive cognitive and behavioral pattern contributes to further enhancing individuals' mental health literacy and makes them more disposed to seek help when they encounter mental health problems. Similarly, the ecological systems theory and the theory of positive psychology also uphold this perspective, believing that the well-being individuals experience in the social environment will have a positive influence on their mental health literacy. A social environment replete with support, understanding, and acceptance can assist individuals in forming positive self-cognition and self-efficacy, thereby improving their mental health literacy level. Based on the above reason, we propose a hypothesis that social well-being has a positive predictive effect on mental health literacy.

In current study, firstly, we used an integrated multidimensional concept of mental health literacy, including self–others, mental health–mental disorders, and knowledge–attitude–behavior, to explore the correlation between mental health literacy and social well-being in the Chinese college students' group. Secondly, cross-lagged analysis was used to explore the prediction direction of mental health literacy and social well-being from the static level. Lastly, a latent change score model was used to further verify the relationship between the two variables, and the interactive relationship between the rate of change of mental health literacy and social well-being was explored at the dynamic level. This study aimed to deepen our comprehension of the relationship between mental health literacy and social well-being, illuminating the potential effects and implications of mental health literacy.

2. Method

2.1. Participants

The G*power software (Version 3.1.9.7) was utilized in this study to conduct a power analysis and calculate the necessary sample size. We aimed for a power of 0.95 and set the α level at 0.05 with an expected effect size of 0.15 (Faul et al., 2007). G*Power eventually determined a total sample size of 107 participants, which provided acceptable statistical power. The final sample size of the study was determined after accounting for potential attrition or missing data during data collection.

The study was carried out with 795 participants from a business college in Shanghai, China, at the T1 time point, which was in the early fall semester. The second test was conducted four months later. Both tests were executed in the form of coursework, and students received corresponding credits. However, due to illness, absence, etc., two participants did not participate in the T2 time point test. After excluding these participants without T2 data, 793 participants were included in the study. The age range of participants at T1 time point was 17–31 ($M = 19.23$, $SD = 0.76$). Among these participants, there were 507 female (63.9%), 285 male; 448 participants were single children (43.5%), 345 participants were non-single children; 621 participants were from urban areas (78.3%), 172 participants were from rural areas.

2.2. Measures

2.2.1. Social Economic Status

The Social Economic Status Scale (SES) included three indicators of parental occupation type, parental education level, and income, with a total of 5 items (Jiang et al., 2021). Among these, the occupation type was divided into 11 categories, the education level into 4 categories, and the income into 6 categories based on the results of the 2022 China's National Economic and Social Development Statistical Bulletin. In this study, SES score was obtained by converting three indicators of parental occupation type, parental education level, and income into rank variables and using factor analysis to carry out weighted transformation. The specific approach was as follows: Firstly, the average values of parental occupation type and parental education level were calculated, respectively. Then, the 10 levels of occupation type (excluding school students) were assigned scores of 1–10 in ascending order of points from low to high. The 4 levels of education were assigned 1–4 points from in the same manner, and the 6 levels of per capita disposable annual income of families were assigned 1–6 points from low to high. Then, the three indexes were converted into standard scores, and principal component analysis was carried out to obtain a principal factor with characteristic root greater than 1, which explained 66.29% of the variance. Finally, using the load coefficients of the three indexes on the principal factors, the calculation formula of SES was made as follows: $SES = (0.856 \times Z_{occupation\ type} + 0.843 \times Z_{education\ level} + 0.738 \times Z_{income})/1.989$. Among them, 0.856, 0.843, and 0.738 were the factor loads of the three factor indexes, respectively, and 1.989 was the characteristic root of the first factor. The higher the SES score, the higher the socioeconomic status.

2.2.2. Mental Health Literacy

Mental health literacy was measured using the Mental Health Literacy Questionnaire (MHLQ) developed by Wu et al. (Wu et al., 2023). This 60-item scale consists of six dimensions: mental illness knowledge (e.g., "People who have good relationships with others do not have mental illness"), mental health knowledge (e.g., "One's mental health state is stable and unchanging"), attitudes towards mental illness (e.g., "Mental illness is a minor problem, and we don't need pay too much attention to it"), attitudes towards mental health (e.g., "I think my mental health is the most important"), behaviors to cope with mental illness (e.g., "When I feel down or lack energy and this doesn't get better for some time, I'll seek professional help"), and behaviors to maintain mental health (e.g., "I know how to find information and knowledge about mental health"). Thirty true/false/don't know items assessed MHL knowledge, of which "True" responses were coded as 1 and other responses were coded as 0. It was scored using a 5-point Likert scale (1 = strongly disagree, 5 = strongly agree) to assess MHL attitude and behavior—the two options in the same correct direction as the score were coded as 1, and the other options were coded as 0. The MHL score is the sum of the values of all items. A higher total score indicates a greater level of mental health literacy. The Cronbach's α coefficient of the scale in this study at two time points were 0.85 and 0.91, respectively.

2.2.3. Social Well-Being

The Social Well-being Scale was employed to measure the participants' level of social well-being (Miao & Wang, 2009), which was revised by Miao and Wang to be suitable for Chinese (Keyes & Shapiro, 2003). This scale comprises 15 items and consists of five dimensions (e.g., "The community I belong to makes me feel good"), including social acceptance, social actualization, social contribution, social coherence, and social integration. The 5-point Likert scoring method was adopted in this scale, and the total score is calculated by summing all items. The higher total score indicates the higher level of social well-being. The Cronbach's α coefficients at two time points in current study were 0.89 and 0.93, respectively.

2.3. Statistical Analyses

The data were statistically analyzed by SPSS 20.0, Mplus 8.3, and R 4.4.1 software. Firstly, SPSS 20.0 was used for data collection, descriptive statistical analysis, correlation analysis, and the common method deviation test. Secondly, Mplus 8.3 was used to construct a cross-lagged model to test the model fit, exploring how a variable affects itself and other variables over time. Finally, we further investigated the relationship between the rate of change among variables and built a bivariate latent change score model through R 4.4.1 software to explore the impact of the initial state of a variable on the subsequent development rate of itself or other variables at a dynamic level (Kievit et al., 2018).

3. Result

3.1. The Common Method Deviation Test

The data in this study were based on self-reported questionnaires, which may lead to common method bias. In the process of testing, the anonymity and confidentiality of data were emphasized to control the common source of method deviation. In addition, the result of Harman's single-factor test showed that there were 23 factors at T1 and 17 factors at T2 with eigenvalues greater than 1, respectively. The total variance explained by the first factor was 13.08% and 18.75%, which was below the critical value of 40% (Podsakoff et al., 2003), indicating that there was no severe common method bias in this study.

3.2. Descriptive and Correlation Analysis

The results of descriptive statistics and correlation analysis are shown in Table 1. The mean scores of mental health literacy and social well-being across the two time points (T1 and T2) ranged from 39.11 to 40.60 and from 51.61 to 54.61, respectively. Correlation analysis of the measured variables in the two time points (T1 and T2) manifested that T1 was significantly positively correlated with T2 both in mental health literacy ($r = 0.58$, $p < 0.05$) and in social well-being ($r = 0.64$, $p < 0.05$). At both time points, mental health literacy and social well-being were significantly positively correlated with each other ($r = 0.31$, $p < 0.05$; $r = 0.35$, $p < 0.05$). Mental health literacy at two time points was significantly negatively associated with gender (T1: $r = -0.17$, $p < 0.05$; T2: $r = -0.23$, $p < 0.05$), and significantly positively associated with single children (T1: $r = 0.08$, $p < 0.05$; T2: $r = 0.08$, $p < 0.05$) and SES (T1: $r = 0.08$, $p < 0.05$; T2: $r = 0.08$, $p < 0.05$). In addition, at any point in time, social well-being was not significantly related to gender, single children, or SES.

Table 1. Descriptive and correlation analysis of all variables.

	M ± SD	**1**	**2**	**3**	**4**	**5**	**6**	**7**
1. T1 MHL	39.11 ± 8.10	-						
2. T1 SW	51.61 ± 10.02	0.31 **	-					
3. T2 MHL	40.60 ± 10.15	0.58 **	0.27 **	-				
4. T2 SW	54.61 ± 11.25	0.25 **	0.64 **	0.35 **	-			
5. Gender	-	−0.17 **	0.02	−0.23 **	−0.01	-		
6. SC	-	0.08 *	−0.04	0.08 *	0.02	0.002	-	
7. SES	-	0.08 *	0.01	0.08 *	0.06	−0.06	0.43 **	-

Note. $N = 793$. * $p < 0.05$, ** $p < 0.01$. Gender is a dummy variable; female = 0, male = 1. SC = single children; SC is a dummy variable: non-single children = 0, single children = 1. SES = social economic status. MHL = mental health literacy. SW = social well-being.

3.3. Longitudinal Cross-Lagged Model Analysis

As shown in Figure 1, a cross-lagged model was used to determine the relationship between mental health literacy and social well-being over time. Controlling for gender, single children, and SES, the model fit of the cross-lagged model had an acceptable fit to the data ($\chi^2/df = 38.31/6$, CFI = 0.94, TLI = 0.89, RMSEA = 0.08, SRMR = 0.05). Cross-lagged paths indicated that all variables at T1 could predict themselves at T2. To be specific, the level of initial mental health literacy could significantly predict the level of subsequent mental health literacy ($\beta = 0.52$, $p < 0.05$), and the level of initial social well-being could significantly predict the level of subsequent social well-being ($\beta = 0.62$, $p < 0.05$). In addition, the results indicated that one variable at T1 can predict another variable at T2.

Social well-being at T1 could significantly and positively predict mental health literacy at T2 ($\beta = 0.12$, $p < 0.05$). However, mental health literacy at T1 could not significantly predict social well-being at T2 ($\beta = 0.05$, $p > 0.05$).

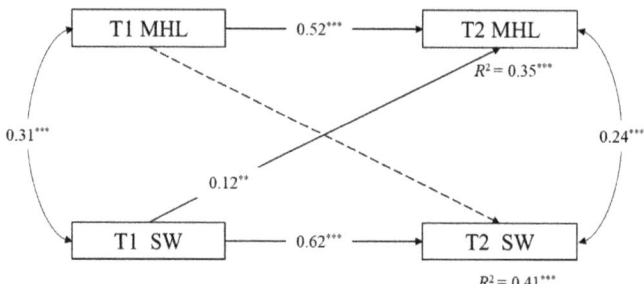

Figure 1. Cross-lagged model. Note. ** $p < 0.01$, *** $p < 0.001$. MHL = mental health literacy. SW = social well-being. Nonsignificant paths are represented by dotted lines. The paths from the covariates gender, single children, and SES are not presented for reasons of clarity. All path coefficients are standardized.

3.4. Latent Change Score Model Analysis

The latent change score model of the relationship between mental health literacy and social well-being is presented in Figure 2. The data obtained a saturated model. The results of self-feedback effect demonstrated that prior levels of mental health literacy could significantly and negatively predict subsequent changes in mental health literacy ($\beta = -0.30$, $p < 0.05$), indicating an overall slowing of growth over time. That is, compared with individuals with a high level of mental health literacy, individuals with a low level of mental health literacy would increase their mental health literacy ability faster in the future. A similar pattern was found for social well-being ($\beta = -0.34$, $p < 0.05$). The results of the cross-domain coupling effect demonstrated that prior levels of social well-being could significantly and positively predict subsequent changes in mental health literacy ($\gamma = 0.12$, $p < 0.05$), indicating that higher levels of social well-being in the previous time point (T1) could facilitate the rate of growth change in mental health literacy. However, the prior levels of mental health literacy could not predict subsequent changes in social well-being ($\gamma = 0.07$, $p > 0.05$). The above results showed that social well-being is a leading variable in the developmental process.

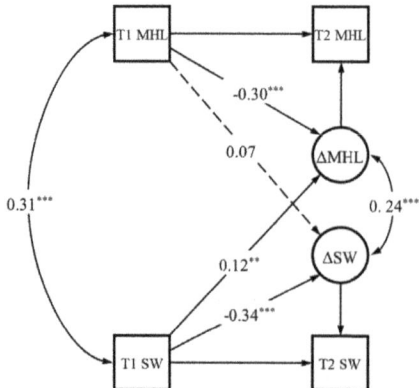

Figure 2. Latent change score model. Note. ** $p < 0.01$, *** $p < 0.001$. MHL = mental health literacy. SW = social well-being. All path coefficients of solid line are standardized, except for unlabeled paths that are constrained to 1. Nonsignificant paths are represented by dotted lines.

4. Discussion

The aim of this study was to investigate the relationship between mental health literacy and social well-being in college students (i.e., early adulthood) and to examine the predicted directivity of relative static and dynamic development changes between the two.

The social well-being and mental health literacy of young adults in China were evaluated in this study, and both scores were higher than half of the total, demonstrating that they are at medium to high levels. Our results found that there was a significant positive correlation between social economic status and mental health literacy; that is, individuals with higher socioeconomic status have higher levels of mental health literacy, which is consistent with the findings of Jiang et al. (Jiang et al., 2021). As China's social and economic development proceeds, people's priorities move from basic material requirements to psychological health demands, resulting in an increased focus on mental health. As a result, as social and economic conditions have improved, so too has mental health literacy. When controlling for age and gender, research shows that socioeconomic disadvantage is strongly related with depression symptoms in early adulthood, implying that higher income levels predict fewer depressed symptoms (Ferschmann et al., 2024). This corresponds to our research findings. It is clear that social and economic development levels can influence individuals' motivations for psychological health needs, hence improving mental health. Meanwhile, the advancement of many parts of society fosters individuals' social relationships and improves social well-being.

In addition, the results of this study show that gender is significantly related to mental health literacy, as shown by females having higher levels of mental health literacy. This result further supports the view of previous studies (Holzinger et al., 2012; Jiang et al., 2021; Tay et al., 2018). A systematic review found gender differences in mental health literacy (Holzinger et al., 2012). On the one hand, for themselves, females were more likely to seek informal and formal help (family, doctors, psychological counselors, etc.) (Furnham et al., 2014) and had a higher propensity to seek help (Tay et al., 2018). On the other hand, females were more likely to recommend professional help for other people (Coles et al., 2016; Holzinger et al., 2012). Mental health literacy is not only the individual's understanding of mental health knowledge, but also includes the knowledge learning, attitude internalization, and behavior performance of their own and others' mental health or disease (Jiang et al., 2021; Wu et al., 2023). Compared with males, females tended to be more accommodating, more helpful, more agreeable, and had more prosocial behavior (Holzinger et al., 2012; Kuhnert et al., 2017). These characteristics make females, while focusing on themselves, often hopeful of improving their mental health literacy by increasing their knowledge of mental health and disease prevention (knowledge level), having a greater willingness to help people around them (such as family, friends, and even strangers) (attitude level), and then adopting corresponding behavioral strategies conducive to mental health (behavior level).

The results in this study indicated that single children had higher levels of mental health literacy. Although there were few studies exploring the mental health literacy of single children, numerous studies have shown that single children are able to receive more family attention (Chen & Zhou, 2019; Liu & Jiang, 2021). Due to the influence of traditional Chinese culture, the single children in China are often favored by parents and grandparents, and have more educational resources, family support, and material foundation. A study of junior high school students in China found that single children tended to have closer relationships with their parents than children from multiple-child families (Liu & Jiang, 2021), and that parents were more concerned about their children's physical and mental health (Chen & Zhou, 2019). This positive family relationship can effectively promote parent–child communication and imperceptibly pass on parents' knowledge, attitude, and behavior of mental health to their children.

Is mental health literacy related to social well-being? The results of this study found that mental health literacy was significantly positively correlated with social well-being to a moderate degree (T1: $r = 0.31$; T2: $r = 0.35$), which is consistent with previous studies (Bjornsen et al., 2019; de Carvalho et al., 2022; Gorczynski et al., 2020; Mahmoodi et al., 2023; Nalipay et al., 2024; Zhang et al., 2023). A study of young and middle-aged people found that individuals with a high level of mental health literacy tended to have higher levels of well-being (Zhang et al., 2023). Similar results were found in the study of 15–21-year-old adolescents, with a significantly positive correlation between mental health literacy and well-being (Bjornsen et al., 2019). It is worth noting that in previous studies, there was only a weak positive correlation between mental health literacy and well-being (Bjornsen et al., 2019; Mahmoodi et al., 2023; Nalipay et al., 2024), or even no significant correlation (Hamzah et al., 2023). The reason may be that these researchers mostly used subjective well-being or psychological well-being (Gorczynski et al., 2020; Mahmoodi et al., 2023), which emphasize individual emotional experience and psychological function, respectively, and reflect the personal characteristics of well-being (Ye et al., 2023). As a social characteristic, social well-being refers to an individual's self-assessment of the quality of their relationships with others, the collective, and society, as well as their living environment and social function (Keyes, 1998). As individuals, we are part of society and cannot function without social connection. Individuals are closely connected with themselves, others, and their environment, and they evaluate their quality of life and personal functioning based on social standards. Mental health literacy refers to the knowledge, attitudes, and behavioral habits developed to promote mental health and cope with mental disorders. It encompasses not only aspects related to oneself but also those related to others (Jiang et al., 2021; Wu et al., 2023). This means that an individual's mental health literacy is not isolated; it is influenced by external factors and, in turn, affects the external environment or others, also possessing social characteristics. Therefore, compared with subjective well-being and psychological well-being, social well-being has a stronger correlation with mental health literacy. Our results confirm that social well-being, subjective well-being, and psychological well-being are distinct components of well-being, sharing commonalities as well as unique aspects (Gallagher et al., 2009). There are varying degrees of correlation between mental health literacy and different subtypes of well-being.

Mental health literacy and social well-being are merely a unidirectional predictive relationship. Our longitudinal cross-lagged study results found that social well-being at T1 can significantly positively predict mental health literacy at T2, but mental health literacy at T1 cannot predict social well-being at T2. This differs from previous cross-sectional study results (Bjornsen et al., 2019; Nalipay et al., 2024). Nalipay and other researchers explored the impact of positive mental health literacy on well-being, and they found that positive mental health literacy can positively predict well-being (Nalipay et al., 2024). Positive mental health literacy mainly focuses on how individuals can acquire and maintain mental health (Carvalho et al., 2022), while neglecting the aspect of coping with mental disorders. But, as Keyes' dual-factor model of mental health suggests, mental health and mental disorder are not a one-dimensional, bipolar potential unity. Mental disorder and mental health do not lie at the ends of this continuum, respectively, but, rather, are two potential continuums (Keyes, 1998). The elimination of mental disorder does not mean the presence of mental health; neither the disease model nor the health model can independently describe the mental health of a population. Mental health and mental disorder are a combined assessment system. When the aspect of addressing mental disorder is integrated into mental health literacy, this excessive focus on mental disorder can trigger negative emotions such as anxiety and depression in individuals, thereby reducing their sense of well-being (Malone & Wachholtz, 2018). Previous studies have focused more on positive aspects of mental health literacy (Bjornsen et al., 2019; de Carvalho et al., 2022; Nalipay et al., 2024). When adopting this mental health literacy that integrates mental health with mental disorders, the effect of individual attention to mental health in promoting increased well-being is, thus, offset; therefore, mental health literacy cannot predict subsequent social well-being. In addition, highly sensitive personality traits may also affect the relationship between mental health literacy and social well-being. The Intense World Theory posits that some individuals have intense and excessive perceptions, attention, memory, and emotional responses to environmental information, and integration deficits further lead to various social withdrawal issues (Markram & Markram, 2010). Some studies have found that highly sensitive personalities often positively predict individuals' internalizing problems (Burgard et al., 2022), and they are more likely to experience anxiety (Dosari et al., 2023). Compared to normal individuals, when these individuals are exposed to an environment with high mental health literacy, their own highly sensitive personality traits make them overly sensitive to mental disorders, resulting in more anxiety, depression, and other negative emotions. This, in turn, affects their social interactions, leading to social withdrawal, decreased satisfaction, and, ultimately, a decline in their sense of social well-being. The diversity of these personality traits may also be one of the reasons why mental health literacy cannot directly predict social well-being.

The cross-lagged model analysis showed results that were different from previous studies, finding that social well-being can predict subsequent mental health literacy. Keyes proposed in 1998 that social well-being has five dimensions, including social integration, social acceptance, social contribution, social actualization, and social coherence (Keyes, 1998). Social integration refers to individuals having a sense of belonging and being able to receive comfort and support from society. Healthy individuals feel like a part of society, and this sense of integration makes them feel a commonality with others who make up society. Therefore, individuals with a good sense of social well-being not only pay attention to their own mental health and mental disorders but also to the mental health and mental disorders of others, thereby having better mental health literacy. Individuals with high social well-being also tend to have stronger social acceptance. These individuals often perceive others as benevolent, have better relationships with others, possess higher levels of mental health literacy, and have a greater willingness to seek help (for themselves) and offer help (to others). Social contribution reflects an individual's recognition of their social value, while also being acknowledged or valued by society and others. This recognition further promotes the development of the individual's social actualization, making them believe that people, collectives, and society have the potential to develop and grow positively. This sense of self-efficacy regarding the positive aspects of society inspires individuals to strive to improve their own mental health literacy and also enhances their desire for society and others to have mental health as well. Thus, while maintaining one's own mental health and addressing personal mental disorder, one should not forget to pay attention to these aspects in others and attempt to help them. Individuals with good social harmony are often interested in life, can find meaning in social life, and have a certain degree of understanding. We experience countless life events every day, some positive and some negative, some predictable and some unpredictable, some involving others and some involving ourselves. This requires individuals to coordinate various aspects well to achieve a degree of harmony (Miao & Zhao, 2009). The concept of mental health literacy aligns with this viewpoint, encompassing the maintenance of mental health (positive aspect) and the coping with mental disorder (negative aspect), self and others, knowledge, attitude, and behavior. Individuals with high social well-being can accept and pay attention to both the positive and negative aspects of things, respond actively to achieve harmony, and possess higher mental health literacy. It can be seen that social well-being can affect the positive development of individual mental health literacy.

The latent change score model reaffirms the conclusions of the cross-lagged model analysis from a dynamic change perspective. First, the higher the initial level of mental health literacy, the slower its subsequent rate of change. Social well-being exhibits the same developmental pattern. Second, only the initial level of social well-being can positively predict the subsequent changes in mental health literacy, meaning that a high level of social well-being can promote the rapid improvement of mental health literacy. Individuals with high social well-being have a better self-concept, self-esteem, and self-acceptance, are more satisfied with their personal lives, and hold a more optimistic attitude towards the future and society (Lluch-Canut et al., 2013). An individual's positive inclination towards society, as well as their acceptance of others and different social characteristics, can encourage them to be willing to understand mental health knowledge, help others cope with mental disorder, and engage in corresponding positive behaviors. Therefore, individuals with high social well-being often experience a faster growth rate in their mental health literacy (Carvalho et al., 2022).

5. Limitations and Future Directions

First, the participants in this study were recruited from a business college in Shanghai, China, with a higher proportion of female students. Social culture, sampling range, and gender ratio may all affect the generalizability of the results. In the future, it is necessary to balance the gender ratio and expand the sampling range to include multiple regions, schools, and age groups to enhance the representability of the results and increase external validity. Furthermore, future research could compare the relationship between mental health literacy and social well-being across different cultural groups to explore whether the conclusions are cross-culturally consistent.

Second, this study only measured two time points, making it difficult to observe more subtle developmental changes in individuals' mental health literacy and social well-being. Future research could further extend the interval and number of test points to explore the developmental changes in the relationship between mental health literacy and social well-being over time.

Third, although there is a unidirectional relationship between mental health literacy and social well-being, the mechanisms of their development are still unclear. Further exploration can be conducted on the roles of other variables in this relationship and the mediating mechanisms involved.

6. Conclusions

Our research expands on the relationship between mental health literacy and well-being, finding a moderate and significant positive correlation between mental health literacy and social well-being. Cross-lagged model analysis shows that mental health literacy at T1 can significantly and positively predict its own level at T2, and social well-being at T1 can similarly and significantly predict its own level at T2. Social well-being at T1 can positively predict mental health literacy at T2, meaning that higher social well-being is associated with higher mental health literacy. But mental health literacy at T1 cannot predict social well-being at T2. The latent change score model analysis shows that the self-feedback effect of mental health literacy is significant, meaning that the higher the initial level of mental health literacy, the smaller the subsequent development changes in mental health literacy. Social well-being exhibits the same pattern of self-feedback effect. Mental health literacy and social well-being only exhibit a unidirectional cross-domain coupling effect. Merely, the initial level of social well-being can positively predict the subsequent development changes in mental health literacy, implying that the higher the initial level of social well-being, the faster the growth rate of mental health literacy. This indicates that social well-being is the leading variable between the two.

Author Contributions: Conceptualization, J.P. and T.X.; methodology, T.X.; software, T.X.; validation, J.P., T.X. and D.L.; formal analysis, T.X.; investigation, J.P.; resources, J.P.; data curation, J.P.; writing—original draft preparation, J.P. and T.X.; writing—review and editing, D.L.; visualization, T.X.; supervision, D.L.; project administration, D.L.; funding acquisition, J.P. All authors have read and agreed to the published version of the manuscript.

Funding: The work was funded by the Shanghai Committee of the Chinese Communist Youth League (Project No. 2024QYKTLX17-7), the Youth League Committee of Shanghai Business School (Project No. QN202404), the Academic Affairs Office of Shanghai Business School (Project No. SBS-2024-XJKCSZ-19), and the Student Affairs Office of Shanghai Business School (Project No. AG24-13006-1301).

Institutional Review Board Statement: The study was conducted in accordance with the Declaration of Helsinki, and approved by the Human Participants Ethics Committee of Shanghai Normal University (protocol code: Shanghai Normal University Ethics [2023] No. 062; date of approval: 9 November 2023).

Informed Consent Statement: Informed consent was obtained from all subjects involved in the study.

Data Availability Statement: The data presented in this study are available on request from the corresponding author (the data are not publicly available due to privacy or ethical restrictions).

Conflicts of Interest: The authors declare no conflicts of interest.

References

Baldwin, C., Vincent, P., Anderson, J., & Rawstorne, P. (2020). Measuring well-being: Trial of the neighbourhood thriving scale for social well-being among pro-social individuals. *International Journal of Community Well-Being*, *3*(3), 361–390. [CrossRef]

BinDhim, N. F., Althumiri, N. A., Ad-Dab'bagh, Y., Alqahtani, M. M. J., Alshayea, A. K., Al-Luhaidan, S. M., Svendrovski, A., Al-Duraihem, R. A., & Alhabeeb, A. A. (2023). Validation and psychometric testing of the Arabic version of the mental health literacy scale among the Saudi Arabian general population. *International Journal of Mental Health Systems*, *17*(1), 42. [CrossRef] [PubMed]

Bjornsen, H. N., Eilertsen, M.-E. B., Ringdal, R., Espnes, G. A., & Moksnes, U. K. (2017). Positive mental health literacy: Development and validation of a measure among Norwegian adolescents. *BMC Public Health*, *17*, 717. [CrossRef] [PubMed]

Bjornsen, H. N., Espnes, G. A., Eilertsen, M.-E. B., Ringdal, R., & Moksnes, U. K. (2019). The relationship between positive mental health literacy and mental well-being among adolescents: Implications for school health services. *Journal of School Nursing*, *35*(2), 107–116. [CrossRef] [PubMed]

Brijnath, B., Protheroe, J., Mahtani, K. R., & Antoniades, J. (2016). Do web-based mental health literacy interventions improve the mental health literacy of adult consumers? Results from a systematic review. *Journal of Medical Internet Research*, *18*(6), e165. [CrossRef]

Bronfenbrenner, U. (1979). *The ecology of human development: Experiments by nature and design* (Vol. 2). Harvard University Press.

Burgard, S. S. C., Liber, J. M., Geurts, S. M., & Koning, I. M. (2022). Youth sensitivity in a pandemic: The relationship between sensory processing sensitivity, internalizing problems, COVID-19 and parenting. *Journal of Child and Family Studies*, *31*(6), 1501–1510. [CrossRef]

Carvalho, D., Sequeira, C., Querido, A., Tomas, C., Morgado, T., Valentim, O., Moutinho, L., Gomes, J., & Laranjeira, C. (2022). Positive mental health literacy: A concept analysis. *Frontiers in Psychology*, *13*, 877611. [CrossRef] [PubMed]

Chen, B.-B., & Zhou, N. (2019). The weight status of only children in China: The role of marital satisfaction and maternal warmth. *Journal of Child and Family Studies*, *28*(10), 2754–2761. [CrossRef]

Cicognani, E., Pirini, C., Keyes, C., Joshanloo, M., Rostami, R., & Nosratabadi, M. (2008). Social participation, sense of community and social well being: A study on American, Italian and Iranian University students. *Social Indicators Research*, *89*(1), 97–112. [CrossRef]

Coles, M. E., Ravid, A., Gibb, B., George-Denn, D., Bronstein, L. R., & McLeod, S. (2016). Adolescent mental health literacy: Young people's knowledge of depression and social anxiety disorder. *Journal of Adolescent Health*, *58*(1), 57–62. [CrossRef]

de Carvalho, M. M., da Luz Vale-Dias, M., Keyes, C., & Carvalho, S. A. (2022). The positive mental health literacy questionnaire-PosMHLit. *Mediterranean Journal of Clinical Psychology*, *10*(2), 2022. [CrossRef]

Diener, E. (2009). *The science of well-being*. Springer.

Dosari, M., Aldayel, S. K., Alduraibi, K. M., Alturki, A. A., Aljehaiman, F., Alamri, S., Alshammari, H. S., & Alsuwailem, M. (2023). Prevalence of highly sensitive personality and its relationship with depression, and anxiety in the Saudi general population. *Cureus Journal of Medical Science*, *15*(12), e49834. [CrossRef] [PubMed]

Faul, F., Erdfelder, E., Lang, A.-G., & Buchner, A. (2007). G*Power 3: A flexible statistical power analysis program for the social, behavioral, and biomedical sciences. *Behavior Research Methods*, *39*(2), 175–191. [CrossRef] [PubMed]

Ferschmann, L., Grydeland, H., MacSweeney, N., Beck, D., Bos, M. G. N., Norbom, L. B., Eira Aksnes, R., Bekkhus, M., Havdahl, A., Crone, E. A., von Soest, T., & Tamnes, C. K. (2024). The importance of timing of socioeconomic disadvantage throughout development for depressive symptoms and brain structure. *Developmental Cognitive Neuroscience*, *69*, 101449. [CrossRef] [PubMed]

Furnham, A., Annis, J., & Cleridou, K. (2014). Gender differences in the mental health literacy of young people. *International Journal of Adolescent Medicine and Health*, *26*(2), 283–292. [CrossRef]

Gabriel, A., & Violato, C. (2010). The development and psychometric assessment of an instrument to measure attitudes towards depression and its treatments in patients suffering from non-psychotic depression. *Journal of Affective Disorders*, *124*(3), 241–249. [CrossRef]

Gallagher, M. W., Lopez, S. J., & Preacher, K. J. (2009). The hierarchical structure of well-being. *Journal of Personality*, *77*(4), 1025–1050. [CrossRef] [PubMed]

Gorczynski, P., Sims-Schouten, W., & Wilson, C. (2020). Evaluating mental health literacy and help-seeking behaviours in UK university students: A country wide study. *Journal of Public Mental Health*, *19*(4), 311–319. [CrossRef]

Hamzah, S. R. a., Musa, S. N. S., Badruldin, M. N. W. B., Amiludin, N. A., Zameram, Q. A., Kamaruzaman, M. J. M., Said, N. N., & Haniff, N. A. A. (2023). Identifying predictors of university students? Mental well-being during the COVID-19 pandemic. *Kontakt-Journal of Nursing and Social Sciences Related to Health and Illness*, *25*(1), 372–378. [CrossRef]

Holzinger, A., Floris, F., Schomerus, G., Carta, M. G., & Angermeyer, M. C. (2012). Gender differences in public beliefs and attitudes about mental disorder in western countries: A systematic review of population studies. *Epidemiology and Psychiatric Sciences*, *21*(1), 73–85. [CrossRef] [PubMed]

Jacka, F. N., O'Neil, A., Opie, R., Itsiopoulos, C., Cotton, S., Mohebbi, M., Castle, D., Dash, S., Mihalopoulos, C., Chatterton, M. L., Brazionis, L., Dean, O. M., Hodge, A. M., & Berk, M. (2017). A randomised controlled trial of dietary improvement for adults with major depression (the 'SMILES' trial). *BMC Medicine*, *15*, 23. [CrossRef] [PubMed]

Jafari, A., Nejatian, M., Momeniyan, V., Barsalani, F. R., & Tehrani, H. (2021). Mental health literacy and quality of life in Iran: A cross-sectional study. *BMC Psychiatry*, *21*(1), 499. [CrossRef] [PubMed]

Jiang, G., Li, D., Ren, Z., Yan, Y., Wu, X., Zhu, X., Yu, L., Xia, M., Li, F., Wei, H., Zhang, Y., Zhao, C., & Zhang, L. (2021). The status quo and characteristics of Chinese mental health literacy. *Acta Psychologica Sinica*, *53*(2), 182–198. [CrossRef]

Jiang, G., Zhao, C., Wei, H., Yu, L., Li, D., Lin, X., & Ren, Z. (2020). Mental health literacy: Connotation, measurement and new framework. *Journal of Psychological Science*, *43*, 232–238. [CrossRef]

Jorm, A. F. (2000). Mental health literacy: Public knowledge and beliefs about mental disorders. *The British Journal of Psychiatry*, *177*(5), 396–401. [CrossRef] [PubMed]

Jorm, A. F. (2012). Mental health literacy: Empowering the community to take action for better mental health. *American Psychologist*, *67*(3), 231–243. [CrossRef]

Jorm, A. F. (2015). Why we need the concept of "mental health literacy". *Health Communication*, *30*(12), 1166–1168. [CrossRef] [PubMed]

Jorm, A. F., Korten, A. E., Jacomb, P. A., Christensen, H., Rodgers, B., & Pollitt, P. (1997). "Mental health literacy": A survey of the public's ability to recognise mental disorders and their beliefs about the effectiveness of treatment. *Medical Journal of Australia*, *166*(4), 182–186. [CrossRef]

Kahneman, D., Diener, E., & Schwarz, N. (1999). *Well-being: Foundations of hedonic psychology*. Russell Sage Foundation.

Kajawu, L., Chingarande, S. D., Jack, H., Ward, C., & Taylor, T. (2016). What do African traditional medical practitioners do in the treatment of mental disorders in Zimbabwe? *International Journal of Culture and Mental Health*, *9*(1), 44–55. [CrossRef]

Keyes, C. L. M. (1998). Social well-being. *Social Psychology Quarterly*, *61*(2), 121–140. [CrossRef]

Keyes, C. L. M. (2003). Complete mental health: An agenda for the 21st century. In *Flourishing: Positive psychology and the life well-lived*. American Psychological Association.

Keyes, C. L. M. (2005). Mental illness and/or mental health? Investigating axioms of the complete state model of health. *Journal of Consulting and Clinical Psychology*, *73*(3), 539–548. [CrossRef] [PubMed]

Keyes, C. L. M. (2007). Promoting and protecting mental health as flourishing: A complementary strategy for improving national mental health. *American Psychologist*, *62*(2), 95–108. [CrossRef]

Keyes, C. L. M., & Shapiro, A. D. (2003). Social well-being in the United States: A descriptive epidemiology. In O. G. Brim, C. D. Ryff, & R. C. Kessler (Eds.), *How healthy are we?* (pp. 350–372) University of Chicago Press.

Kievit, R. A., Brandmaier, A. M., Ziegler, G., van Harmelen, A.-L., de Mooij, S. M. M., Moutoussis, M., Goodyer, I. M., Bullmore, E., Jones, P. B., Fonagy, P., Consortium, N. S. P. N., Lindenberger, U., & Dolan, R. J. (2018). Developmental cognitive neuroscience using latent change score models: A tutorial and applications. *Developmental Cognitive Neuroscience, 33*, 99–117. [CrossRef] [PubMed]

Kuhnert, R.-L., Begeer, S., Fink, E., & de Rosnay, M. (2017). Gender-differentiated effects of theory of mind, emotion understanding, and social preference on prosocial behavior development: A longitudinal study. *Journal of Experimental Child Psychology, 154*, 13–27. [CrossRef]

Kutcher, S., Bagnell, A., & Wei, Y. (2015). Mental health literacy in secondary schools: A Canadian approach. *Child and Adolescent Psychiatric Clinics of North America, 24*(2), 233–244. [CrossRef]

Kutcher, S., Wei, Y., & Coniglio, C. (2016). Mental health literacy: Past, present, and future. *Canadian Journal of Psychiatry-Revue Canadienne De Psychiatrie, 61*(3), 154–158. [CrossRef]

Larson, J. S. (1993). The measurement of social well-being. *Social Indicators Research, 28*(3), 285–296. [CrossRef]

Liu, Y., & Jiang, Q. (2021). Who benefits from being an only child? A study of parent-child relationship among Chinese junior high school students. *Frontiers in Psychology, 11*, 608995. [CrossRef] [PubMed]

Lluch-Canut, T., Puig-Llobet, M., Sanchez-Ortega, A., Roldan-Merino, J., Ferre-Grau, C., & Positive Mental Hlth Res, G. (2013). Assessing positive mental health in people with chronic physical health problems: Correlations with socio-demographic variables and physical health status. *BMC Public Health, 13*, 928. [CrossRef] [PubMed]

Mahmoodi, S. M. H., Rasoulian, M., Khodadoust, E., Jabari, Z., Emami, S., & Ahmadzad-Asl, M. (2023). The well-being of Iranian adult citizens; is it related to mental health literacy? *Frontiers in Psychiatry, 14*, 1127639. [CrossRef] [PubMed]

Malone, C., & Wachholtz, A. (2018). The relationship of anxiety and depression to subjective well-being in a mainland Chinese sample. *Journal of Religion & Health, 57*(1), 266–278. [CrossRef]

Markram, K., & Markram, H. (2010). The intense world theory: A unifying theory of the neurobiology of autism. *Frontiers in Human Neuroscience, 4*, 224. [CrossRef]

Miao, Y., & Wang, Q. (2009). An empirical study on social well-being. *Journal of Gannan Normal University, 30*(4), 76–81. [CrossRef]

Miao, Y., & Zhao, S. (2009). From social well-being to positive mental health model: Keyes's introduction and assessment. *Psychological Research, 2*(5), 13–16+25.

Ming, Z. J., & Chen, Z. Y. (2020). Mental health literacy: Concept, measurement, intervention and effect. *Advances in Psychological Science, 28*(1), 1–12. [CrossRef]

Morales-Torres, R., Carrasco-Gubernatis, C., Grasso-Cladera, A., Cosmelli, D., Parada, F. J., & Palacios-Garcia, I. (2023). Psychobiotic effects on anxiety are modulated by lifestyle behaviors: A randomized placebo-controlled trial on healthy adults. *Nutrients, 15*(7), 1706. [CrossRef] [PubMed]

Moser, G. (2009). Quality of life and sustainability: Toward person–environment congruity. *Journal of Environmental Psychology, 29*(3), 351–357. [CrossRef]

Nalipay, M. J. N., Chai, C.-S., Jong, M. S.-Y., King, R. B., & Mordeno, I. G. (2024). Positive mental health literacy for teachers: Adaptation and construct validation. *Current Psychology, 43*(6), 4888–4898. [CrossRef]

O'Connor, M., & Casey, L. (2015). The mental health literacy scale (MHLS): A new scale-based measure of mental health literacy. *Psychiatry Research, 229*(1–2), 511–516. [CrossRef] [PubMed]

Podsakoff, P. M., MacKenzie, S. B., Lee, J.-Y., & Podsakoff, N. P. (2003). Common method biases in behavioral research: A critical review of the literature and recommended remedies. *Journal of Applied Psychology, 88*(5), 879–903. [CrossRef]

Ryan, R. M., & Deci, E. L. (2001). On happiness and human potentials: A review of research on hedonic and eudaimonic well-being. *Annual Review of Psychology, 52*(1), 141–166. [CrossRef] [PubMed]

Ryff, C. D., & Keyes, C. L. M. (1995). The structure of psychological well-being revisited. *Journal of Personality and Social Psychology, 69*(4), 719–727. [CrossRef]

Seligman, M. E., & Csikszentmihalyi, M. (2000). *Positive psychology: An introduction* (Vol. 55). American Psychological Association.

Son, J., & Wilson, J. (2012). Volunteer work and hedonic, eudemonic, and social well-being. *Sociological Forum, 27*(3), 658–681. [CrossRef]

Spiker, D. A., & Hammer, J. H. (2019). Mental health literacy as theory: Current challenges and future directions. *Journal of Mental Health, 28*(3), 238–242. [CrossRef]

Tambling, R. R., D'Aniello, C., & Russell, B. S. (2023). Mental health literacy: A critical target for narrowing racial disparities in behavioral health. *International Journal of Mental Health and Addiction, 21*(3), 1867–1881. [CrossRef] [PubMed]

Tang, Z., Yang, X., Tan, W., Ke, Y., Kou, C., Zhang, M., Liu, L., Zhang, Y., Li, X., Li, W., & Wang, S. B. (2024). Patterns of unhealthy lifestyle and their associations with depressive and anxiety symptoms among Chinese young adults: A latent class analysis. *Journal of Affective Disorders, 352*, 267–277. [CrossRef]

Tay, J. L., Tay, Y. F., & Klainin-Yobas, P. (2018). Mental health literacy levels. *Archives of Psychiatric Nursing*, 32(5), 757–763. [CrossRef] [PubMed]

Wang, J., He, Y., Jiang, Q., Cai, J., Wang, W., Zeng, Q., Miao, J., Qi, X., Chen, J., Bian, Q., Cai, C., Ma, N., Zhu, Z., & Zhang, M. (2013). Mental health literacy among residents in Shanghai. *Shanghai Archives of Psychiatry*, 25(4), 224–235. [CrossRef]

Waterman, A. S. (1993). Two conceptions of happiness: Contrasts of personal expressiveness (eudaimonia) and hedonic enjoyment. *Journal of Personality and Social Psychology*, 64(4), 678–691. [CrossRef]

Wei, Y., McGrath, P. J., Hayden, J., & Kutcher, S. (2015). Mental health literacy measures evaluating knowledge, attitudes and help-seeking: A scoping review. *BMC Psychiatry*, 15, 291. [CrossRef]

Winding, T. N., Nielsen, M. L., & Grytnes, R. (2023). Perceived stress in adolescence and labour market participation in young adulthood-a prospective cohort study. *BMC Public Health*, 23(1), 186. [CrossRef] [PubMed]

Wu, J., Wang, C., Lu, Y., Zhu, X., Li, Y., Liu, G., & Jiang, G. (2023). Development and initial validation of the mental health literacy questionnaire for Chinese adults. *Current Psychology*, 42(10), 8425–8440. [CrossRef]

Ye, Y., Zhang, L., Zhao, J., & Kong, F. (2023). The relationship between gratitude and social well-being: Evidence from a longitudinal study and a daily diary investigation. *Acta Psychologica Sinica*, 55(7), 1087–1098. [CrossRef]

Zeng, F., John, W. C. M., Qiao, D., & Sun, X. (2023). Association between psychological distress and mental help-seeking intentions in international students of national university of Singapore: A mediation analysis of mental health literacy. *BMC Public Health*, 23(1), 2358. [CrossRef]

Zhang, Z., Chen, S., Wang, X., Liu, J., Zhang, Y., Mei, Y., & Zhang, Z. (2023). The relationship between mental health literacy and subjective well-being of young and middle-aged residents: Perceived the mediating role of social support and its urban-rural differences. *International Journal of Mental Health Promotion*, 25(4), 471–483. [CrossRef]

Zhong, S.-L., Wang, S.-B., Ding, K.-R., Tan, W.-Y., & Zhou, L. (2024). Low mental health literacy is associated with depression and anxiety among adults: A population-based survey of 16,715 adults in China. *BMC Public Health*, 24(1), 2721. [CrossRef]

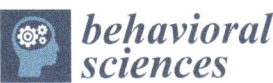

Article

Interplay between Children's Electronic Media Use and Prosocial Behavior: The Chain Mediating Role of Parent–Child Closeness and Emotion Regulation

Xiaocen Liu [1,*,†], Shuliang Geng [1,†] and Donghui Dou [2]

[1] College of Preschool Education, Capital Normal University, Beijing 100048, China; 2223102004@cnu.edu.cn
[2] School of Sociology and Psychology, Central University of Finance and Economics, Beijing 100081, China; psychaos@126.com
* Correspondence: cindyliu@cnu.edu.cn
† These authors contributed equally to this work.

Abstract: In the contemporary digital milieu, children's pervasive engagement with electronic media is ubiquitous in their daily lives, presenting complex implications for their socialization. Prosocial behavior, a cornerstone of social interaction and child development, is intricately intertwined with these digital experiences. This relation gains further depth, considering the significant roles of parent–child relationships and emotion regulation in shaping children's social trajectories. This study surveyed 701 families to examine the association between children's electronic media use and prosocial behavior, specifically exploring the mediating roles of parent–child closeness and emotion regulation. Structural equation modeling was employed for the analysis. Children's electronic media use negatively correlated with prosocial behavior, parent–child closeness, and emotion regulation. In contrast, a positive association emerged between parent–child closeness, emotion regulation, and prosocial behavior. Emotion regulation also correlated positively with prosocial behavior. Statistical analyses revealed that parent–child closeness and emotion regulation function as both individual and sequential mediators in the relation between electronic media use and prosocial behavior. The study's analyses reveal that fostering children's prosocial behavior in the digital era requires strong family ties, effective emotional management, and balanced digital exposure, which are pivotal for their comprehensive development.

Keywords: electronic media; parent–child relationship; emotion regulation; prosocial behavior; social interaction; children

1. Introduction

The post-pandemic era has witnessed a significant rise in electronic media use among children, altering their daily interactions and educational methodologies. The rapid spread of coronavirus disease 2019 (COVID-19) has exerted a profound impact on human life across the globe [1]. To mitigate the spread of the virus, educational institutions from kindergartens to secondary schools universally embraced online learning [2], thereby integrating electronic media deeply into children's conventional living and learning paradigms. Research has highlighted a downturn in children's physical and social activities during the pandemic, coupled with a noticeable increase in time allocated to electronic devices such as televisions, computers, and mobile phones [3]. Nagata et al. discovered that adolescents' average daily screen time soared to 7.70 h during the early pandemic period, markedly higher than pre-pandemic figures, within a cohort of 5412 U.S. adolescents aged 12 and 13 [4]. Additionally, Carroll et al. found that, based on parent-reported data, 87% of Canadian children experienced a screen time surge [5]. This change in children's electronic media consumption did not recede. Rather, it persisted beyond the reopening of schools [6], indicating a potential long-term shift in their media use patterns.

Electronic media use encompasses a spectrum of digital platforms, extending beyond traditional mediums like television and DVDs to include mobile phones, computers, tablets, and an array of interactive and streaming services [7]. This expansion reflects a broader societal pivot toward digital integration. The diverse implications of electronic media on children's development have been extensively studied, yielding many outcomes across various domains. Feng et al. have noted potential benefits, such as enhancing spatial attention and reducing gender disparities in spatial cognition through action video games [8]. Conversely, findings by Zoromba et al. suggest that excessive media exposure may be associated with hyperactivity, anxiety, and learning difficulties in children [9]. Similarly, research by Raheem et al. has shown negative correlations between the duration of electronic media exposure and developmental aspects such as attention and language [10]. Given these varied findings, there is a pressing need for focused inquiry into electronic media use by children who have experienced the COVID-19 pandemic, to guide the development of informed media usage behaviors.

As digital technology entrenches itself in the fabric of childhood, a deeper understanding of electronic media use and its association with critical developmental outcomes like prosocial behavior becomes increasingly important. Prosocial behavior, characterized by voluntary actions intended to benefit others, such as care, help, consideration, comfort, and sharing, is a vital indicator of healthy social development in children [11]. Notably, positive social development, including prosocial behavior, is linked to enhanced interpersonal relationships, academic achievement, and cognitive abilities later in life [12,13]. Prosocial behaviors emerge early, around 1–2 years, and become more varied and frequent between ages 3 and 6, a critical period for social norm internalization [14]. The Social Context Model further emphasizes the significance of normative behaviors like prosocial actions for group acceptance and integration, underscoring their importance for social development [15]. This study delves into the complex association between electronic media use and the development of prosocial behavior in children, with particular attention to the roles of parent–child closeness and emotion regulation. In examining these relations, the research highlights the need for supporting prosocial development in children, particularly in an era where digital interactions are increasingly shaping their experiences and social dynamics.

1.1. Electronic Media Use and Prosocial Behavior in Children

The interplay between electronic media use and children's prosocial behavior is multifaceted, drawing continued attention and scholarly debate. A segment of this research suggests a positive correlation. For example, Coyne et al. conducted a meta-analysis that uncovered a substantial relation between multidimensional prosocial media content and an increase in children's prosocial behaviors [16]. Additionally, Stone et al. noted that the multiplayer collaborative nature of many video games could enhance cooperative skills, such as social interaction and information sharing [17]. Prot et al. similarly reported a positive association between prosocial media use and helpful behaviors in children, suggesting that certain types of electronic media use could support the development of prosocial tendencies [18]. Furthermore, Ostrov et al. found that among a sample of children of relatively high socio-economic status who were frequently exposed to educational programming like PBS Kids, there was an association between the amount of television viewed and concurrent prosocial behavior [19].

In contrast, other studies have offered a more nuanced view, suggesting potential negative outcomes associated with extensive electronic media use. Poulain et al. identified a link between excessive media use in children and reduced prosocial behavior [20]. Guo observed a negative correlation between media violence exposure and prosocial behaviors [21], resonating with earlier findings by Veraksa et al., who noted a relation between electronic media use, increased aggressive behavior, and decreased prosocial behavior [22]. Adding to this perspective, Lissak provided psychoneurological evidence indicating an inverse correlation between screen time and social skills [23]. Moreover, Christensen discussed how instant rewards in video games, enhancing gaming pleasure and triggering dopamine release, can lead to electronically mediated addictive behaviors and frontal lobe structure changes [24], impacting cognitive processes crucial for prosocial behaviors like empathy [25]. The General Learning Model (GLM) suggests that escalating electronic media use might lead to addiction-like relationships, potentially hindering social development [12,26]. Wiegman and van Schie highlighted a significant negative correlation between video game use and prosocial behavior [27]. Such evidence implies that the nature of media content and the extent of its use play significant roles in influencing children's prosocial behavior.

Based on these findings, Hypothesis H1 is formulated in this study: There is a negative correlation between children's electronic media use and prosocial behavior. It is postulated that increased engagement with electronic media may correspond to diminished real-world prosocial interactions among children.

1.2. Relations among Children's Electronic Media Use, Parent–Child Closeness, and Prosocial Behavior

The construct of parent–child closeness, characterized by support, warmth, and a shared willingness for open communication, is a cornerstone of the parent–child dynamic [28,29]. Empirical evidence has illuminated the significant impact of children's electronic media use on the quality of this relationship. Studies such as those by Zhu et al., Horita et al., and Ahmadian et al. have consistently shown that higher levels of problematic internet use among children are linked to poorer parent–child relationships [30–32]. The Displacement Hypothesis posits that excessive use of electronic media may supplant meaningful face-to-face interactions, eroding intimacy and satisfaction within familial relationships [33]. Similarly, Sampasa-Kanyinga et al. reported that intensive social media use can diminish parent–child communication and weaken the positive bonds within these relationships [34]. Adding to this, Nergiz et al. found that excessive screen time is positively associated with parental neglect, potentially leading to a decrease in parent–child closeness [35].

Conversely, a robust body of research underscores a positive association between parent–child closeness and children's prosocial behavior. The Attachment Inner Work Model suggests that the quality of the parent–child bond lays the groundwork for the child's interpersonal relationships and behaviors [36]. Xu et al. demonstrated that nurturing parent–child relationships is fundamental to preschoolers' social interactions and significantly influences their subsequent social development [37]. Confirming this, Liu and Wang found a positive correlation between parent–child closeness and prosocial behaviors in a study encompassing 507 young children, with considerations for genetic factors [28]. Furthermore, research conducted in Ireland on 1,151 families illustrated that parent–child closeness significantly predicted prosocial behaviors in children, even when controlling for a spectrum of demographic variables [38]. This positive trend continues into adolescence, as indicated by Padilla-Walker et al., who observed that warmth and connection in the parent–child relationship are positively related to adolescents' prosocial behavior [39]. Similarly, Ferreira et al. emphasized the link between the quality of early caregiver relationships and children's prosocial behavior [11].

Therefore, this study introduces Hypothesis H2, which posits that parent–child closeness acts as a mediating factor in the relation between children's electronic media use and their prosocial behavior. Specifically, it is hypothesized that increased electronic media use among children may be associated with decreased parent–child closeness, which may reduce prosocial behaviors. This mediation hypothesis suggests that parent–child closeness is a critical mediator that could explain the link between children's electronic media use and prosocial conduct.

1.3. Interconnections among Children's Electronic Media Use, Emotion Regulation, and Prosocial Behavior

Emotion regulation is pivotal for maintaining both physical and mental well-being. It involves modulating one's emotional responses adaptively through various strategies to alter the intensity and duration of emotions [7,40]. The nexus between electronic media use and emotion regulation has increasingly become scrutinized with the rise in media accessibility. Lobel et al. found in their longitudinal study of 7 to 11-year-olds that children's gaming on electronic devices correlated with heightened emotional difficulties [41]. Günaydin et al. and Özer et al. corroborated this by identifying a significant link between problematic internet use and challenges in emotion regulation [42,43]. Moreover, Oflu et al. emphasized that excessive screen time was associated with the negative development of emotional regulation in early childhood [44]. Echoing these findings, Hidayatullah et al. reported that internet-addicted individuals exhibited significant difficulties with emotion regulation [45]. This trend persisted across various demographic groups, including differences in gender, age, and educational level [46].

The relation between children's emotion regulation and prosocial behavior has been extensively studied, revealing a consistent pattern of associations. Dunfield noted that individual differences in emotion regulation abilities significantly influence children's propensity for prosocial actions [47]. This finding aligns with Benita et al., who identified effortful control, an essential aspect of emotion regulation, as facilitating empathy and prosocial behavior in social contexts [48]. Fabes et al. further elucidated that positive emotion regulation aids children in being attentive to and empathetic towards others' suffering, thereby enhancing their prosocial inclinations [49]. Additionally, effective emotion regulation enables children to better manage their responses in distressing scenarios, making them more likely to offer help and support [50]. Similarly, Song et al. found in their study with 4–8-year-old children that the ability to regulate grief was positively associated with mother-reported prosocial behavior [51].

Based on these observations, Hypothesis H3 is proposed: children's use of electronic media is negatively associated with their capacity for emotion regulation, which in turn is positively associated with prosocial behavior. The hypothesis further suggests that emotion regulation may mediate the relation between electronic media use and prosocial behavior in children.

1.4. Associative Patterns among Children's Electronic Media Use, Parent–Child Closeness, Emotion Regulation, and Prosocial Behavior

Research has shed light on the relation between parent–child closeness and emotion regulation in children. Dysfunctional family environments or negative parent–child relationships have been shown to disrupt emotion regulation, leading to increased insecurity in individuals [52,53]. In contrast, children with secure attachment, which fosters improved emotion regulation, are likely to exhibit enhanced empathic responding and prosocial behavior [54]. Strong parent–child bonds, characterized by quality interactions, are essential for developing effective emotion regulation. These interactions often involve emotional synchronization, positively contributing to children's emotional growth [55,56]. Zhao et al. emphasized how early mother–child interactions develop synchrony across physiological, neurological, and behavioral aspects, influencing children's emotion regulation abilities [57].

Building on Bowlby's Attachment Theory, Ainsworth introduced an emotional dimension to the parent–child attachment relationship, emphasizing its profound influence on children's emotion regulation and social adjustment [58]. This early childhood relationship is crucial in forming children's self-perception and understanding of others. Bronfenbrenner and Morris further demonstrated that positive parent–child relationships are instrumental in nurturing children's socio-emotional regulation, influencing their ability to form healthy interpersonal relationships [59]. On the other hand, negative parent–child interactions can lead to emotional dysregulation and foster negative perceptions in children about interpersonal relationships, potentially leading to a reduction in prosocial behaviors such as cooperation and helping [28,60].

Considering the insights gained from the preceding review, a chain mediation hypothesis is proposed. This hypothesis, Hypothesis H4, suggests that parent–child closeness and emotion regulation play sequential mediating roles in the relation between children's electronic media use and prosocial behaviors. Specifically, this hypothesis considers the possibility of an association where higher levels of children's electronic media use might be related to lower parent–child closeness. In turn, lower parent–child closeness might be associated with less-effective emotion regulation, which could correlate with decreased prosocial behaviors among children.

1.5. The Present Study

In the burgeoning field of child development research, the comprehensive effects of electronic media have become increasingly prominent. Despite extensive exploration, the majority of existing studies predominantly focus on the adverse developmental outcomes associated with children's electronic media use, such as problematic behaviors. However, there is a noticeable dearth of research delving into the positive aspects of development, particularly prosocial behavior, concerning children's electronic media engagement. This gap is significant considering the pivotal role of early childhood in cultivating social and emotional competencies, often nurtured through family interactions. Our study seeks to fill this gap by investigating the specific impact of children's media use within the family context, exploring its relation with parent–child closeness, emotion regulation, and the development of prosocial behaviors.

Moreover, the previous literature has frequently concentrated on the impact of parental media habits on the parent–child relationship. In contrast, our study focuses on how children's interactions with media contribute to this dynamic, providing a more comprehensive understanding of the family media environment. We frame our exploration using Knafo and Plomin's Individual–Environment Interaction theory [61]. This theory suggests that children's development is influenced by a blend of individual characteristics, such as media use and emotion regulation, and environmental factors, like parent–child closeness. Additionally, we integrate the concept of the Bi-Directionality of Parent–Child Relationships theory, highlighting the reciprocal nature of these interactions. This perspective emphasizes the co-contributory roles of both parents and children in shaping their relationship dynamics. Through our research, we aim to illuminate how children's electronic media use, within the context of their family environment, influences and is influenced by their emotional and social development.

Our study addresses a critical knowledge gap by exploring the positive developmental outcomes associated with electronic media use in children, particularly focusing on prosocial behavior. Employing chain mediation analysis and grounded in established theories, our research delves into the associations and interrelationships between children's use of electronic media, their prosocial behaviors, and the roles of parent–child closeness and emotion regulation as mediators. This study aims to provide a deeper understanding of these associations within the digital age context. The chain mediation model, depicted in Figure 1, is designed to elucidate these interconnections, offering insights into the complex dynamics of electronic media's role in children's social and emotional development.

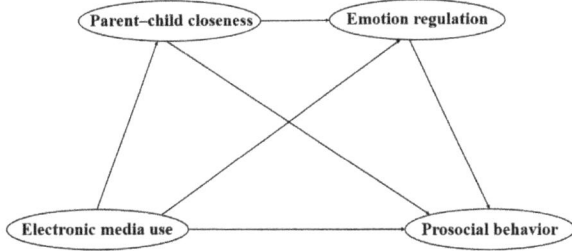

Figure 1. Hypothetical chain mediation model.

2. Materials and Methods

2.1. Participants and Procedure

For this study, we collaborated with teachers from kindergartens and primary schools across northern China to facilitate the distribution of questionnaires. From December 2022 to February 2023, these questionnaires were administered to parents via an online survey platform. The selection criteria included ensuring that the children and their parents were free from any psychiatric or neurological conditions, as reported by the teachers. Before participants filled out the questionnaire, we provided them with a comprehensive briefing. This briefing included detailed definitions and the scope of electronic media use to ensure a common understanding of the terms used in the study. Informed consent was obtained from all participants, affirming their voluntary participation and awareness of the study's objectives and procedures.

We conducted rigorous screening to ensure data integrity and the relevance of the responses. The initial phase of our study involved the distribution of 796 questionnaires. Questionnaires were excluded if they contained inconsistencies, such as affirmative responses to the lie detector statement "My child never blinks", which served to identify non-serious responses. We also excluded questionnaires with contradictory responses (e.g., claiming "The child has never been exposed to electronic media" but later reporting media usage), incomplete entries, or those not filled out by the child's primary caregivers. After applying these criteria, we obtained 701 valid questionnaires for our final analysis.

To validate the robustness of our statistical conclusions, we conducted a post hoc power analysis using G*Power 3.1.9.7 software. We aimed for an effect size of at least a small magnitude ($f^2 = 0.02$) with an alpha level (α) set at 0.05. This analysis showed that our sample of 701 participants provides a power value of 0.84, surpassing the commonly accepted threshold of 0.80 [62]. The power analysis result confirmed that the sample size of 701 is sufficiently large to detect small effect sizes, thus ensuring adequate statistical power for the statistical tests employed. Moreover, according to guidelines by Bentler et al., the sample size for structural equation modeling should ideally range from 5 to 10 times the number of estimable parameters [63]. With 47 estimable parameters in our model, the recommended sample size would be between 235 and 470. Thus, our sample size meets and comfortably exceeds these recommendations, enhancing our findings' reliability and validity and ensuring the structural equation model's robustness.

The final participant pool comprised 190 fathers (27.1%), with an average age of 34.09 years (SD = 5.11), and 511 mothers (72.9%), with an average age of 32.33 years (SD = 4.63). The predominance of mothers in the sample can be attributed to the traditional gender roles prevalent within Chinese families. Historically, societal expectations have designated men as the primary breadwinners, involved chiefly in the public sphere. At the same time, women are typically seen as the principal caregivers, responsible for domestic roles, including child-rearing. This cultural norm has naturally led mothers to assume a more substantial role in managing children's daily needs and activities, resulting in their deeper involvement and understanding of the children's routines and challenges [64]. However, contemporary societal shifts and changes in family dynamics are gradually altering these traditional roles. An increasing number of fathers are now actively engaging in parenting, spending more time with their children, and sharing the responsibilities traditionally held by mothers. It is important to note that all participants in this study were primary caregivers who resided with the children, ensuring they were well-informed about their daily lives and capable of providing reliable responses.

Further enriching the demographic profile, the educational qualifications of the participants vary significantly, offering a broad perspective on parental influence. Concerning the educational qualifications of the children's mothers, 2.8% attained junior high school level or below, 8.5% completed high school or junior college, 78.4% held a college or bachelor's degree, and 10.3% were postgraduate students. Similarly, for the fathers, 2.7% had a junior high school education or below, 9.4% had completed high school or junior college, 70.4% had a college or undergraduate degree, and 17.5% had postgraduate qualifications.

Additionally, family structure within the sample was split between 54.6% nuclear families and 45.4% extended families, illustrating the diversity of family setups influencing child development.

The children involved in this study had a mean age of 5.20 years ($SD = 1.87$), consisting of 339 boys (48.4%) and 362 girls (51.6%). The sample included 547 singletons (78.0%) and 154 children with siblings (22.0%). Concerning their educational settings, 6.7% of the children were not enrolled in any educational institution, 81.7% attended kindergartens, and 11.6% were enrolled in primary schools. To ensure the reliability of our findings, we only included children and parents with no psychiatric or neurological conditions, as verified by the teachers at the time of recruitment. This careful selection was crucial to ensure that the observed behaviors and interactions were typical of the general child population, unaffected by underlying health issues.

2.2. Measures

2.2.1. Electronic Media Use

Our recent study assessed children's interaction with electronic media using an adjusted version of the Children's Electronic Media Use Questionnaire. Building upon foundational work by Huang et al. [65], further elaborated on by Geng et al. [66], this instrument consists of 14 items designed to evaluate various aspects of children's media usage. For example, it includes questions such as "My child throws tantrums because I limit her/his time to use electronic media", highlighting emotional reactions to restricted media access. Responses to these items were recorded on a 5-point scale to quantify the extent of media engagement. The questionnaire's reliability in our study was evident, with a Cronbach's α value of 0.93, indicating high internal consistency.

2.2.2. Parent–Child Closeness

In assessing the parent–child intimacy, our study utilized the closeness subscale from the Child–Parent Relationship Scale, originally conceptualized by Pianta [29] and later adapted by Xu and Wang [67]. The closeness aspect of this scale is particularly insightful, encompassing ten items that gauge the warmth and affection in the parent–child relationship (e.g., "My child values his/her relationship with me"). These items are rated on a 5-point scale, where higher scores indicate a stronger, more positive bond between parent and child. In our study, the closeness subscale exhibited strong internal consistency, as evidenced by a Cronbach's α value of 0.85.

2.2.3. Emotion Regulation

In this study, we utilized the Emotion Regulation Checklist, originally developed by Shields and Cicchetti [68] and later revised by Xing et al. [69], with a particular emphasis on its emotion regulation subscale for assessing this facet of children's abilities. The subscale comprises eight items that measure children's adaptability and response to emotional challenges. An example is the item "Can recover quickly from upset or distress (for example, doesn't pout or remain sullen, anxious, or sad after emotionally distressing events)". These items were rated on a 4-point scale, with higher scores indicating more effective emotion regulation. In our research, the emotion regulation subscale demonstrated sound internal consistency, as reflected by Cronbach's α value of 0.73.

2.2.4. Prosocial Behavior

The Strengths and Difficulties Questionnaire (SDQ), known for its robust reliability in assessing mental health across various child age groups, was employed to evaluate children's prosocial behavior. Formulated initially by Goodman [70] and adapted for broader applicability by Aarø et al. [71], this questionnaire includes 21 items spanning three key dimensions: prosocial behavior, externalizing problems, and internalizing problems. For this research, we selectively focused on seven items from the prosocial behavior dimension. For example, my child shares readily with other children (treats, toys, pencils etc.). These items were rated on a 3-point scale, where 0 signifies "not true" and 2 denotes "certainly true". A higher tally on this subscale suggests a more frequent occurrence of prosocial behaviors like sharing. The Cronbach's α value for this specific subscale in our research was 0.80, indicating a satisfactory level of internal consistency.

2.3. Data Analysis

In this study, SPSS software (version 23.0) served as the primary tool for the initial stages of data handling, encompassing input, organization, and preliminary assessments such as checking for common method bias, evaluating data normality, and verifying scale reliability. We then conducted descriptive and correlational analyses to ascertain the scores of each variable and explore their interrelationships. Subsequently, to build upon this initial data exploration, structural equation modeling (SEM) was employed using AMOS (version 26.0). This advanced technique detailed the associations among children's electronic media use, parent–child closeness, emotion regulation, and prosocial behavior.

3. Results

3.1. Common Method Bias and The Normality of the Data

To address potential common method bias due to the self-reported nature of our data, we implemented measures such as anonymous response collection and the inclusion of reverse-scored items. In further evaluating common method bias, we applied Harman's single-factor test, as Podsakoff et al. suggested [72]. The exploratory factor analysis results revealed six factors with eigenvalues exceeding one. Notably, the variance attributed to the most substantial common factor was 25.48%, falling below the threshold of 40%. This finding suggests that common method bias did not significantly influence our study's results. Regarding data normality, we utilized Q–Q plots for assessment. The alignment of most data points close to the diagonal line in these plots substantiates our research's assumption of data normality.

3.2. Descriptive Statistics and Correlation Analysis

This section provides a comprehensive overview of the demographic data and distribution characteristics of our study sample, detailing the socio-economic, familial, and individual attributes along with their associations with the study's outcomes. To accurately categorize families and analyze their potential influence on child development, we calculated Family Socio-Economic Status (SES) using Reng's formula [73]. This calculation incorporates the highest educational level of the parents, their occupation, and monthly family income as key indicators: $SES = \beta_1 \times Z_{\text{higher education level}} + (\beta_2 \times Z_{\text{higher occupation}} + \beta_3 \times Z_{\text{monthly family income}}) / \varepsilon f$.

Following this foundational classification, Table 1 provides a detailed breakdown of the children's and families' sociodemographic characteristics alongside the children's scores for electronic media use and prosocial behavior. Notable findings include significant differences in prosocial behavior scores between genders, with boys scoring lower than girls ($p < 0.001$). Children under three years of age displayed significantly lower prosocial behavior scores compared to those aged 3–6 years and older than 6 years, with all comparisons yielding $p < 0.001$. However, no significant differences were observed between other sociodemographic characteristics and scores for electronic media use and prosocial behavior.

Building upon the demographic and socio-economic profiles outlined, we delve deeper into the data to explore various interactions and correlations, as detailed in Table 2. Notably, a negative correlation existed between children's electronic media use and key variables such as parent–child closeness, emotion regulation, and prosocial behavior. In contrast, parent–child closeness positively correlated with emotion regulation and prosocial behavior in children. Additionally, children's emotion regulation was positively correlated with their prosocial behavior. Furthermore, children's age positively correlated with electronic media use and prosocial behavior. Intriguingly, the correlation between children's gender and prosocial behavior was positive, suggesting that girls exhibited more prosocial behavior than boys. Given these insights, children's age and gender, informed by the results above, were subsequently included as control variables in the model.

Table 1. Associations between sociodemographic features and scores for children's electronic media use and prosocial behavior.

	n (%)	Electronic Media Use Score				p	Prosocial Behavior Score				p
		Median	Mean	SD	IQR		Median	Mean	SD	IQR	
		Family structure									
Nuclear families	383 (54.64%)	2.29	2.33	0.71	1.14	0.370	1.43	1.37	0.41	0.71	0.304
Extended families	318 (45.36%)	2.36	2.38	0.78	1.14		1.43	1.40	0.40	0.57	
		Family socio-economic status (SES)									
Low SES	224 (32.0%)	2.43	2.43	0.74	1.00	0.064	1.29	1.34	0.42	0.71	0.071
Middle SES	213 (30.4%)	2.29	2.36	0.75	1.00		1.43	1.38	0.40	0.57	
High SES	264 (37.7%)	2.29	2.27	0.74	1.14		1.43	1.42	0.39	0.57	
		Situation of siblings									
Singletons	547 (78.03%)	2.29	2.34	0.74	1.07	0.514	1.43	1.40	0.40	0.57	0.157
Children with siblings	154 (21.97%)	2.36	2.38	0.77	1.21		1.29	1.34	0.42	0.71	
		Children'sgender									
Boys	339 (48.36%)	2.36	2.39	0.76	1.14	0.116	1.29	1.33	0.40	0.71	0.000
Girls	362 (51.64%)	2.29	2.31	0.73	1.07		1.43	1.44	0.40	0.61	
		Children'sage									
<3 years	46 (6.56%)	2.07	2.12	0.78	1.20	0.055	1.14	1.13	0.48	0.61	0.000
3–6 years	495 (70.61%)	2.29	2.35	0.74	1.07		1.43	1.40	0.39	0.57	
>6 years	160 (22.82%)	2.43	2.42	0.72	1.13		1.43	1.42	0.40	0.57	

Table 2. Descriptive statistics and correlations of the main variables.

Variables	M	SD	1	2	3	4	5	6
1. Age	5.20	1.87	-					
2. Gender	0.52	0.50	-	-				
3. Electronic media use	2.35	0.74	0.11 **	−0.06	-			
4. Parent–child closeness	3.73	0.65	0.06	0.04	−0.15 ***	-		
5. Emotion regulation	3.32	0.47	0.05	0.07	−0.21 ***	0.64 ***	-	
6. Prosocial behavior	1.39	0.41	0.11 **	0.13 ***	−0.16 ***	0.59 ***	0.62 ***	-

Notes. Boy = 0, Girl = 1, ** $p < 0.01$, *** $p < 0.001$.

3.3. Chain Mediation Model Test

To analyze the structural equation model, AMOS 26.0 was employed to validate the mediating roles of parent–child closeness and emotion regulation. We implemented a bias-corrected confidence interval Bootstrap test for examining the model paths. This test involved 5000 resamples and set 95% confidence intervals, ensuring robustness in our findings. In line with the guidelines suggested by Little et al. [74] and Rogers and Schmitt [75] for item parceling in structural modeling, we adopted specific approaches for different scales. For the Electronic Media Use questionnaire, which contains multiple subscales, we used isolated parceling to combine these subscales into a single indicator. Conversely, a factorial algorithm approach was applied for scales with a single dimension, such as the parent–child closeness and emotion regulation subscales. Given the limited number of items in the prosocial behavior subscale, we opted not to employ the parceling strategy for this measure.

The initial stage of our mediation analysis was to investigate the relation between children's usage of electronic media and their display of prosocial behavior, considering age and gender as potential influencing factors. The model fit, as measured by several indices, showed an appropriate level: $\chi^2/df = 1.85$, RMSEA = 0.03, NFI = 0.97, GFI = 0.98,

IFI = 0.98, RFI = 0.96, CFI = 0.98, and TLI = 0.98. A statistically significant negative link was found between children's electronic media usage and prosocial behavior (β = −0.19, *p* < 0.001, 95% CI [−0.27, −0.10]), implying that increased electronic media use tends to correspond with reduced prosocial behavior.

In further exploring the model, we included parent−child closeness and emotion regulation to understand their roles as mediators. The revised model also demonstrated a satisfactory fit (χ^2/df = 2.35, RMSEA = 0.04, NFI = 0.94, GFI = 0.95, IFI = 0.97, RFI = 0.93, CFI = 0.97, and TLI = 0.96). Interestingly, the direct association between children's electronic media use and prosocial behavior became non-significant (β = 0.04, *p* = 0.290, and 95% CI [−0.03, 0.12]) upon introducing parent−child closeness and emotion regulation into the model. However, as depicted in Figure 2, negative paths emerged from electronic media use to both parent−child closeness (β = −0.15, *p* < 0.001, and 95% CI [−0.23, −0.07]) and emotion regulation (β = −0.19, *p* < 0.001, and 95% CI [−0.26, −0.12]). Positive and significant pathways were observed from parent–child closeness to emotion regulation (β = 0.74, *p* < 0.001, and 95% CI [0.68, 0.79]) and prosocial behavior (β = 0.19, *p* < 0.05, and 95% CI [0.03, 0.32]), as well as from emotion regulation to prosocial behavior (β = 0.66, *p* < 0.001, and 95% CI [0.52, 0.82]). These findings indicate a complete mediation effect, suggesting the pivotal role of parent−child closeness and emotion regulation in the link between electronic media use and prosocial behavior.

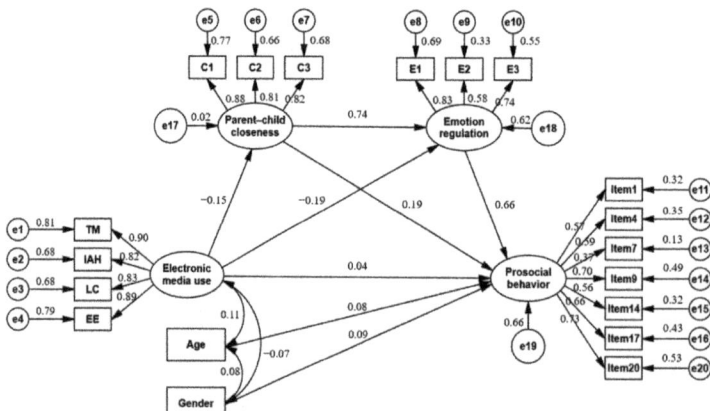

Figure 2. Standardized path diagram of relations.

To substantiate these mediating roles, we employed Bootstrap analysis for a more accurate estimation of confidence intervals (see Table 3). The mediating effect is significant if the 95% confidence interval does not include zero. The results showed a significant mediated effect from children's electronic media use to prosocial behavior via parent–child closeness (standardized effect = −0.0282 and 95% CI [−0.06, −0.01]) and via emotion regulation (standardized effect = −0.1249 and 95% CI [−0.19, −0.07]). Moreover, the chain-mediated pathway—from electronic media use through parent–child closeness and emotion regulation to prosocial behavior—was also significant (standardized effect = −0.0744 and 95% CI [−0.12, −0.03]). This outcome illustrates the significance of the chain-mediated effect, suggesting a cascading influence: higher electronic media use in children is associated with reduced parent–child closeness and increased emotional challenges, adversely affecting prosocial behavior.

Table 3. Bootstrap analysis of the mediation effect significance in the proposed model.

	Effect Value	95% Confidence Interval	
		Boot LLCI	Boot ULCI
Electronic media us→Parent–child closeness→Prosocial behavior	−0.0282	−0.06	−0.01
Electronic media us→Emotion regulation→Prosocial behavior	−0.1249	−0.19	−0.07
Electronic media us→Parent–child closeness→Emotion regulation→Prosocial behavior	−0.0744	−0.12	−0.03
Total indirect effect	−0.2275	−0.30	−0.15

Notes. When parent−child closeness and emotion regulation are included as mediators in the model, the direct effect of electronic media use on prosocial behavior is not significant ($\beta = 0.04$, $p = 0.290$, and 95% CI [−0.03, 0.12]). However, without accounting for these mediating variables, the direct effect is significant ($\beta = −0.19$, $p < 0.001$, and 95% CI [−0.27, −0.10]), suggesting full mediation within the tested model.

4. Discussion

This study aimed to validate the association between children's electronic media use and prosocial behavior and explore the mediating role of parent–child closeness and emotion regulation in this connection. Our findings support the complexity of this interplay, revealing that electronic media use is intricately linked with prosocial behavior through both direct and mediated pathways involving parent–child closeness and emotion regulation.

4.1. Children's Electronic Media Use and Prosocial Behavior

Consistent with the first hypothesis (H1), our analysis found a negative association between children's electronic media use and prosocial behavior. Structural equation modeling unveiled that prosocial behavior tends to diminish as electronic media use escalates. This phenomenon may be attributed to the pervasive nature of electronic media, which, as documented by Ding et al., is becoming a significant health concern globally, increasingly affecting younger populations [76]. The World Health Organization, in the 11th edition of the International Classification of Diseases (ICD) published in 2018, has recognized video game addiction as a mental health disorder. Children, with their developmental cognitive and neural mechanisms, are particularly vulnerable to the adverse impacts of electronic media [23,76]. Excessive engagement with electronic media may disrupt crucial real-life interactions that foster the development of communication skills and prosocial behaviors such as empathy, sharing, and cooperation [22,77]. The displacement of face-to-face interaction time is particularly concerning, as it is through these direct social engagements that children learn and practice prosocial behaviors [78]. Such interpersonal experiences, often cultivated through real-life experiences and direct social engagement, may not be adequately stimulated in digitally mediated environments. Furthermore, the immersive qualities of electronic media can engender escapism, potentially diminishing children's willingness to engage with real-world challenges and respond with prosocial behaviors [79].

4.2. Mediation of Parent–Child Closeness

Our investigation, corresponding to the second hypothesis (H2), indicated that parent–child closeness appears to mediate the relation between children's electronic media use and prosocial behavior. The data suggest a pattern where elevated use of electronic media aligns with reduced levels of parent–child closeness, which is concurrently associated with lower indications of prosocial behavior in children. Insights into the association between children's electronic media use and the quality of parent–child closeness emerge from examining the Displacement Hypothesis. This theory, as outlined by Hong et al., suggests that time spent engaging in electronic media might encroach upon and diminish valuable real-life interactions, leading to reduced intimacy in interpersonal relationships [33]. Supporting this theory, research by Nergiz et al. indicates that excessive access to electronic media could exacerbate parental neglect and undermine the development of parent–child closeness [35]. Furthermore, high media engagement levels might conflict with parental expectations for their children's active involvement in real-life activities, leading to an "expectation deviation" that can negatively impact the parent–child bond [66]. Additionally, Beyens and Beullens noted the negative impact of extensive tablet computer use on developing a positive parent–child relationship [80].

The linkage between parent–child closeness and prosocial behavior can be understood through various psychological frameworks. The Emotional Security Hypothesis suggests that secure parent–child relationships are fundamental to children's emotional well-being and social adaptation, while insecure relationships may contribute to difficulties in social adjustment [81]. This view is supported by the Attachment Inner Work Model, which posits parent–child closeness as foundational for an individual's interpersonal relationships and behaviors [36]. Consistent with these perspectives, positive parent–child interactions have been shown to significantly predict children's prosocial behavior, as seen in the findings of Liu and Wang [28]. Moreover, Attachment Theory provides a compelling framework for understanding the impact of parent–child relationships on children's social development. Secure attachments, characterized by warmth and responsiveness, are essential for children's development of empathy and cooperative behaviors, which are key components of prosocial conduct [82]. Conversely, insecure attachments may hinder these competencies. Supporting these findings, Katsantonis and Mclellan have demonstrated that high-quality parent–child relationships foster prosocial behaviors in children, underscoring the importance of positive family interactions in developing social competencies [83].

4.3. Mediation of Children's Emotion Regulation

Hypothesis 3 (H3) of our study posited that emotion regulation may mediate the relation between children's electronic media use and prosocial behavior. Confirmatory results from structural equation modeling indicated a notable association, suggesting that as children's electronic media use increases, their capacity for emotion regulation may be compromised, which is associated with a lower propensity for prosocial behavior. This finding contributes to understanding how electronic media, which often require rapid and reactive attention shifts, may influence children's emotional development. The cognitive load imposed by many electronic media tasks may tax children's developing neural systems, leaving less capacity for the reflective control necessary for emotion regulation [84–86]. These findings align with the work of Lobel et al., which associated extensive gameplay on electronic devices with increased emotional problems among children [41]. von der Heiden et al. also reported that problematic video game use was moderately negatively associated with emotional and psychological well-being, further highlighting the potential impact of electronic media on children's emotional competencies [87].

Beyond psychological explanations, recent research has revealed the physiological underpinnings that strengthen the association between emotion regulation and prosocial behavior in children. Eisenberg accentuated the role of cardiac vagal tone—a physiological marker of emotion regulation—in nurturing prosocial behavior, suggesting that a calm and well-regulated emotional state is likely instrumental in promoting prosocial actions [88]. In support of this notion, Song et al. provided complementary evidence, showing that children who excel in emotion regulation tend to exhibit more prosocial behaviors [51]. Likewise, Elhusseini et al. found that children skilled in managing their emotions demonstrate a heightened ability to attend to others' needs and show an increased propensity for helping behaviors in difficult situations [50].

4.4. Sequential Mediation of Parent–Child Closeness and Children's Emotion Regulation

Our investigation substantiates Hypothesis 4 (H4), suggesting that parent–child closeness and emotion regulation sequentially mediate the relation between children's electronic media use and prosocial behaviors. Specifically, this hypothesis considers a pathway wherein elevated levels of electronic media engagement in children may correlate with diminished parent–child intimacy. This observed decrease in closeness is associated with a corresponding decrease in children's emotion regulation capabilities, which may be related to a reduction in prosocial behaviors. The Parent–Child Emotion Regulation Dynamics model, developed by Morris and colleagues, provides a framework for understanding the association between parent–child relationships and children's emotion regulation [89]. It emphasizes the dynamic, reciprocal processes of emotion regulation within the parent–child interaction, where both parties influence each other's emotional states. This model is enhanced by neurobiological research, such as that by Ratliff et al., which includes cross-brain associations in dyadic emotion regulation during social-emotional interactions, highlighting the role of coordinated brain responses in shaping children's emotion regulation [90]. Supporting this, studies like Liu et al.'s associate negative parent–child interactions with negative emotion regulation outcomes in children [91].

In the nuanced interplay between electronic media use and children's prosocial behavior, the chain mediation effect of parent–child closeness and emotion regulation emerges as a pivotal factor. Geng et al. highlight how children's intensified use of electronic media may clash with parental expectations, potentially diminishing parent–child intimacy and increasing the likelihood of conflict [66]. This disruption in closeness is a critical precursor to the observed impairments in emotion regulation as outlined by Cummings and Davies [52] and Fabes et al. [53], which, in turn, can lead to decreased prosocial behaviors among children. The findings of Criss et al. reinforce this cascade by delineating the strong link between the quality of parent–child relationships and children's emotion regulation and subsequent behavior patterns [92]. Secure attachments, foundational for the development of effortful control as described by Gross et al., enable children to engage in other-oriented behavior, a cornerstone of prosocial action [93]. By eroding these attachments, excessive electronic media use may decrease positive parent–child interactions, reducing closeness and fostering emotional dysregulation. This sequence—beginning with electronic media use and flowing through diminished parent–child closeness and impaired emotion regulation—culminates in reduced prosocial behavior, outlining a clear chain-mediating pathway.

4.5. Limitations and Future Research Directions

In the present study, we explored how children's electronic media use might inversely relate to their prosocial behaviors and how this relation is potentially mediated by parent–child closeness and the children's ability to regulate emotions. These connections offer insights into the multifaceted influences of digital media consumption on the healthy development of children. Nevertheless, acknowledging the limitations enhances the robustness of the research.

Turning to the constraints of our study, we acknowledge that our analysis did not differentiate between various types of electronic media content such as video games, internet usage, or TV programs. While programs like "Baby Einstein" and "Sesame Street" are intentionally designed for children, providing educational content and themes suitable for their developmental stages, our study did not precisely control for these distinctions. Future studies should incorporate a comprehensive content analysis to deepen our understanding of how media influences children's social and emotional well-being. Such an analysis would examine how various types of media—educational, entertainment, and social networking—differentially affect children's development. By exploring the specific intentions behind media design, such as whether they aim to enhance learning or foster social skills, researchers can better assess how these influences contribute to or detract from children's prosocial behaviors.

Beyond the content analysis, the methodological design of our research also warrants further discussion. Our study's methodology is rooted in cross-sectional analysis, which provides a snapshot of the complex relations between children's electronic media use and prosocial behavior. While useful, this approach is limited in its ability to ascertain the directionality or causality of these relationships. The intricate dynamics of how children's media consumption patterns might be shaped by, and potentially shape, the quality of parent–child interactions call for a deeper, temporal examination. In light of this, adopting a longitudinal research design would be highly valuable, enabling observation of the long-term dynamics between children's electronic media use and prosocial development and providing the evolution of these relations over time.

Additionally, while considering the data's validity, the nature of its collection necessitates scrutiny. Parental self-reports, which served as the primary data source for this study, are susceptible to biases such as social desirability, where respondents may answer in a manner they perceive to be more favorable rather than reflecting their actual behaviors or feelings. Such biases can particularly distort insights into sensitive areas such as parent–child relationships. Thus, future research should adopt a multifaceted data collection strategy to mitigate these limitations and enhance the reliability of the findings. An improved research methodology would incorporate objective measures like digital usage logs and behavioral observations to complement self-reported data. Additionally, collecting data from multiple informants, including teachers and healthcare providers, could broaden the perspective and enrich the data quality. Furthermore, directly engaging with children alongside their parents would offer deeper insights into family dynamics and their impact on children's prosocial behaviors and interactions with media. This comprehensive approach would provide a more holistic understanding of the factors influencing children's development in a digital world.

In addition to the methodological enhancements, the development of children's prosocial behavior is influenced by multiple factors, including temperament, which plays a crucial role. While the emotion regulation examined in this study partially reflects temperament, it is clear that a more detailed control of variables such as children's temperament types is necessary for future studies to provide a more comprehensive understanding of prosocial development in the digital media era. Additionally, replicating this study with parents of older children would be insightful, particularly by comparing groups with preschoolers, school-aged children, and adolescents. This approach would allow us to explore how prosocial behavior evolves with age and how different stages of childhood might interact differently with media use.

4.6. Practical Implications

Drawing on the findings of our study, the practical implications for children's development in the context of digital media are multifaceted. These implications, integrating the research outcomes, provide a framework for informed interventions and strategies to support children's healthy development in the digital age.

Parent–child closeness is a critical factor in mediating the impact of electronic media use on children's prosocial behavior. This finding underscores the importance of fostering strong parent–child relationships. Parents can be encouraged to engage more actively with their children's media use, supervising and participating in their digital activities. This active involvement can provide opportunities for bonding, understanding each other's perspectives, and guiding children toward positive digital practices.

Emotion regulation emerged as a crucial mediator between electronic media use and prosocial behavior. Educational interventions can be designed in schools and communities to enhance children's emotional awareness and management skills. These programs can be integrated into the curriculum or offered as extracurricular activities, focusing on teaching children effective strategies for understanding and regulating their emotions, which are necessary for developing prosocial behaviors.

Considering the complex interplay between electronic media use and children's development, promoting a balanced approach to digital consumption is essential. Parents and educators can collaborate to set reasonable limits on screen time while encouraging children to engage in various activities that support their social and emotional development. This balanced approach should include outdoor activities, reading, and face-to-face social interactions, pivotal for holistic growth.

In summary, the practical implications of our research highlight the need for comprehensive strategies involving parents and educators to support children's development in the digital age. By enhancing parent–child closeness, improving emotion regulation skills, and promoting a balanced media diet, we can guide children toward positive developmental outcomes in the era of digital media.

5. Conclusions

Our study found a notable association between children's electronic media use and prosocial behavior, underscoring the complex dynamics of digital media in the context of child development. The research not only highlighted the individual mediating roles of parent–child closeness and emotion regulation but also importantly confirmed their interconnected, sequential mediation effect in this relation. The results suggest that extensive involvement in electronic media might be linked to decreased parent–child closeness and could be associated with challenges in emotion regulation, which in turn appears to correlate with reduced prosocial behaviors in children.

Author Contributions: Conceptualization, X.L. and S.G.; methodology, S.G.; software, S.G.; validation, X.L. and S.G.; formal analysis, S.G.; investigation, X.L.; resources, X.L. and D.D.; data curation, S.G.; writing—original draft preparation, S.G.; writing—review and editing, X.L. and D.D.; visualization, S.G.; supervision, X.L. and D.D.; project administration, X.L.; funding acquisition, X.L. All authors have read and agreed to the published version of the manuscript.

Funding: This research was funded by the Beijing Social Science Foundation Project, grant number 22GJB017, and the R&D Program of the Beijing Municipal Education Commission, grant number SZ202310028013.

Institutional Review Board Statement: The study was conducted in accordance with the Declaration of Helsinki, and approved by the Institutional Review Board of Capital Normal University (No. IRB-2023-0617), approved on 10 December 2023.

Informed Consent Statement: Informed consent was obtained from all subjects involved in the study.

Data Availability Statement: The data from this study can be obtained by contacting the corresponding author.

Acknowledgments: We would like to express our deepest gratitude to the editors and reviewers for their invaluable guidance and constructive suggestions. Their expertise and detailed feedback have been instrumental in enhancing the overall quality of this manuscript.

Conflicts of Interest: The authors declare no conflicts of interest.

References

1. Pitol, N.S.; Patwary, M.M.; Aurnob, S.; Ahmed, S.; Islam, M.A.; Dash, H.K.; Hasan, T.; Ruhani, A.; Islam, A.; Saha, C. Exploring media consumption and mental health among young adults during the second wave of COVID-19 in Bangladesh. *Heliyon* **2023**, *9*, e20371. [CrossRef] [PubMed]
2. Chen, Q.N.; Liang, M.N.; Li, Y.M.; Guo, J.C.; Fei, D.X.; Wang, L.; He, L.; Sheng, C.H.; Cai, Y.W.; Li, X.J.; et al. Mental health care for medical staff in China during the COVID-19 outbreak. *Lancet Psychiatry* **2020**, *7*, E15–E16. [CrossRef]
3. Nugroho, F.A.; Ruchaina, A.N.; Wicaksono, A.G.L. Effects of COVID-19 Pandemic on Changes in Nutritional Status and Physical Activities of School-Age Children: A Scoping Review. *J. Gizi Pangan* **2022**, *17*, 139–148. [CrossRef]
4. Nagata, J.M.; Cortez, C.A.; Cattle, C.J.; Ganson, K.T.; Iyer, P.; Bibbins-Domingo, K.; Baker, F.C. Screen Time Use among US Adolescents During the COVID-19 Pandemic Findings from the Adolescent Brain Cognitive Development (ABCD) Study. *JAMA Pediatr.* **2022**, *176*, 94–96. [CrossRef] [PubMed]
5. Carroll, N.; Sadowski, A.; Laila, A.; Hruska, V.; Nixon, M.; Ma, D.W.L.; Haines, J.; Guelph Family Hlth, S. The Impact of COVID-19 on Health Behavior, Stress, Financial and Food Security among Middle to High Income Canadian Families with Young Children. *Nutrients* **2020**, *12*, 2352. [CrossRef] [PubMed]
6. So, H.K.; Chua, G.T.; Yip, K.M.; Tung, K.T.S.; Wong, R.S.; Louie, L.H.T.; Tso, W.W.Y.; Wong, I.C.K.; Yam, J.C.; Kwan, M.Y.W.; et al. Impact of COVID-19 Pandemic on School-Aged Children's Physical Activity, Screen Time, and Sleep in Hong Kong: A Cross-Sectional Repeated Measures Study. *Int. J. Environ. Res. Public Health* **2022**, *19*, 10539. [CrossRef]

7. Liu, X.C.; Geng, S.L.; Lei, T.; Cheng, Y.; Yu, H. Connections between Parental Phubbing and Electronic Media Use in Young Children: The Mediating Role of Parent-Child Conflict and Moderating Effect of Child Emotion Regulation. *Behav. Sci.* **2024**, *14*, 119. [CrossRef]
8. Feng, J.; Spence, I.; Pratt, J. Playing an action video game reduces gender differences in spatial cognition. *Psychol. Sci.* **2007**, *18*, 850–855. [CrossRef] [PubMed]
9. Zoromba, M.A.A.; Abdelgawad, D.; Hashem, S.; El-Gazar, H.; El Aziz, M.A.A. Association between media exposure and behavioral problems among preschool children. *Front. Psychol.* **2023**, *14*, 1080550. [CrossRef] [PubMed]
10. Raheem, A.; Khan, S.G.; Ahmed, M.; Alvi, F.J.; Saleem, K.; Batool, S. Impact of Excessive Screen Time on Speech and Language in Children. *J. Liaquat Univ. Med. Health Sci.* **2023**, *22*, 155–159. [CrossRef]
11. Ferreira, T.; Cadima, J.; Matias, M.; Vieira, J.M.; Leal, T.; Matos, P.M. Preschool Children's Prosocial Behavior: The Role of Mother-Child, Father-Child and Teacher-Child Relationships. *J. Child Fam. Stud.* **2016**, *25*, 1829–1839. [CrossRef]
12. Xu, K.; Geng, S.L.; Dou, D.H.; Liu, X.C. Relations between Video Game Engagement and Social Development in Children: The Mediating Role of Executive Function and Age-Related Moderation. *Behav. Sci.* **2023**, *13*, 833. [CrossRef] [PubMed]
13. Zhao, Q.; Wang, Z.H.; Wang, D.F.; Yuan, Y.Y.; Yin, X.Y.; Li, Z.H. Developmental trajectory of prosocial behavior in impoverished children during early adolescence: The effects of gender and parenting style heterogeneity. *Psychol. Dev. Educ.* **2023**, *39*, 323–332. [CrossRef]
14. Zahnwaxler, C.; Radkeyarrow, M.; Wagner, E.; Chapman, M. Development of concern for others. *Dev. Psychol.* **1992**, *28*, 126–136. [CrossRef]
15. Duffy, M.K.; Scott, K.L.; Shaw, J.D.; Tepper, B.J.; Aquino, K. A Social context model of envy and social undermining. *Acad. Manag. J.* **2012**, *55*, 643–666. [CrossRef]
16. Coyne, S.M.; Padilla-Walker, L.M.; Holmgren, H.G.; Davis, E.J.; Collier, K.M.; Memmott-Elison, M.K.; Hawkins, A.J. A Meta-Analysis of Prosocial Media on Prosocial Behavior, Aggression, and Empathic Concern: A Multidimensional Approach. *Dev. Psychol.* **2018**, *54*, 331–347. [CrossRef] [PubMed]
17. Stone, B.G.; Mills, K.A.; Saggers, B. Online multiplayer games for the social interactions of children with autism spectrum disorder: A resource for inclusive education. *Int. J. Incl. Educ.* **2019**, *23*, 209–228. [CrossRef]
18. Prot, S.; Gentile, D.A.; Anderson, C.A.; Suzuki, K.; Swing, E.; Lim, K.M.; Horiuchi, Y.; Jelic, M.; Krahé, B.; Wei, L.Q.; et al. Long-Term Relations among Prosocial-Media Use, Empathy, and Prosocial Behavior. *Psychol. Sci.* **2014**, *25*, 358–368. [CrossRef]
19. Ostrov, J.M.; Gentile, D.A.; Crick, N.R. Media exposure, aggression and prosocial behavior during early childhood: A longitudinal study. *Soc. Dev.* **2006**, *15*, 612–627. [CrossRef]
20. Poulain, T.; Ludwig, J.; Hiemisch, A.; Hilbert, A.; Kiess, W. Media Use of Mothers, Media Use of Children, and Parent-Child Interaction Are Related to Behavioral Difficulties and Strengths of Children. *Int. J. Environ. Res. Public Health* **2019**, *16*, 4651. [CrossRef]
21. Guo, X. Research on the Influence of Media Violence on Youth. *Adv. Soc. Sci. Educ. Humanit.* **2022**, *631*, 1170–1173. [CrossRef]
22. Veraksa, A.N.; Bukhalenkova, D.A.; Chichinina, E.A.; Almazova, O.V. Relationship Between the Use of Digital Devices and Personal and Emotional Development in Preschool Children. *Psikhologicheskaya Nauka Obraz.-Psychol. Sci. Edu.* **2021**, *26*, 27–40. [CrossRef]
23. Lissak, G. Adverse physiological and psychological effects of screen time on children and adolescents: Literature review and case study. *Environ. Res.* **2018**, *164*, 149–157. [CrossRef] [PubMed]
24. Christensen, J.F. Pleasure junkies all around! Why it matters and why 'the arts' might be the answer: A biopsychological perspective. *Proc. Biol. Sci.* **2017**, *284*, 20162837. [CrossRef] [PubMed]
25. Masten, C.L.; Morelli, S.A.; Eisenberger, N.I. An fMRI investigation of empathy for 'social pain' and subsequent prosocial behavior. *Neuroimage* **2011**, *55*, 381–388. [CrossRef] [PubMed]
26. Gentile, D.; Groves, C.; Gentile, J. The general learning model: Unveiling the teaching potential of video games. In *Learning by Playing: Video Gaming in Education*; Blumberg, F., Ed.; Oxford University Press: New York, NY, USA, 2014; pp. 121–142.
27. Wiegman, O.; van Schie, E.G.M. Video game playing and its relations with aggressive and prosocial behaviour. *Br. J. Soc. Psychol.* **1998**, *37*, 367–378. [CrossRef] [PubMed]
28. Liu, Q.W.; Wang, Z.H. The interactive effects of parent-child relationship, sensory processing sensitivity, and the COMT Val158Met polymorphism on preschoolers' prosocial behaviors. *Acta Psychol. Sin.* **2023**, *55*, 711–725. [CrossRef]
29. Pianta, R.C. Child-parent relationship scale. *J. Early Child. Infant Psychol.* **1992**, *427*, 1–3.
30. Zhu, Y.L.; Deng, L.Y.; Wan, K. The association between parent-child relationship and problematic internet use among English- and Chinese-language studies: A meta-analysis. *Front. Psychol.* **2022**, *13*, 885819. [CrossRef]
31. Horita, H.; Seki, Y.; Shimizu, E. Parents? Perspectives on Their Relationship with Their Adolescent Children with Internet Addiction: Survey Study. *JMIR Pediatr. Parent.* **2022**, *5*, e35466. [CrossRef]
32. Ahmadian, M.; Namnabati, M.; Joonbakhsh, F. Investigation of correlation between internet addiction and parent-child relationship in girls' adolescence in the COVID-19 pandemic. *J. Educ. Health Promot.* **2022**, *11*, 340. [CrossRef] [PubMed]
33. Hong, W.; Liu, R.D.; Ding, Y.; Oei, T.P.; Zhen, R.; Jiang, S.Y. Parents' Phubbing and Problematic Mobile Phone Use: The Roles of the Parent-Child Relationship and Children's Self-Esteem. *Cyberpsychol. Behav. Soc. Netw.* **2019**, *22*, 779–786. [CrossRef] [PubMed]
34. Sampasa-Kanyinga, H.; Goldfield, G.S.; Kingsbury, M.; Clayborne, Z.; Colman, I. Social media use and parent-child relationship: A cross-sectional study of adolescents. *J. Community Psychol.* **2020**, *48*, 793–803. [CrossRef]

35. Nergiz, M.E.; Çaylan, N.; Yalçin, S.S.; Oflu, A.; Tezol, Ö.; Özdemir, D.F.; Ciçek, S.; Yildiz, D. Excessive screen time is associated with maternal rejection behaviours in pre-school children. *J. Paediatr. Child Health* **2020**, *56*, 1077–1082. [CrossRef] [PubMed]
36. Yan, J.; Feng, X.; Schoppe-Sullivan, S.J. Longitudinal Associations Between Parent-Child Relationships in Middle Childhood and Child-Perceived Loneliness. *J. Fam. Psychol.* **2018**, *32*, 841–847. [CrossRef]
37. Xu, L.Y.; Liu, L.S.; Li, Y.F.; Liu, L.J.; Huntsinger, C.S. Parent-child relationships and Chinese children's social adaptations: Gender difference in parent-child dyads. *Pers. Relatsh.* **2018**, *25*, 462–479. [CrossRef]
38. Calatrava, M.; Swords, L.; Spratt, T. Socio-emotional adjustment in children attending family centres: The role of the parent-child relationship. *Br. J. Soc. Work* **2023**, *53*, 2725–2741. [CrossRef]
39. Padilla-Walker, L.M.; Carlo, G.; Christensen, K.J.; Yorgason, J.B. Bidirectional Relations between Authoritative Parenting and Adolescents' Prosocial Behaviors. *J. Res. Adolesc.* **2012**, *22*, 400–408. [CrossRef]
40. Gross, J.J. Emotion regulation: Past, present, future. *Cogn. Emot.* **1999**, *13*, 551–573. [CrossRef]
41. Lobel, A.; Engels, R.; Stone, L.L.; Burk, W.J.; Granic, I. Video Gaming and Children's Psychosocial Wellbeing: A Longitudinal Study. *J. Youth Adolesc.* **2017**, *46*, 884–897. [CrossRef]
42. Günaydin, N.; Arici, Y.K.; Kutlu, F.Y.; Demir, E.Y. The relationship between problematic internet use in adolescents and emotion regulation difficulty and family Internet attitude. *J. Community Psychol.* **2022**, *50*, 1135–1154. [CrossRef] [PubMed]
43. Özer, D.; Altun, Ö.; Avsar, G. Investigation of the relationship between internet addiction, communication skills and difficulties in emotion regulation in nursing students. *Arch. Psychiatr. Nurs.* **2023**, *42*, 18–24. [CrossRef]
44. Oflu, A.; Tezol, O.; Yalcin, S.; Yildiz, D.; Caylan, N.; Ozdemir, D.F.; Cicek, S.; Nergiz, M.E. Excessive screen time is associated with emotional lability in preschool children. *Arch. Argent. Pediatr.* **2021**, *119*, 106–113. [CrossRef] [PubMed]
45. Hidayatullah, A.; Naz, F.; Niazi, S. Internet Addiction: Predictor of Disturbed Emotion Regulation, Sleep quality and General Health in University Students. *FWU J. Soc. Sci.* **2023**, *17*, 78–89. [PubMed]
46. Lin, P.Y.; Lin, H.C.; Lin, P.C.; Yen, J.Y.; Ko, C.H. The association between emotional regulation and internet gaming disorder. *Psychiatry Res.* **2020**, *289*, 113060. [CrossRef]
47. Dunfield, K.A. A construct divided: Prosocial behavior as helping, sharing, and comforting subtypes. *Front. Psychol.* **2014**, *5*, 958. [CrossRef]
48. Benita, M.; Levkovitz, T.; Roth, G. Integrative emotion regulation predicts adolescents' prosocial behavior through the mediation of empathy. *Learn. Instr.* **2017**, *50*, 14–20. [CrossRef]
49. Fabes, R.A.; Eisenberg, N.; Karbon, M.; Troyer, D.; Switzer, G. The relations of children's emotion regulation to their vicarious emotional responses and comforting behaviors. *Child Dev.* **1994**, *65*, 1678–1693. [CrossRef]
50. Elhusseini, S.; Rawn, K.; El-Sheikh, M.; Keller, P.S. Attachment and prosocial behavior in middle childhood: The role of emotion regulation. *J. Exp. Child Psychol.* **2023**, *225*, 105534. [CrossRef]
51. Song, J.H.; Colasante, T.; Malti, T. Helping Yourself Helps Others: Linking Children's Emotion Regulation to Prosocial Behavior Through Sympathy and Trust. *Emotion* **2018**, *18*, 518–527. [CrossRef]
52. Cummings, E.M.; Davies, P. Emotional security as a regulatory process in normal development and the development of psychopathology. *Dev. Psychopathol.* **1996**, *8*, 123–139. [CrossRef]
53. Fabes, R.A.; Leonard, S.A.; Kupanoff, K.; Martin, C.L. Parental coping with children's negative emotions: Relations with children's emotional and social responding. *Child Dev.* **2001**, *72*, 907–920. [CrossRef] [PubMed]
54. Paulus, M. The multidimensional nature of early prosocial behavior: A motivational perspective. *Curr. Opin. Psychol.* **2018**, *20*, 111–116. [CrossRef]
55. Reindl, V.; Gerloff, C.; Scharke, W.; Konrad, K. Brain-to-brain synchrony in parent-child dyads and the relationship with emotion regulation revealed by fNIRS-based hyperscanning. *Neuroimage* **2018**, *178*, 493–502. [CrossRef] [PubMed]
56. Feldman, R. Mutual influences between child emotion regulation and parent-child reciprocity support development across the first 10 years of life: Implications for developmental psychopathology. *Dev. Psychopathol.* **2015**, *27*, 1007–1023. [CrossRef] [PubMed]
57. Zhao, H.; Cheng, T.; Zhai, Y.; Long, Y.H.; Wang, Z.Y.; Lu, C.M. How Mother-Child Interactions are Associated with a Child's Compliance. *Cereb. Cortex* **2021**, *31*, 4398–4410. [CrossRef]
58. Ainsworth, M.D.S. Bowlby-Ainsworth attachment theory. *Behav. Brain Sci.* **1978**, *1*, 436–438. [CrossRef]
59. Bronfenbrenner, U.; Morris, P.A. The ecology of developmental processes. In *Handbook of Child Psychology: Theoretical Models of Human Development*, 5th ed.; Damon, W., Lerner, R.M., Eds.; John Wiley & Sons Inc.: Hoboken, NJ, USA, 1998; Volume 1, pp. 993–1028.
60. Acar, I.H.; Evans, M.Y.Q.; Rudasill, K.M.; Yildiz, S. The contributions of relationships with parents and teachers to Turkish children's antisocial behaviour. *Educ. Psychol.* **2018**, *38*, 877–897. [CrossRef]
61. Knafo, A.; Plomin, R. Parental discipline and affection and children's prosocial behavior: Genetic and environmental links. *J. Pers. Soc. Psychol.* **2006**, *90*, 147–164. [CrossRef]
62. Faul, F.; Erdfelder, E.; Buchner, A.; Lang, A.G. Statistical power analyses using G*Power 3.1: Tests for correlation and regression analyses. *Behav. Res. Methods* **2009**, *41*, 1149–1160. [CrossRef]
63. Bentler, P.M.; Chou, C.P. Practical issues in structural modeling. *Sociol. Methods Res.* **1987**, *16*, 78–117. [CrossRef]
64. Liu, X.J.; Li, Y. The influence of mother's perception of coparenting on behavior problems among children: A moderated mediation model. *Psychol. Dev. Educ.* **2022**, *38*, 626–634. [CrossRef]

65. Huang, H.Q.; Zhou, Y.; Qu, F.B.; Liu, X.C. The Role of Parenting Styles and Parents' Involvement in Young Children's Videogames Use. In Proceedings of the HCI in Games: Second International Conference, Copenhagen, Denmark, 19–24 July 2020.
66. Geng, S.L.; Xu, K.; Liu, X.C. Association between Electronic Media Use and Internalizing Problems: The Mediating Effect of Parent-Child Conflict and Moderating Effect of Children's Age. *Behav. Sci.* **2023**, *13*, 694. [CrossRef]
67. Xu, H.Y.; Wang, X.Y. Home chaos and prosocial behavior of young children in two-child families: The chain mediating role of parent-child and sibling relationship. *Chin. J. Clin. Psychol.* **2023**, *31*, 1391–1394. [CrossRef]
68. Shields, A.; Cicchetti, D. Emotion regulation among school-age children: The development and validation of a new criterion Q-sort scale. *Dev. Psychol.* **1997**, *33*, 906–916. [CrossRef]
69. Xing, X.P.; Zhao, X.Y.; Hu, X. Reciprocal relation between executive function and emotion regulation in preschoolers: A cross-lagged and random intercept cross-lagged analysis. *J. Psychol. Sci.* **2024**, *47*, 80–88. [CrossRef]
70. Goodman, R. The strengths and difficulties questionnaire: A research note. *J. Child Psychol. Psychiatry* **1997**, *38*, 581–586. [CrossRef]
71. Aarø, L.E.; Davids, E.L.; Mathews, C.; Wubs, A.G.; Smith, O.R.F.; de Vries, P.J. Internalizing problems, externalizing problems, and prosocial behavior—Three dimensions of the strengths and difficulties questionnaire (SDQ): A study among South African adolescents. *Scand. J. Psychol.* **2022**, *63*, 415–425. [CrossRef]
72. Podsakoff, P.M.; MacKenzie, S.B.; Lee, J.Y.; Podsakoff, N.P. Common method biases in behavioral research: A critical review of the literature and recommended remedies. *J. Appl. Psychol.* **2003**, *88*, 879–903. [CrossRef]
73. Reng, C.R. Measurement methodology on social economic status index of students. *J. Educ. Stud.* **2010**, *673*, 77–82. [CrossRef]
74. Little, T.D.; Cunningham, W.A.; Shahar, G.; Widaman, K.F. To parcel or not to parcel: Exploring the question, weighing the merits. *Struct. Equ. Model.* **2002**, *9*, 151–173. [CrossRef]
75. Rogers, W.M.; Schmitt, N. Parameter recovery and model fit using multidimensional composites: A comparison of four empirical parceling algorithms. *Multivar. Behav. Res.* **2004**, *39*, 379–412. [CrossRef]
76. Ding, K.Y.; Shen, Y.N.; Liu, Q.M.; Li, H.; Giansanti, D. The Effects of Digital Addiction on Brain Function and Structure of Children and Adolescents: A Scoping Review. *Healthcare* **2024**, *12*, 15. [CrossRef]
77. Kattein, E.; Schmidt, H.; Witt, S.; Joerren, H.L.; Menrath, I.; Rumpf, H.J.; Wartberg, L.; Pawils, S.; Connelly, M.A. Increased Digital Media Use in Preschool Children: Exploring the Links with Parental Stress and Their Problematic Media Use. *Children* **2023**, *10*, 1921. [CrossRef]
78. Hauser, D.J.; Preston, S.D.; Stansfield, R.B. Altruism in the Wild: When Affiliative Motives to Help Positive People Overtake Empathic Motives to Help the Distressed. *J. Exp. Psychol. Gen.* **2014**, *143*, 1295–1305. [CrossRef]
79. Marques, L.M.; Uchida, P.M.; Aguiar, F.O.; Kadri, G.; Santos, R.I.M.; Barbosa, S.P. Escaping through virtual gaming-what is the association with emotional, social, and mental health? A systematic review. *Front. Psychiatry* **2023**, *14*, 1257685. [CrossRef]
80. Beyens, I.; Beullens, K. Parent-child conflict about children's tablet use: The role of parental mediation. *New Media Soc.* **2017**, *19*, 2075–2093. [CrossRef]
81. Davies, P.T.; Cummings, E.M. Marital conflict and child adjustment—An emotional security hypothesis. *Psychol. Bull.* **1994**, *116*, 387–411. [CrossRef]
82. Bretherton, I. Attachment theory: Retrospect and prospect. *Monogr. Soc. Res. Child Dev.* **1985**, *50*, 3–35. [CrossRef]
83. Katsantonis, I.; McLellan, R. The role of parent-child interactions in the association between mental health and prosocial behavior: Evidence from early childhood to late adolescence. *Int. J. Behav. Dev.* **2024**, *48*, 59–70. [CrossRef]
84. Demir, Y.P.; Sümer, M.M. Effects of smartphone overuse on headache, sleep and quality of life in migraine patients. *Neurosciences* **2019**, *24*, 115–121. [CrossRef] [PubMed]
85. Alqassim, A.Y.; Alharbi, A.A.; Muaddi, M.A.; Makeen, A.M.; Shuayri, W.H.; Safhi, A.M.; Alfifa, A.Y.; Samily, I.H.; Darbashi, N.A.; Otayn, M.A.; et al. Associations of Electronic Device Use and Physical Activity with Headaches in Saudi Medical Students. *Medicina-Lithuania* **2024**, *60*, 299. [CrossRef]
86. Rathod, A.S.; Ingole, A.; Gaidhane, A.; Choudhari, S.G. Psychological Morbidities Associated with Excessive Usage of Smart-phones among Adolescents and Young Adults: A Review. *Cureus J. Med. Sci.* **2022**, *14*, e30756. [CrossRef] [PubMed]
87. von der Heiden, J.M.; Braun, B.; Müller, K.W.; Egloff, B. The Association Between Video Gaming and Psychological Functioning. *Front. Psychol.* **2019**, *10*, 1731. [CrossRef]
88. Eisenberg, N. Emotion, regulation, and moral development. *Annu. Rev. Psychol.* **2000**, *51*, 665–697. [CrossRef] [PubMed]
89. Morris, A.S.; Cui, L.X.; Criss, M.M.; Simmons, W.K. Emotion regulation dynamics during parent–child interactions: Implications for research and practice. In *Emotion Regulation: A Matter of Time*, 1st ed.; Cole, P.M., Hollenstein, T., Eds.; Routledge: London, UK; New York, NY, USA, 2018; pp. 70–90.
90. Ratliff, E.L.; Kerr, K.L.; Cosgrove, K.T.; Simmons, W.K.; Morris, A.S. The Role of Neurobiological Bases of Dyadic Emotion Regulation in the Development of Psychopathology: Cross-Brain Associations Between Parents and Children. *Clin. Child Fam. Psychol. Rev.* **2022**, *25*, 5–18. [CrossRef] [PubMed]
91. Liu, X.C.; Geng, S.L.; Xu, K.; Huang, H.Q. Parental phubbing and parent-children relationship: Chain mediation effects of preschooler's emotional instability and externalizing problem behavior. *J. Tianjin Norm. Univ. (Soc. Sci.)* **2023**, *6*, 121–128.

92. Criss, M.M.; Cui, L.X.; Wood, E.E.; Morris, A.S. Associations between Emotion Regulation and Adolescent Adjustment Difficulties: Moderating Effects of Parents and Peers. *J. Child Fam. Stud.* **2021**, *30*, 1979–1989. [CrossRef]
93. Gross, J.T.; Stern, J.A.; Brett, B.E.; Cassidy, J. The multifaceted nature of prosocial behavior in children: Links with attachment theory and research. *Soc. Dev.* **2017**, *26*, 661–678. [CrossRef]

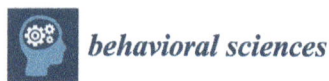 *behavioral sciences*

Article

Developmental Trajectories of Loneliness Among Chinese Early Adolescents: The Roles of Early Peer Preference and Social Withdrawal

Wanfen Chen [1,*,†] and Bowen Xiao [2,†]

1   School of Education, Suzhou University of Science and Technology, Suzhou 215009, China
2   Faculty of Education, The University of British Columbia, Vancouver, BC V6T 1Z4, Canada;
     bowen.xiao@ubc.ca
*   Correspondence: chenwf827@163.com or 2871@mail.usts.edu.cn
†   These authors contributed equally to this work.

Abstract: This study aimed to examine distinct loneliness trajectories and to explore the roles of group-level peer preference and individual-level social withdrawal (i.e., unsociability and shyness) as predictors of these trajectories. Participants were 1134 Chinese elementary school students (Mage = 10.44 years; 565 boys). Data were collected from self-reports and peer nominations. Latent class growth analysis (LCGA) was employed to identify distinct trajectories of loneliness, and multinomial logistic regression was subsequently used to examine the relationships between these trajectories and their predictors. Results showed that three loneliness trajectories were identified: high increasing, moderate decreasing, and low decreasing. Participants at baseline with higher peer preference were more likely to belong to the low decreasing trajectory subgroup rather than the other two subgroups. Furthermore, those at Time 1 with higher unsociability had lower odds of being classified into the moderate or low decreasing trajectory subgroup compared to the high increasing trajectory subgroup. Additionally, participants at baseline with higher shyness had reduced likelihoods of following the low decreasing trajectory subgroup as opposed to the other two subgroups. These results have implications for how we understand both the different subgroups of loneliness trajectories and the predictions of peer preference and social withdrawal on these trajectories in Chinese early adolescents.

Keywords: loneliness; peer preference; unsociability; shyness; social withdrawal; developmental heterogeneity

1. Introduction

Loneliness is commonly defined as a negative emotional response arising from the discrepancy between one's ideal and actual perceptions of their interpersonal relationships [1]. Most people experience different levels of loneliness during their lifetimes [2]. Although temporary loneliness may be adaptive and normative, chronic loneliness poses a significant risk during the early years of life [3]. Chronic loneliness during childhood and adolescence has been linked to a range of psychological issues, including depressive symptoms, suicidal ideation, anxiety, and low self-esteem [4–6], as well as an increased risk for physical health problems, including poor general health, great sleep disturbance, morbidity, and mortality [4,7]. Therefore, it is essential to conduct longitudinal research to identify the factors that contribute to chronic loneliness among children and adolescents. However, existing studies in this field have primarily concentrated on Western societies [4,5]. To our knowledge, little research has examined distinct trajectories of loneliness in Chinese samples or explored predictors of these trajectories [8]. Thus, the current research aims to address these gaps by examining the developmental trajectories of loneliness among Chinese early adolescents, taking into account peer preference and social withdrawal factors such as unsociability and shyness.

1.1. Development of Loneliness from Childhood to Adolescence

Previous empirical research on the developmental trends of loneliness was inconsistent. For example, Heinrich and Gullone summarized that the prevalence of loneliness was the highest during adolescence [2]. However, Brennan suggested that there was no significant difference in loneliness incidences between childhood and adolescent age groups [9]. Additionally, Liu et al. claimed that Chinese children's loneliness decreased over time from grade 2 to grade 5 [10]. Furthermore, a recent meta-analysis of longitudinal studies revealed that, in terms of mean-level development, loneliness tends to decrease throughout childhood and remains relatively stable from adolescence into the oldest old age [11].

These contradictory findings stem from comparisons based on mean-level loneliness, which assume that all individuals within the samples follow the same pattern of changes in loneliness. However, not all children and adolescents are able to successfully form and maintain satisfying social relationships to fulfill their need for belonging [12]. Therefore, individual differences may emerge in the development of loneliness, as not all children and adolescents experience the same patterns of social connection and support [6]. According to Bauer and Curran, researchers may not be able to obtain accurate and adequate information that appeared in distinct subgroups if developmental heterogeneity is not taken into account [13]. Indeed, Western studies have suggested that there existed subgroups in which individuals followed different developmental courses. For instance, Qualter et al. identified four loneliness trajectories in people aged 7–17 (data gathered at 2-year intervals), namely, a low stable (37% of the sample), a moderate decreasing (23%), a moderate increasing (18%), and a relatively high stable subgroup (22%) [4]. Schinka et al. found five discrete trajectories of loneliness (each wave at the age of 9, 11, and 15). These trajectory classes were referred to as low stable (49.1%), moderate increasing (31.6%), decreasing (10.7%), high increasing (4.5%), and chronic (4.1%) [5]. Additionally, Liu et al. found that Chinese children's mean-level loneliness was initially low and decreased in a non-linear (i.e., quadratic) trend from grade 2 to grade 5 [10]. Given the differences in the sample's age range (Mage = 10.44 years at wave 1) and the longitudinal intervals (once a year) in this study compared to previous research, it is reasonable to expect heterogeneity in the developmental trajectories of loneliness among Chinese early adolescents. We anticipate that most will follow a low, decreasing trajectory of loneliness. Additionally, we expect to observe moderate decreasing and high increasing loneliness trajectories as well.

1.2. Peer Preference and Developmental Trajectories of Loneliness

Peer preference refers to the extent to which a child is accepted and liked by their peer group [14]. Loneliness occurs when individuals perceive deficiencies in the quantity and/or quality of their social connections [11]. Peer relationships are among the most important social connections in early adolescence. Positive peer interactions significantly fulfill the need for security and belonging, both of which are essential for the development of socioemotional functioning, including the prevention of loneliness [15]. Moreover, Parkhurst and Hopmeyer's developmental theory on the sources of loneliness suggests that a lack of prestige, popularity, and acceptance among peers can lead to feelings of loneliness in upper-grade elementary and middle school students [16].

Previous longitudinal studies have supported these theoretical perspectives, showing that children who are more popular among their peers tend to experience less loneliness [10,17]. For instance, Liu et al. reported that peer preference as a time-variant variable in latent growth curve modeling reduced loneliness among Grades 2–5 children [10]. In the research of Liu et al., results from the developmental cascade model indicated that peer preference could negatively predict children's later loneliness [17]. Additionally, research on distinct trajectories of loneliness and its predictors among 7–17-year-old individuals showed that low peer preference was a predictor for highly stable and moderately increasing trajectories [4]. Taken together, guided by both theoretical and empirical evidence, we inferred that low peer preference serves as a risk factor for increasing loneliness during early adolescence.

1.3. Social Withdrawal and Developmental Trajectories of Loneliness

Socially withdrawn children and adolescents often remove themselves from peer interactions [18]. We proposed that two subtypes of social withdrawal—unsociability and shyness—might influence the developmental trajectories of loneliness. Unsociability refers to a non-fearful preference for solitude [19]. Unsociable individuals enjoy and value their alone time [20]. Nonetheless, researchers have suggested that unsociability may negatively impact the socioemotional development of older children and early adolescents [20,21]. Individuals who spend excessive time alone miss out on many opportunities for social interactions and skill development, which can negatively affect their social and emotional adjustment, leading to poor social skills, depressive symptoms, and loneliness [15,18]. Moreover, based on Maslow's Hierarchy of Needs [22], humans have strong needs and motivations to form and maintain interpersonal relationships and to gain a sense of belonging, but unsociability may lead to a lack of social connections, which can cause emotional maladjustment such as loneliness [21,23].

Furthermore, researchers have suggested that cultural values influence the implications of different subtypes of social withdrawal [24]. Specifically, Chinese culture is a collectivist culture that focuses on maintaining harmony [25]. Thus, intentionally withdrawing from the social group is viewed as eccentric and abnormal within this cultural context [25]. Therefore, unsociability has been associated with a range of internalizing problems, particularly loneliness, within Chinese culture [21,24]. For instance, Bullock et al. [26] and Xiao et al. [21] both revealed that unsociability was positively related to loneliness in Chinese older children and early adolescents. Additionally, a short-term longitudinal study showed that unsociability perhaps acted as a risk factor for later loneliness among 10–14-year-old children [23]. Despite the consistently detrimental effects of unsociability on Chinese children, to our knowledge, no research has examined whether or how unsociability influences the trajectories of loneliness over time. Based on the aforementioned factors, we hypothesized that high levels of unsociability may serve as a risk factor for increasing loneliness over time among Chinese early adolescents.

Shyness is another subtype of social withdrawal, which refers to a temperamental trait characterized by anxiety and wariness in the face of social interaction [19]. In Western culture, shy children are perceived as deviant, immature, and incompetent [18]. From early childhood to adulthood, shyness is concurrently and predicatively linked to maladjustment [18], such as loneliness, depression, and peer difficulties [27,28]. As discussed before, in traditional Chinese society, being sensitive to others, wariness, and behavioral restraint are positively valued and viewed as social maturity and accomplishment [25]. In this cultural context, shy children may obtain support and encouragement from peers and adults, which in turn would help them develop socioemotional adjustment [25]. However, China has undergone massive economic reform and societal change over the past four decades. In the competitive and fast-paced urban environment, temperament and behavioral traits such as bravery, proactiveness, goal orientation, and expressiveness have become more adaptive for achieving progress and success [25]. This shift has led to a significant decrease in the adaptability of shyness. Indeed, recent research has shown that shyness in children and early adolescents is positively associated with internalizing problems, such as loneliness and depression, in contemporary urban China [28].

Specifically, recent cross-sectional and longitudinal studies have demonstrated that shy children and preadolescents are more likely to experience both concurrent and subsequent loneliness in suburban and urban Chinese areas [24,28]. For instance, Yang et al. indicated that Chinese children's shyness had significant contributions to later internalizing problems (including loneliness) in a four-wave longitudinal study [28]. Therefore, we hypothesized that early adolescents with high levels of shyness are less likely to follow a decreasing trajectory of loneliness and are more likely to follow a high increasing trajectory of loneliness.

1.4. The Present Study

The aim of this study was to describe the developmental trajectories of loneliness and examine the differential effects of peer preference and social withdrawal (i.e., unsociability and shyness) on these trajectories among Chinese early adolescents. Gender was controlled for due to inconsistent findings in previous research regarding gender differences in loneliness trajectories. Based on the aforementioned literature, we hypothesized that the majority of participants would follow low or moderate decreasing loneliness trajectories while a minority would exhibit high increasing loneliness trajectories. Additionally, we posited that participants with high initial peer preference would be more likely to belong to the low decreasing trajectory group, whereas those with high initial levels of shyness would be more likely to follow a high increasing trajectory. Similarly, participants with high initial levels of unsociability were expected to have a higher probability of following the high increasing loneliness trajectory.

2. Materials and Methods

2.1. Participants

Participants were a sample of early adolescents from a large longitudinal study on the development of socioemotional functioning. They were recruited from 19 classes in five public elementary schools in Anhui Province, China. At Time 1 (T1), participants were 1134 fourth-grade students (Mage = 10.44 years, SD = 0.65 years; 565 boys).

Almost all participants in this sample identified their ethnicity as Han, which is the primary ethnic group (about 91% of the whole population) in China. Most of the subjects were from families with low socioeconomic status. Among their parents, about 28.71% of the fathers and 42.23% of the mothers received a junior high school or lower education, 64.77% of the fathers and 52.77% of the mothers received a high school education, and 6.52% of the fathers and 5.00% of the mothers received an education above high school.

Longitudinal data were annually gathered for two years in the same schools. At Time 2 (T2) and Time 3 (T3), 1045 and 1048 participants provided effective data, respectively. We utilized Little's Missing Completely at Random test to examine missing data [29], with $\chi^2 (106) = 130.365$, $p = 0.054$, suggesting that there were no significant differences in main study variables between subjects who participated in all waves and those who did not.

2.2. Measures

2.2.1. Loneliness

Participants rated their loneliness with a Chinese version of the self-report measure, revised by Asher et al. [30]. This single factor measure comprises 16 items (e.g., "Nobody talks to me") employing a 5-point scale (1 meaning not true at all and 5 meaning always true). The mean score of the answers was computed, with higher scores meaning a higher degree of loneliness. This measure has been demonstrated to be valid and reliable in prior research in Chinese children and early adolescents [28]. The internal consistency reliabilities were 0.86 to 0.90 at T1-T3 in the current investigations.

2.2.2. Peer Preference

Each participant nominated a maximum of 3 classmates with whom he/she preferred to be and 3 classmates with whom he/she preferred not to be (i.e., positive and negative nominations). As recommended by previous researchers [31], nominations were permitted for both same-gender and different-gender individuals. The number of nominations for each student received from every classmate was added up and subsequently standardized within each class to enable suitable comparisons. In line with previous research, an index of peer preference was calculated by subtracting negative nomination scores from positive nomination scores [31]. Higher scores on peer preference indicated higher peer likability in the class. This measure has been proven to be valid and reliable in Chinese children and adolescents [17,32].

2.2.3. Unsociability

Unsociability was assessed by a peer nomination measure modified from the Revised Class Play [32,33]. In accordance with the prior procedure [33], each participant nominated up to three classmates who were most suitable for playing the specific role in a class play. Each specific role corresponds to one item. Four items were used to measure unsociability (e.g., "prefer to play alone rather than with others"). Subjects can nominate both same-gender and different-gender classmates. One's nominations received from each classmate for each item were summed and then standardized within the class to account for differences in class size. Previous research demonstrated that this measure is a valid and reliable assessment of unsociability among Chinese children and adolescents [21]. In this research, the Alpha coefficient of this measure was 0.70 at T1.

2.2.4. Shyness

The shyness of participants was assessed by a Chinese version of the Children's Shyness Questionnaire [34], revised by Crozier [35]. This measure consists of 12 self-statements (e.g., "I feel shy when the teacher talks to me") rated on a 3-point scale (1 = yes, 2 = sometimes, 3 = no). The example item and the other nine items were reverse-coded, after which the mean score of the responses was calculated. Higher scores indicated greater levels of shyness. In this study, the Alpha coefficient was 0.74 at T1.

2.3. Procedure

We annually administered a self-report measure of loneliness around the end of the academic year for 3 years. The data were collected in June 2022, June 2023, and June 2024. During data collection of this study, the participants studied and lived normally as they did before the COVID-19 pandemic. Additionally, at T1, we gathered data on peer acceptance rejection (for peer preference) and unsociability from peer nominations, and participants rated their own shyness. Participants were given the necessary explanations during the data collection. There was no indication that the participants encountered any challenges in comprehending the measures or procedures of this study. Ethical approval for the current study was obtained from the institutional review board of the first author's affiliation. Informed consents were obtained from all subjects and their parents via the schools.

2.4. Statistical Analytic Strategy

Data analyses were performed with SPSS 23 and Mplus 7.2. Preliminary analysis was first performed, which mainly included descriptive statistics such as means, standard deviations, and correlation coefficients of the main study variables.

To test our primary hypothesis regarding the various developmental trajectories of loneliness and the predictive influence of peer preference and social withdrawal (i.e., unsociability and shyness) on these trajectories, we conducted the data analysis in three phases. Firstly, to examine the overall pattern in the trajectory of loneliness, we utilized latent growth curve modeling (LGCM) [36], which offers both mean level (referred to as intercept) and mean rate of change (referred to as slope). To evaluate model fit, we employed several statistical indicators, such as the chi-square index (χ^2), in which smaller values are preferred, the Comparative Fit Index (CFI), which should exceed 0.90, and both the Standardized Root Mean Square Residual (SRMR) and the Root Mean Square Error of Approximation (RMSEA), which should be below 0.08 for an acceptable fit [37].

Secondly, to identify distinct classes of loneliness trajectories while accounting for gender differences, we utilized latent class growth analysis (LCGA) [38]. The LCGA method combines both variable-centered and person-centered approaches, allowing for the summarization of longitudinal data by modeling individual variability in developmental trajectories. It identifies a small number of trajectory classes based on differences between individuals (intercepts) and changes within individuals over time (slopes) [38]. Based on LGCM results, a series of LCGAs was performed, and model fit was evaluated using Bayesian Information Criteria (BIC), sample-size adjusted BIC (ABIC), Akaike Information Criteria (AIC), entropy, Lo–Mendell–Rubin likelihood ratio test (LMR-LRT), Vuong–Lo–Mendell–Rubin likelihood ratio test (VLMR-LRT), Bootstrapped LRT (BLRT), and practical usefulness [39]. Lower BIC, ABIC, and AIC values indicated better fit, while entropy values above 0.70 suggested good classification accuracy. LMR-LRT, VLMR-LRT, and BLRT tested whether models with more classes fit better, with BLRT being the most reliable [40]. Practical considerations, such as trajectory shape and class size (no less than 1%), were also factored into model selection [39].

Thirdly, after determining the optimal number of latent classes, we estimated the effects of the predictors (i.e., peer preference, unsociability, and shyness) on class membership using a multinomial logit model. One class was designated as the reference class, and the log odds ratios of belonging to the other classes were compared to this reference, allowing us to assess how each predictor distinguished class membership. Missing data were handled using the full information maximum likelihood method in Mplus 7.2.

3. Results

3.1. Preliminary Analysis

Means, standard deviations, and correlation coefficients for gender, loneliness, peer preference, unsociability, and shyness are shown in Table 1. We then conducted LGCM analyses to assess the mean-level trajectory of loneliness, with results displayed in Table 2 indicating an acceptable model fit. The general trajectory of loneliness showed a decreasing pattern over time. The significant variance in the intercept suggested that there was enough variability to justify exploring interindividual differences in loneliness trajectories using LCGA. Additionally, to determine whether there were any gender-based differences in the overall trend of loneliness, we performed a linear regression analysis of the intercept and slope of the loneliness trajectory on gender. The results showed that gender had no statistically significant effect on the intercept or slope of the loneliness trajectory (B = −0.03, 0.02, $p > 0.1$, respectively), indicating that the average loneliness trajectories for boys and girls were similar in this study.

Table 1. Correlation coefficients, means, and standard deviations of main study variables.

	1	2	3	4	5	6	7
1. Gender	1						
2. Loneliness G4	−0.00	1					
3. Loneliness G5	−0.05	0.50 **	1				
4. Loneliness G6	0.02	0.43 **	0.48 **	1			
5. Peer preference G4	0.09 **	−0.25 **	−0.22 **	−.022 **	1		
6. Unsociability G4	−0.04	0.18 **	0.19 **	0.19 **	−0.32 **	1	
7. Shyness G4	0.08 *	0.31 **	0.22 **	0.17 **	−0.03	0.05	1
Mean	1.50	2.13	1.98	1.89	0.02	−0.01	1.82
Standard deviations	0.50	0.66	0.66	0.67	1.51	0.98	0.37

Note: Gender, 1 = boys, 2 = girls; G, grade; * $p < 0.05$. ** $p < 0.01$.

Table 2. Model fit, means, and variances of intercept and slope in LGCM of loneliness.

Model	Model Fit					Mean		Variance	
	χ^2 (*df*)	*p*	CFI	RMSEA	SRMR	Intercept	Slope	Intercept	Slope
LGCM	3.38 (11)	0.066	0.99	0.05	0.01	2.13 ***	−0.12 ***	0.25 ***	0.03 +

Note: LGCM, latent growth curve model; + $p < 0.1$. *** $p < 0.001$.

3.2. Unconditional LCGA of Loneliness

As shown in Table 3, we estimated models with one to four classes, and the three-class model provided the best fit for the data. We selected the three-class model over the two-class model because it had lower BIC, ABIC, and AIC values, and the additional class represented a distinct group comprising 5.82% of the sample. The three-class model was preferred over the four-class model since the latter included a trajectory with only 0.53% of the sample, which reduced its practical usefulness. Furthermore, compared to the two- and four-class models, the three-class model offered the best balance of interpretability, model parsimony, and goodness-of-fit, as indicated by a significant and replicable BLRT value [41].

Table 3. Results of different latent class growth analyses (LCGA) of loneliness.

Class	BIC	ABIC	AIC	Entropy	LMR-LRT	VLMR-LRT	BLRT	Class Probability
1	6192.285	6176.404	6167.118	N/A	N/A	N/A	N/A	1
2	5640.996	5615.586	5600.728	0.747	<0.001	<0.001	<0.001	0.749/0.251
3	5529.961	5495.022	5474.593	0.732	0.010	0.008	<0.001	0.631/0.058/0.311
4	5502.984	5458.516	5432.515	0.762	0.004	0.003	<0.001	0.005/0.605/0.320/0.070

Note: N, 1134; BIC, Bayesian information criterion; ABIC, sample-size adjusted BIC; AIC, Akaike information criterion; LMR-LRT, Lo–Mendell–Rubin likelihood ratio test; VLMR-LRT, Vuong–Lo–Mendell–Rubin likelihood ratio test; BLRT, bootstrap likelihood ratio test; N/A, Not Available.

Three different trajectories of loneliness were illustrated, and the estimated means of the corresponding trajectories were marked in Figure 1. These trajectories included (1) a high increasing trajectory (intercept = 2.89, SE = 0.14, t = 21.03, $p < 0.001$; slope = 0.26, SE = 0.12, t = 2.20, $p = 0.03$; 66 students, 5.82% of the sample): this trajectory began with the highest level of loneliness in grade 4 and gradually increased throughout these three years; (2) a moderate decreasing trajectory (intercept = 2.56, SE = 0.06, t = 41.96, $p < 0.001$; slope = −0.17, SE = 0.04, t = −3.97, $p < 0.001$; 353 students, 31.13% of the sample): students following this trajectory presented a moderate initial level of loneliness in grade 4 and experienced a decrease within this duration; and (3) a low decreasing trajectory (intercept = 1.81, SE = 0.04, t = 46.14, $p < 0.001$; slope =−0.13, SE = 0.02, t = −6.47, $p < 0.001$; 715 students, 63.05% of the sample): students following this trajectory started with the lowest level of loneliness in grade 4, continued to decrease, and maintained the lowest level throughout the three-year span.

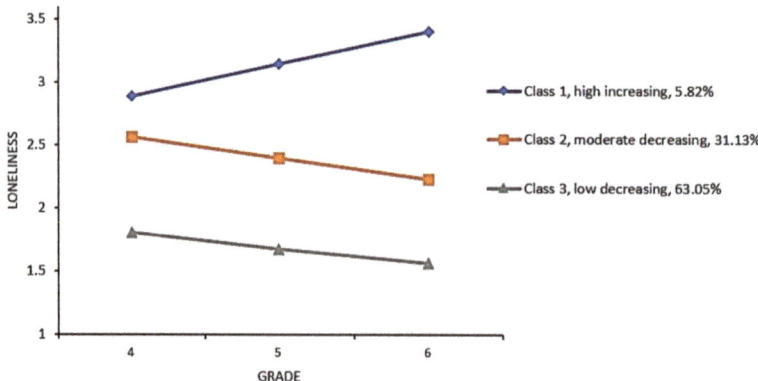

Figure 1. Estimated loneliness trajectories from the three-class LCGA model.

3.3. Conditional LCGA with Covariates Predicting Class Membership

We added covariates (i.e., peer preference, unsociability, and shyness) to the optimal model to examine potential differences among the three class memberships while controlling for gender. To obtain the coefficients of multinomial logistic regression for the predictors on latent class, the high increasing (HI) subgroup was set as a reference group (refer to Table 4). In comparison to the HI subgroup, early adolescents with higher initial levels of peer preference had higher likelihoods (1.73 times) of being categorized into the low decreasing (LD) subgroup, whereas those with higher initial unsociability were less likely to be classified into either the moderate decreasing (MD) subgroup (odds ratio, OR = 0.74) or LD subgroup (OR = 0.59). Additionally, early adolescents with higher initial shyness were significantly less likely to fall into the LD subgroup (OR = 0.11).

Table 4. Multinomial logistic analyses of the relationships between loneliness trajectory class membership and covariates.

| Covariate | Moderate Decreasing | | | Low Decreasing | | | Low Decreasing | | |
| | vs. High Increasing | | | | | | vs. Moderate Decreasing | | |
	Est.	S.E.	OR	Est.	S.E.	OR	Est.	S.E.	OR
Gender	0.04	0.35	1.04	−0.02	0.33	0.98	−0.06	0.21	0.94
Peer Preference	0.11	0.12	1.11	0.55 ***	0.13	1.73	0.44 ***	0.08	1.55
Unsociability	−0.30 *	0.12	0.74	−0.53 **	0.16	0.59	−0.23	0.14	0.79
Shyness	−0.32	0.50	0.73	−2.25 ***	0.48	0.11	−1.93 ***	0.30	0.15

Note: Est., estimate; S.E., standard error; OR, odds ratio. All values are unstandardized estimates. * $p < 0.05$. ** $p < 0.01$. *** $p < 0.001$.

Furthermore, when the MD subgroup was assigned as the reference group, early adolescents with higher scores on initial peer preference had 1.55 times greater probabilities of belonging to the LD subgroup. Relative to the MD subgroup, early adolescents who had higher initial levels of shyness had a considerably lower probability of following the LD subgroup (OR = 0.15).

4. Discussion

Chronic loneliness has numerous negative effects on children's and adolescents' physical and mental health [2,3]. However, there is limited long-term longitudinal research on loneliness trajectories, particularly in non-Western contexts. Therefore, this study primarily focused on examining different trajectories of loneliness and exploring how early peer preference, unsociability, and shyness were related to these trajectories in a substantial sample of Chinese early adolescents.

4.1. Distinct Trajectories of Loneliness

In this study, three distinct loneliness trajectory classes were identified: low decreasing, moderate decreasing, and high increasing. These patterns are somewhat similar to those found in previous research, which also demonstrated developmental heterogeneity in loneliness during early adolescence [4,5,7].

Results revealed that most of the participants followed a low decreasing (63.05%) or moderate decreasing (31.13%) trajectory of loneliness. These findings were partly in line with previous studies that reported large ratios of low stable or moderate decreasing subgroups (37%, 23%, respectively; 49.1%, 10.7%, respectively; 81.5% in low stable subgroup) in children and adolescents [4,5,8]. Notably, in this study, the low level of loneliness was not stable but gradually decreased over the investigation period. Additionally, the two decreasing trajectories began at different initial levels, which aligned with the mean-level changes in loneliness over time. Peer groups play a critical role in providing children and early adolescents with a sense of belonging and intimacy [10,16]. In the upper grades of primary school, older children and early adolescents begin to place greater importance on their acceptance by peers, along with their status and reputation within peer groups [16]. However, the formation and consolidation of peer groups is a gradual process. During the initial stages of forming stable peer groups, individuals encounter various changes and uncertainties, which can increase their likelihood of experiencing loneliness [10]. As the group structure gradually stabilizes, individuals begin to integrate into the group and adapt to the social dynamics. As a result, their feelings of loneliness may decrease over time [10].

Finally, a minority of individuals (5.82% of the sample) in this study were in the high increasing subgroup. This result was in line with previous loneliness studies [4,5] and might be associated with one's social competence. If early adolescents consistently lack a sense of belonging, they may experience chronic or increasing loneliness, putting them at risk for a variety of problems, including emotional, social, psychological, and physical issues [4–7].

4.2. Predictive Associations Between Peer Preference and Loneliness Trajectories

Peer preference promotes a high sense of popularity and prestige among peers [2,16], which can act as a protective factor against loneliness in early adolescents. In line with the previous study [4], the current research discovered that, generally, early adolescents getting higher scores on initial peer preference were more inclined to belong to the low decreasing subgroup compared to the other two subgroups. Early adolescents who initially displayed high levels of peer preference were less likely to experience loneliness following a moderate decreasing or high increasing trajectory. These findings suggest that, in Chinese culture, early peer preference is a key predictor of loneliness trajectory class membership among early adolescents. Being highly accepted and preferred by peers helps early adolescents fulfill their need for belonging and desire for interpersonal attachments [12,22], which may prevent or reduce loneliness over time.

4.3. Predictive Associations Between Social Withdrawal and Loneliness Trajectories

Consistent with the research on solitary activities and loneliness trajectories among Western children and early adolescents [4], our findings revealed that Chinese early adolescents with high initial levels of unsociability were more likely to belong to the high increasing loneliness trajectory rather than the other two classes. This suggests that unsociability at an early developmental stage is a key predictor for the development of loneliness. Children and adolescents who intentionally withdraw from their peer groups and spend excessive time alone are likely to experience a lack of social connectedness and a diminished sense of belonging [21]. However, within the context of Chinese culture, group orientation and social connectedness are traditionally emphasized and continue to be highly valued in recent years [25]. In fact, Chinese children are encouraged and supported by their mothers to demonstrate social connectedness and attachment from a very young age [42]. Taken together, it is not surprising that early adolescents' initial unsociability may lead to high and increasing levels of loneliness over time.

Additionally, our results revealed that early adolescents with higher initial shyness were less likely to be classified into the low decreasing loneliness trajectory and more likely to belong to the moderate decreasing or high increasing subgroups. These findings suggest that early shyness is a significant predictor of loneliness trajectories. This aligns with recent research showing a positive relationship between shyness and loneliness among Chinese children and early adolescents [24]. Researchers also found that shyness can positively predict loneliness one year later in Chinese children and early adolescents [28]. Shy early adolescents often lack social skills due to their fear or wariness of challenging social situations [41], and this can lead to the development of more negative self-perceptions. As a result, they may experience increasing loneliness over time.

4.4. Limitations and Future Directions

It is important to acknowledge some limitations of this research. First, the study was conducted with a sample of Chinese early adolescents, and given the specific historical and cultural context, caution is necessary when extrapolating the findings to other societies. Additionally, China exhibits significant regional differences in social, economic, and cultural development. Therefore, researchers should be cautious when generalizing the results to other regions of China, including major urban centers or remote rural areas. Future studies should consider cross-cultural comparisons (e.g., between Chinese and Western societies) and cross-regional studies (e.g., urban vs. remote rural areas in China) to provide a broader understanding of these issues.

Second, this research only revealed how peer preference and social withdrawal predicted loneliness trajectories. Given that previous studies have shown that parent–child relationships [8,43], teacher–child relationships [8,44], and peer relationships, such as peer victimization [45] and friendship quality [26], have impacts on loneliness, it would be intriguing to explore the relationships between these factors and loneliness in future research. Additionally, intrapersonal and interpersonal factors may interact throughout development, influencing loneliness trajectories [8,15]. Future researchers may find it particularly interesting to investigate how these factors interplay in predicting the developmental trajectories of loneliness over time.

Third, this study did not examine how changes in loneliness affect psychological and physical health during early adolescence. Although previous research has suggested that individuals on high stable or increasing loneliness trajectories tend to report more socioemotional problems, such as depressive symptoms, anxiety, social skills deficits, and suicidal ideation [7], these findings have yet to be explored in a non-Western context. Future research could explore how these health indicators vary across different developmental trajectories of loneliness, which may help us gain a deeper understanding of the impact of loneliness on psychological and physical well-being.

Finally, one possible limitation of the present study is the potential conceptual overlap among the measurement dimensions. Although the constructs of peer preference, unsociability, and shyness were treated as distinct predictors of loneliness trajectories, these dimensions may share some conceptual similarities, potentially influencing the interpretation of our findings. Future research should consider using more refined measures or conducting factor analyses to better distinguish these dimensions.

4.5. Strengths and Implications

The present study integrated person-centered and variable-centered analyses in a large sample to identify distinct developmental trajectories of loneliness among early adolescents in a Chinese cultural context. In addition to the overall decrease in loneliness over time, the study revealed substantial heterogeneity in these trajectories. Three developmental trajectory classes were identified, and they were significantly predicted by peer preference, unsociability, and shyness in different ways. These findings underscore the importance of applying a combination of variable-centered and person-centered approaches to study the development of loneliness.

Moreover, the current study has important implications for designing effective prevention and intervention strategies for early adolescents vulnerable to chronic or increasing loneliness. First, researchers and educators should place greater emphasis on identifying the high increasing loneliness subgroup and encourage their participation in interventions that address not only loneliness but also other aspects of psychosocial maladjustment. Such interventions can have broad benefits, as highlighted in meta-analyses of loneliness interventions [46]. Second, implementing social skills training programs for early adolescents with low peer preference and/or high social withdrawal may reduce the likelihood of them following a high increasing loneliness trajectory. Third, schools and teachers should create an inclusive classroom climate and culture to promote peer interaction that meets students' need for relatedness [47]. Meanwhile, incorporating evidence-based social and emotional learning (SEL) programs into standard educational curricula may significantly improve students' social and emotional skills, attitudes, and behaviors, which would be helpful for reducing social difficulties and loneliness among early adolescents [48].

Author Contributions: Conceptualization, data curation, funding acquisition, investigation, project administration, writing—original draft, review, and editing, W.C.; formal analysis, investigation, methodology, project administration, writing—review and editing, B.X. All authors have read and agreed to the published version of the manuscript.

Funding: This research was funded by the Jiangsu Institute of Education Sciences (C-c/2021/03/09).

Institutional Review Board Statement: The study was conducted in accordance with the Declaration of Helsinki, and approved by Suzhou University of Science and Technology (No. 2021066, 1 August 2021).

Informed Consent Statement: Informed consent was obtained from all subjects and their parents in this study.

Data Availability Statement: The datasets involved in the present study are available from the corresponding author upon reasonable request.

Conflicts of Interest: The authors assert that they do not have any competing interests.

References

1. Peplau, L.A.; Perlman, D. Perspectives on loneliness. In *Loneliness: A Sourcebook of Current Theory, Research, and Therapy*; John Wiley & Sons: New York, NY, USA, 1982; pp. 1–18.
2. Heinrich, L.M.; Gullone, E. The clinical significance of loneliness: A literature review. *Clin. Psychol. Rev.* **2006**, *26*, 695–718. [CrossRef] [PubMed]
3. Vanhalst, J.; Luyckx, K.; Van Petegem, S.; Soenens, B. The Detrimental Effects of Adolescents' Chronic Loneliness on Motivation and Emotion Regulation in Social Situations. *J. Youth Adolesc.* **2018**, *47*, 162–176. [CrossRef] [PubMed]
4. Qualter, P.; Brown, S.L.; Rotenberg, K.J.; Vanhalst, J.; Harris, R.A.; Goossens, L.; Bangee, M.; Munn, P. Trajectories of loneliness during childhood and adolescence: Predictors and health outcomes. *J. Adolesc.* **2013**, *36*, 1283–1293. [CrossRef] [PubMed]
5. Schinka, K.C.; Van Dulmen, M.H.M.; Mata, A.D.; Bossarte, R.; Swahn, M. Psychosocial predictors and outcomes of loneliness trajectories from childhood to early adolescence. *J. Adolesc.* **2013**, *36*, 1251–1260. [CrossRef] [PubMed]
6. Vanhalst, J.; Goossens, L.; Luyckx, K.; Scholte, R.H.J.; Engels, R.C.M.E. The development of loneliness from mid- to late adolescence: Trajectory classes, personality traits, and psychosocial functioning. *J. Adolesc.* **2013**, *36*, 1305–1312. [CrossRef]
7. Harris, R.A.; Qualter, P.; Robinson, S.J. Loneliness trajectories from middle childhood to pre-adolescence: Impact on perceived health and sleep disturbance. *J. Adolesc.* **2013**, *36*, 1295–1304. [CrossRef]
8. Wu, X.; Huebner, E.S.; Tian, L. Developmental trajectories of loneliness in Chinese children: Environmental and personality predictors. *J. Affect. Disord.* **2024**, *367*, 453–461. [CrossRef]
9. Brennan, T. Loneliness at adolescence. In *Loneliness: A Sourcebook of Current Theory, Research, and Therapy*; Peplau, L.A., Perlman, D., Eds.; John Wiley & Sons: New York, NY, USA, 1982; pp. 269–290.
10. Liu, J.; Zhou, Y.; Li, D. Developmental Trajectories of Loneliness During Middle and Late Childhood: A Latent Growth Curve Analysis. *Acta Psychol. Sin.* **2013**, *45*, 179–192. [CrossRef]
11. Mund, M.; Freuding, M.M.; Möbius, K.; Horn, N.; Neyer, F.J. The Stability and Change of Loneliness Across the Life Span: A Meta-Analysis of Longitudinal Studies. *Personal. Soc. Psychol. Rev.* **2020**, *24*, 24–52. [CrossRef]
12. Baumeister, R.F.; Leary, M.R. The need to belong: Desire for interpersonal attachments as a fundamental human motivation. *Psychol. Bull.* **1995**, *117*, 497–529. [CrossRef]
13. Bauer, D.J.; Curran, P.J. Distributional assumptions of growth mixture models: Implications for overextraction of latent trajectory classes. *Psychol. Methods* **2003**, *8*, 338–363. [CrossRef] [PubMed]
14. Bukowski, W.M.; Hoza, B. Popularity and friendship: Issues in theory, measurement, and outcome. In *Peer Relationships in Child Development*; Berndt, T., Ladd, G., Eds.; John Wiley & Sons: New York, NY, USA, 1989; pp. 15–45.
15. Rubin, K.H.; Bukowski, W.M.; Bowker, J.C. Children in peer groups. In *Ecological Settings and Processes in Developmental Systems: Vol. 4. Handbook of Child Psychology and Developmental Science*, 7th ed.; Lerner, R.M., Bornstein, M.H., Leventhal, T., Eds.; Wiley-Blackwell: New York, NY, USA, 2015; pp. 175–222.
16. Parkhurst, J.T.; Hopmeyer, A. Developmental change in the sources of loneliness in childhood and adolescence: Constructing a theoretical model. In *Loneliness in Childhood and Adolescence*; Rotenberg, K.J., Hymel, S., Eds.; Cambridge University Press: Cambridge, UK, 1999; pp. 56–79. [CrossRef]
17. Liu, J.; Xiao, B.; Hipson, W.E.; Coplan, R.J.; Li, D.; Chen, X. Self-control, peer preference, and loneliness in Chinese children: A three-year longitudinal study. *Soc. Dev.* **2017**, *26*, 876–890. [CrossRef]
18. Rubin, K.H.; Coplan, R.J.; Bowker, J.C. Social withdrawal in childhood. *Annu. Rev. Psychol.* **2009**, *60*, 141–171. [CrossRef] [PubMed]
19. Asendorpf, J. Beyond social withdrawal: Shyness, unsociability and peer avoidance. *Hum. Dev.* **1990**, *33*, 250–259. [CrossRef]
20. Coplan, R.J.; Ooi, L.L.; Baldwin, D. Does it matter when we want to Be alone? Exploring developmental timing effects in the implications of unsociability. *New Ideas Psychol.* **2019**, *53*, 47–57. [CrossRef]
21. Xiao, B.; Bullock, A.; Liu, J.; Coplan, R. Unsociability, peer rejection, and loneliness in Chinese early adolescents: Testing a cross-lagged model. *J. Early Adolesc.* **2021**, *41*, 865–885. [CrossRef]

22. Maslow, A.H. A theory of human motivation. *Psychol. Rev.* **1943**, *50*, 370–396. [CrossRef]
23. Liu, J.; Coplan, R.J.; Chen, X.; Li, D.; Ding, X.; Zhou, Y. Unsociability and shyness in Chinese children: Concurrent and predictive relations with indices of adjustment. *Soc. Dev.* **2014**, *23*, 119–136. [CrossRef]
24. Liu, J.; Chen, X.; Coplan, R.J.; Ding, X.; Zarbatany, L.; Ellis, W. Shyness and Unsociability and Their Relations With Adjustment in Chinese and Canadian Children. *J. Cross-Cult. Psychol.* **2015**, *46*, 371–386. [CrossRef]
25. Chen, X. Socioemotional development in Chinese children. In *Handbook of Chinese Psychology*; Bond, M.H., Ed.; Oxford University Press: New York, NY, USA, 2010; pp. 37–52.
26. Bullock, A.; Xiao, B.; Xu, G.; Liu, J.; Coplan, R.; Chen, X. Unsociability, peer relations, and psychological maladjustment among children: A moderated-mediated model. *Soc. Dev.* **2020**, *29*, 1014–1030. [CrossRef]
27. Bowker, J.C.; Richard, C.L.; Stotsky, M.V.; Weingarten, J.P.; Shafik, M.I. Understanding shyness and psychosocial difficulties during early adolescence: The role of friend shyness and self-silencing. *Personal. Individ. Differ.* **2023**, *209–215*, 112209. [CrossRef]
28. Yang, F.; Chen, X.; Wang, L. Shyness-Sensitivity and Social, School, and Psychological Adjustment in Urban Chinese Children: A Four-Wave Longitudinal Study. *Child Dev.* **2015**, *86*, 1848–1864. [CrossRef]
29. Little, R.J.A. A test of missing completely at random for multivariate data with missing values. *J. Am. Stat. Assoc.* **1988**, *83*, 1198–1202. [CrossRef]
30. Asher, S.; Hymel, S.; Renshaw, P.D. Loneliness in children. *Child Dev.* **1984**, *55*, 1456–1464. [CrossRef]
31. Coie, J.; Terry, R.; Lenox, K.; Lochman, J.; Hyman, C. Childhood peer rejection and aggression as predictors of stable patterns of adolescent disorder. *Dev. Psychopathol.* **1995**, *7*, 697–713. [CrossRef]
32. Chen, X.; Rubin, K.H.; Sun, Y. Social reputation and peer relationships in Chinese and Canadian children: A cross-cultural study. *Child Dev.* **1992**, *63*, 1336–1343. [CrossRef]
33. Masten, A.S.; Morison, P.; Pellegrini, D.S. A revised class play method of peer assessment. *Dev. Psychol.* **1985**, *21*, 523–533. [CrossRef]
34. Ding, X.; Liu, J.; Coplan, R.J.; Chen, X.; Li, D.; Sang, B. Self-reported shyness in Chinese children: Validation of the Children's Shyness Questionnaire and exploration of its links with adjustment and the role of coping. *Personal. Individ. Differ.* **2014**, *68*, 183–188. [CrossRef]
35. Crozier, W.R. Shyness and self-esteem in middle childhood. *Br. J. Educ. Psychol.* **1995**, *65*, 85–95. [CrossRef]
36. Duncan, T.E.; Duncan, S.C.; Strycker, L.A. Specification of the LGM. In *An Introduction to Latent Variable Growth Curve Modeling: Concepts, Issues, and Application*, 2nd ed.; Routledge: New York, NY, USA, 2006; pp. 16–38. [CrossRef]
37. Kline, R.B. Model testing and indexing. In *Principles and Practice of Structural Equation Modeling*, 5th ed.; Guilford Press: New York, NY, USA, 2023; pp. 156–177.
38. Nagin, D.S. Laying out the basic model. In *Group-Based Modeling of Development*; Harvard University Press: Cambridge, MA, USA, 2005; pp. 23–78. [CrossRef]
39. Muthén, B.O.; Muthén, L.K. Integrating person-centered and variable-centered analyses: Growth mixture modeling with latent trajectory classes. *Alcohol. Clin. Exp. Res.* **2000**, *24*, 882–891. [CrossRef]
40. Muthén, B.O. Latent variable analysis: Growth mixture modeling and related techniques for longitudinal data. In *Handbook of Quantitative Methodology for the Social Sciences*; Kaplan, D., Ed.; Sage: Newbury Park, UK, 2004; pp. 345–368.
41. Masi, C.M.; Chen, H.Y.; Hawkley, L.C.; Cacioppo, J.T. A meta-analysis of interventions to reduce loneliness. *Personal. Soc. Psychol. Rev.* **2011**, *15*, 219–266. [CrossRef] [PubMed]
42. Liu, M.; Chen, X.; Rubin, K.H.; Zheng, S.; Cui, L.; Li, D.; Chen, H.; Wang, L. Autonomy- vs. connectedness-oriented parenting behaviours in Chinese and Canadian mothers. *Int. J. Behav. Dev.* **2005**, *29*, 489–495. [CrossRef]
43. Wiseman, H.; Mayseless, O.; Sharabany, R. Why are they lonely? Perceived quality of early relationships with parents, attachment, personality predispositions and loneliness in first-year university students. *Personal. Individ. Differ.* **2006**, *40*, 237–248. [CrossRef]
44. Zhang, F.; Jiang, Y.; Lei, X.; Huang, S. Teacher power and children's loneliness: Moderating effects of teacher-child relationships and peer relationships. *Psychol. Sch.* **2019**, *56*, 1455–1471. [CrossRef]
45. Kochenderfer-Ladd, B.; Wardrop, J.L. Chronicity and instability of children's peer victimization experiences as predictors of loneliness and social satisfaction trajectories. *Child Dev.* **2001**, *72*, 134–151. [CrossRef]
46. Chen, X.; Fu, R.; Li, D.; Liu, J. Developmental Trajectories of Shyness-Sensitivity from Middle Childhood to Early Adolescence in China: Contributions of Peer Preference and Mutual Friendship. *J. Abnorm. Child Psychol.* **2019**, *47*, 1197–1209. [CrossRef]
47. Miller, C.F.; Kochel, K.P.; Wheeler, L.A.; Updegraff, K.A.; Fabes, R.A.; Martin, C.L.; Hanish, L.D. The efficacy of a relationship building intervention in 5th grade. *J. Sch. Psychol.* **2017**, *61*, 75–88. [CrossRef]
48. Durlak, J.A.; Weissberg, R.P.; Dymnicki, A.B.; Taylor, R.D.; Schellinger, K.B. The impact of enhancing students' social and emotional learning: A meta-analysis of school-based universal interventions. *Child Dev.* **2011**, *82*, 405–432. [CrossRef]

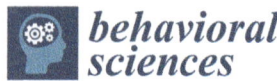

Review

Ineffective Learning Behaviors and Their Psychological Mechanisms among Adolescents in Online Learning: A Narrative Review

Ji Li [1,†], Li Fang [2,†], Yu Liu [3], Jiayu Xie [2] and Xiaoyu Wang [4,*]

[1] West China School of Nursing, Sichuan University, Chengdu 610041, China; 1977liji_1226@scu.edu.cn
[2] Students' Affairs Division, Sichuan Agricultural University, Chengdu 611830, China;
73222@sicau.edu.cn (L.F.); jiayuxie831@gmail.com (J.X.)
[3] College of Psychology, Sichuan Normal University, Chengdu 610066, China; 20212093056@stu.sicnu.edu.cn
[4] West China Hospital, Sichuan University, Chengdu 610041, China
* Correspondence: wangxiaoyu@scu.edu.cn
[†] These authors contributed equally to this work as co-first authors.

Abstract: During the COVID-19 pandemic, many countries and regions experienced a surge in online learning, but the public complained about and questioned its effectiveness. One of the most important reasons for this was the inadequate metacognitive abilities of adolescents. Studies in learning sciences have identified various inefficient learning behaviors among students in online learning, including help abuse, help avoidance, and wheel spinning; all closely related to metacognition. Despite concerns about ecological validity, researchers in psychology have proposed the agenda-based regulation framework, the COPES model, and MAPS model, which may help explain the inefficient learning behaviors among adolescents in online learning. Future studies should aim to verify these theoretical frameworks within the context of online learning and elucidate the causes of inefficient learning behaviors; the design and optimization of online learning systems should be informed by theories in cognitive psychology.

Keywords: online learning; inefficient learning behaviors; metacognition; adolescents

1. Introduction

During the COVID-19 pandemic, many countries and regions experienced a surge in online learning. However, some parents, teachers, and students complained about and questioned the effectiveness of online learning [1]. The inadequate self-learning abilities of children and adolescents were identified as one of the crucial reasons for the suboptimal outcomes in online learning [2]. Represented by Flavell, the cognitive constructivist believes that self-learning is essentially metacognitive monitoring of learning, where students actively adjust learning strategies and effort based on their own learning abilities and the requirements of the learning task [3]. Unfortunately, children and adolescents often exhibit poor metacognitive abilities and are unable to effectively monitor and regulate their own learning behaviors, especially at a younger age, leading to ineffective learning behaviors. For example, children tend to be overly optimistic about their performance, displaying the overconfidence effect by overestimating their performance and placing themselves above others [4,5]. Such misjudgments lead learners to believe they have mastered the content, discouraging reflection after making mistakes and limiting seeking help from external sources. These ineffective learning behaviors have a severe negative impact on the effectiveness of online learning for youngsters, and metacognition is closely linked to this issue. Therefore, it is necessary to explore the manifestation and underlying mechanisms of ineffective learning behaviors in online learning from a metacognitive perspective, aiming to enhance students' self-learning abilities, improve the quality of online learning, and transform students into expert learners.

In the field of learning science, psychologists excel in using true experiments to explore internal mechanisms, while researchers in computer science often use educational big data for machine learning modeling studies. Although different perspectives enrich the study of ineffective learning behaviors, the difficulty of dialogue between these fields has become increasingly apparent, resulting in a trend where the trees are seen but the forest is not. For instance, research on intelligent tutoring systems (ITS) often lags behind in its use of fundamental psychological theories compared to applied research. On one hand, ITS is highly practical, with data models focusing solely on predictive accuracy, while neglecting interpretability [6]. On the other hand, the urgent need for teaching drives researchers to propose numerous intervention strategies, mostly based on past teaching experience or system design experience, lacking theoretical guidance [7]. Therefore, this narrative review comprehensively discusses ineffective learning behaviors among adolescents and their psychological mechanisms in online learning environments from a metacognitive perspective, exploring the limitations of existing research and suggesting future research directions to address the current state of fundamental theory lagging behind applied research.

2. Ineffective Learning Behaviors among Adolescents in Online Learning

The behaviorist psychologist Skinner pioneered teaching machines in the 1950s [8]. Subsequently, digital learning environments gradually emerged, but early digital environments simply digitized instructional content, leaving learners passively receiving knowledge [8]. Intelligent learning environments are transformative products for digital education, with ITS being one of the most widely used intelligent learning environments, representing the application of artificial intelligence in education. ITS simulates one-on-one cognitive apprenticeship teaching by human teachers through a human–computer interaction interface [9]. Today, ITS is widely applied in various fields of teaching, such as medical education, mathematics, computer science, and reading and writing [10]. Its basic mode involves students inputting specified objects on the interactive interface, and the system's teaching agent guides students step by step. For example, when solving an equation, the system provides an electronic canvas for learners to detail the calculation steps, known as substeps. The system guides students step by step in writing substeps to solve the equation through various human–computer interaction interfaces. In recent years, researchers have found various ineffective learning behaviors among children and adolescents in such systems, with the most typical being help avoidance, help abuse, wheel spinning, and gaming the system. While these behaviors may be related to metacognition [11,12], the lack of a systematic review weakens the theoretical foundation of educational data mining research.

2.1. Help Avoidance and Help Abuse

In ITS, each item/step is accompanied by hints or scaffolding of different granularity, which students can view at any time. The presentation order of hints goes from abstract to concrete, culminating in the final answer, aiming to facilitate students' thinking and deepen learning. For example, in a problem like "What is the slope of the line graphed above?", if the student answer incorrectly, the problem will be divided into a set of scaffolding items, which would ask students to complete each step required to solve the original problem. Substep1: "Slope is a number that measures the steepness of a straight line. We measure slope by picking 2 points and dividing the change along the y-axis by the change along the x-axis. What is the change along the y-axis for this line from point A to point B?". Substep2: "What is the change in x for this line from point A to point B?". If substep2 was answered correctly, "Good, Remember, the slope is the change in y divided the change in x. What is the slope for this line?" [13]. Despite providing carefully designed hints and scaffolding, students often fail to use them effectively [14]. They either ignore the hints or frequently click them to quickly obtain the final answer [15]. In fact, the students who need help the most are often the least willing to seek assistance. Therefore, examining students' help-seeking behavior is crucial, as it may reflect their metacognitive level and help understand their academic failures, providing insights for optimizing and improving ITS.

In the practice and research into ITS, the two most common types of help-seeking deviations are help avoidance and help abuse. Help avoidance occurs when learners purposefully refrain from seeking assistance or support from the available resources, such as hints, explanations, or feedback provided by the educational system. Help abuse, on the other hand, involves an excessive reliance on or misuse of the available help features within the educational system [16,17]. Aleven et al. found that 36% of adolescent students showed help abuse and 19% exhibited help avoidance [16]. These help-seeking deviations were significantly negatively correlated with learning performance. For example, help avoidance was significantly negatively correlated with students' transfer learning scores. Previous studies used Bayesian knowledge tracing algorithms to calculate learners' probabilities of mastering a certain skill, where Kai et al. considered students as not having mastered a skill if the probability was below 0.6, marking students who did not seek help as having help avoidance [18]. Specifically, help avoidance manifested in two points: first, learners did not master the skill but did not click hints; second, students only had a slight understanding of the skill but did not consult the system's glossary. Help abuse typically involved students who had not mastered a skill but continuously clicked hints or consulted the glossary, even when they had completely mastered the skill. Overall, more than 70% of ITS users in Aleven et al.'s study exhibited help-seeking deviations [16], indicating an urgent need to improve students' metacognitive levels. Furthermore, these help-seeking deviations to some extent explained why online education is challenging. It places high demands on students' metacognition and self-control, which many children and adolescents cannot meet.

2.2. Wheel Spinning

Persistence and self-control in learning are often significantly positively correlated with academic performance [18,19]. However, not all persistence is effective, and meaningless persistence may hinder learning and even lead to learned helplessness [18]. Beck and Gong first identified a type of meaningless persistence behavior among adolescent students in online learning, which they termed "wheel-spinning" [20]. It refers to learners spending a considerable amount of time on a learning topic without mastering it, neither reflecting nor seeking help, and persistently answering without reconsideration.

It is noteworthy that the definition of wheel-spinning varies among different learning systems, due to design differences. For instance, Matsuda et al. defined it as attempting a task more than five times without achieving mastery and without seeking help from the system. A machine learning model of wheel-spinning had a recall rate of 79%, but a precision of only 25% [21]. Flores and Rodrigo identified wheel-spinning as attempting a task more than five times without mastery and making four or more consecutive errors [16–23]. Similarly, ASSISTments considers answering three consecutive items correctly on the same skill as mastery [18], while Cognitive Tutor relies on Bayesian knowledge tracing to calculate the probability of learners mastering a specific skill, considering probabilities equal to or greater than 95% as mastery.

In summary, learners' persistence in the learning process is meaningful, but there is a risk that this may transform into wheel-spinning and harming learning [24]. Therefore, a learning system capable of automatically distinguishing meaningful persistence from meaningless persistence behaviors (i.e., wheel-spinning) would be beneficial for providing timely feedback and conducting real-time interventions. Previous studies have attempted to differentiate between these types of persistence behaviors based on students' actions and cognitive levels, such as students' actions in the system or the number of practice attempts, as well as students' mastery of knowledge points [18,25]. We argue that considering students' metacognition is crucial, as it could potentially enhance the predictive effectiveness of machine learning models. Students' decision to persist is often based on their metacognitive monitoring of their own knowledge mastery, i.e., metacognitive monitoring. Ineffective persistence by students may result from biased metacognitive monitoring, where students erroneously believe they can master the learning content without seeking external help.

2.3. Gaming the System

Gaming the system is defined as students leveraging the features and rules of online learning platforms to achieve success in a learning task without thoroughly contemplating the learning content [26]. For instance, students may engage in activities such as "flooding" the discussion forum, guessing correct answers to obtain higher scores, or intentionally quickly making errors [26–28]. These behaviors are prevalent among children and adolescence in online learning environments. Baker et al. suggested that gaming the system is related to learners' self-regulated learning and metacognition [12]. Research indicates that students selectively engage in gaming behaviors; for example, some may avoid specific steps in a task, while others target areas where their mastery is weaker, and some may focus on well-mastered content [29]. Thus, gaming the system involves learners making behavioral decisions through cognitive monitoring.

Baker et al. categorized gaming the system into "Harmful gaming" and "Non-harmful gaming". Non-harmful gaming behaviors primarily refer to students employing gaming behaviors in familiar and time-consuming problem-solving steps, allocating a significant amount of time to what they genuinely need to learn [12]. Alternatively, students may rapidly click hints to view answers and then engage in self-explanation or reflection [30]. However, both types of gaming behaviors are significantly correlated with poorer academic performance [12]. The present study tends to view gaming the system as an ineffective learning behavior resulting from learners' cognitive monitoring bias. It is noteworthy that gaming the system is associated with emotional states and motivation; it may be perceived by students as a self-regulatory behavior to escape learning, especially when they experience boredom, confusion, or frustration [31].

3. Psychological Mechanisms of Ineffective Learning Behaviors in Online Learning

The various ineffective learning behaviors among children and adolescents mentioned earlier are closely related to metacognition, self-regulation, and self-control. Therefore, it is essential to review relevant theoretical models to explain the psychological mechanisms of ineffective learning behaviors. This paper focuses on Dunlosky et al.'s agenda-based regulation (ABR) framework [32], Winne and Hadwin's COPES theory [24,33], and Frazier et al.'s MAPS model [34]. The reason for selecting these theories is that metacognitive monitoring plays a crucial role among these theories, with metacognitive monitoring being the core content of the ABR framework and COPES theory, while the MAPS theory emphasizes the control of metacognition by agency. In addition, they tend to focus more on a micro-level analysis compared to other concepts and theories, such the self-directed learning and community of inquiry framework. This is particularly evident given that the inefficient learning behaviors discussed in this paper are all examined through microanalytic measures of a temporal process (i.e., event measures), meaning that the analysis of these behaviors relies entirely on detailed log data from online learning systems. These theories can effectively guide future research in discovering factors contributing to the decline in students' self-regulated learning performance and providing timely suggestions for improvement.

3.1. ABR Framework and Its Precursor Models

Before the ABR framework, Dunlosky and colleagues proposed several theoretical models for revealing the metacognitive mechanisms of learning time allocation. These precursor models laid the foundation for the ABR framework. They included the discrepancy-reduction model [35], the hierarchical model of self-regulated study [36], and the hypothesis of a region of proximal learning [37]. The discrepancy-reduction model focuses on the gap between the target state and the current state, leading learners to choose difficult items to narrow this gap [35,38]. The hierarchical model of self-regulated study constructs higher-level plans based on the target state and the current state, to optimize learning plans [36]. This model explains why learners may allocate less time to difficult items, where time-pressed learning groups tend to focus on simple items, while time-unconstrained groups lean towards difficult items [36]. However, these models still do not address the core issue of "dynamic learning processes". Morehead et al. and Li et al. suggested that learners prioritize learning content they have not encountered or have not mastered [39,40]. This supports Metcalfe's hypothesis of a region of proximal learning, where learners allocate time to unfamiliar and easily mastered items first, gradually increasing difficulty [37]. For example, experts allocate more time to difficult items than novices, and as proficiency deepens, the learner's region of proximal learning gradually increases to a higher level. This indicates a close relationship between domain knowledge and the individual's region of proximal learning, affecting learners' time allocation, and reflects the dynamic changes in the learning process. Although research has closely related the region of proximal learning to domain knowledge, common measurement methods like self-reporting are inadequate for gauging changes in the region of proximal learning, making operationalization challenging. Additionally, while this hypothesis emphasizes the dynamic changes in learning, it does not specify the mechanisms of these changes or the impact of learner traits and external factors, etc., on the learning process.

Therefore, researchers proposed the agenda-based regulation (ABR) theoretical framework (Figure 1). The ABR model suggests that learners construct learning agendas/plans based on various factors such as their characteristics and the nature of the task, to maximize learning goals [32]. Similarly to information processing, task-relevant internal and external stimuli activate long-term memory representations, then enter the working memory, triggering the learner's attention to similar stimuli. The central executive system monitors and maintains attention focus, while inhibiting the influence of other irrelevant stimuli. If inhibition fails, learners will be dominated by habitual responses, making it difficult to complete the learning task.

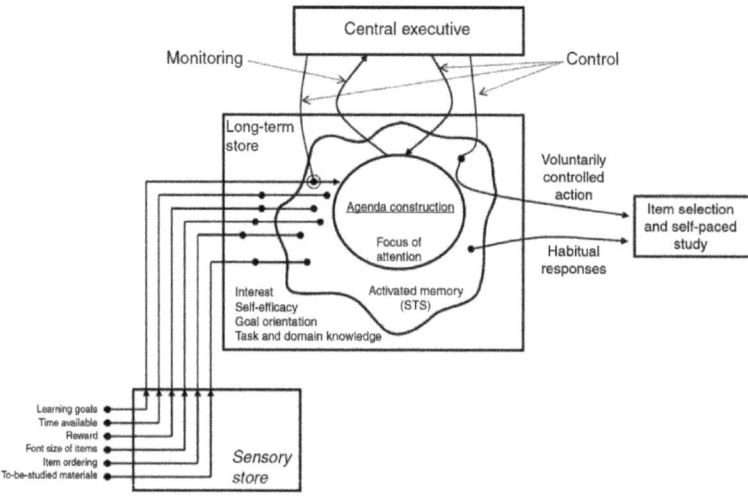

Figure 1. The agenda-based regulation (ABR) theoretical framework (adapted from [32]).

According to the ABR framework, two main causes can lead to ineffective learning behaviors in online learning: (1) learners struggle to construct appropriate learning agendas or plans, and (2) the central executive system struggles to inhibit irrelevant stimuli. The ABR framework suggests that learners are influenced by various factors, such as their characteristics and the nature of the task, when constructing learning plans, but it does not specify how the construction of learning plans is influenced. Thus, our focus is primarily on the relationship between ineffective learning behaviors and the central executive system, such as monitoring bias, cognitive load, attention deficits, etc. For instance, help avoidance and wheel-spinning may be related to cognitive load; when learners' cognitive resources are entirely focused on challenging tasks, they may lack additional cognitive resources to make help-seeking decisions [17]. Additionally, research has found that conspicuous system interface layouts (such as help-seeking signs) can make learners aware that they can seek help [17,41]. In this process, a conspicuous help-seeking sign serves as a perceptual cue, preventing learners from being influenced by habitual responses (such as help avoidance). However, the impact of perceptual cues on metacognitive monitoring is not always effective; one study found that learners tend to use perceptual cues that do not affect learning outcomes to monitor metacognitive processes, resulting in metacognitive errors [42]. We speculate that perceptual cues with low relevance to help seeking or learning outcomes may affect metacognitive monitoring processes, thereby promoting habitual responses (such as help avoidance).

Most of the precursor models of ABR framework focused on two aspects: item difficulty and time allocation, viewing the learning process as a static state, and considering the influence of other factors and dynamic changes in the learning process less. The ABR framework not only provides a possible explanation for ineffective learning behaviors, but also overcomes the limitations of task difficulty. It can more comprehensively consider other factors. Of course, the ABR framework also has its limitations, such as when the cognitive load or memory capacity is limited in the ABR framework, the mechanism of the central executive system will be affected accordingly, as well as how effectively it can inhibit irrelevant stimuli. Additionally, the factors that trigger habitual responses are not sufficiently explained, making interventions challenging.

3.2. COPES Model

Winne and Hadwin proposed that learning occurs in four fundamental stages: task definition, goal setting and planning, studying tactics, and adaptation [33]. Each stage is influenced by both cognitive and metacognitive factors. They categorized factors interacting with these stages into five aspects: condition, operation, product, evaluation, and standard, collectively referred to as the COPES theoretical model (Figure 2). When learners receive task stimuli, they engage in cognitive operations (SMART processes) based on task-related conditions (internal conditions such as domain knowledge, learning strategies, motivation, and external conditions) and perceived environmental features. The cognitive operations involve forming definitions and standards for tasks, developing goals and plans based on declarative knowledge, and selecting appropriate learning strategies [43]. The content relevant to goals and the results of metacognitive evaluation generated throughout the cognitive process are collectively referred to as products.

Monitoring is one of the decisive conditions for self-regulated learning [44,45], and the COPES theory is no exception. Winne mentioned two dominant relationships in metacognitive evaluation: control and monitoring, and two hierarchical levels: meta-level and object-level [46]. For learners, the cognitive operations in the early stages of learning are exploratory, and with the accumulation of practical experience, the cognitive operation process becomes faster, gradually forming an automated cognitive pattern. If metacognitive monitoring detects differences between meta-level and object-level, metacognition will search for an effective cognitive form to modify the cognitive operations at the object level.

Taking wheel-spinning as an example, it can be considered an ineffective self-regulation behavior, and one of its underlying mechanisms may be a lack of metacognitive knowledge, making it difficult for learners to find effective cognitive patterns. They may produce results based on past experiences that cannot meet current learning requirements. For instance, compared to mixed training, learners in non-mixed training and control groups find it more difficult to transfer knowledge, and their metacognitive strategy levels are relatively lower [47,48]. This suggests that a lack of metacognitive knowledge may lead individuals to ineffectively apply a past cognitive pattern in a new environment. Secondly, Winne and Baker et al. found that, as the difficulty level of a task increases, learners' metacognitive monitoring ability decreases [17,49]. This is likely because metacognitive monitoring struggles to identify differences between meta-level and object-level, thus maintaining the original cognitive operation. Motivation may play a crucial role in this; overly confident learners often have lower metacognitive monitoring levels [50].

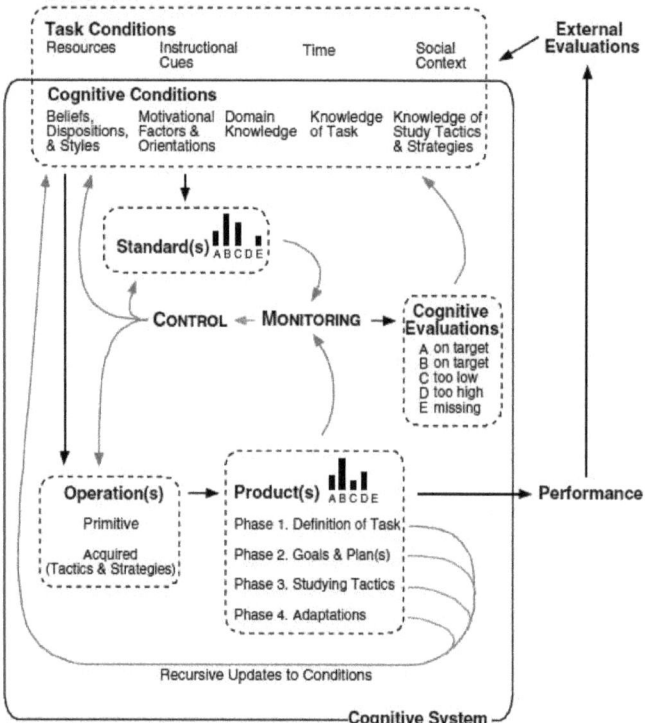

Figure 2. COPES model (adapted from [33]).

Winne believes that motivation and emotions are essential regulatory factors that can influence the information of cognitive operations and metacognitive knowledge [43]. The behavior of gaming the system is likely an external manifestation of changes in learners' motivation. Engelschalk et al. argued that when learners face tasks that are too difficult or too boring, they adjust their strategies for that specific task [51]. Additionally, Ocumpaugh et al. mentioned that when learners experience negative emotions such as boredom and frustration, they are likely to game the system [31]. This negative academic emotional experience may also lead students to avoid seeking help. For example, performance-oriented students may be reluctant to seek help when they do not understand the learning content or materials, fearing that seeking help will trigger negative reactions to their perceived abilities [52]. Help abuse can manifest in various ways (mastery vs. non-mastery), requiring a case-by-case analysis. We believe it is essential to first determine the motivation and goals of learners with help abuse, in order to further consider potential deviations in their overall self-regulation process.

In summary, the ABR framework seems more like a cognitive processing process that incorporates learner and task characteristics. Each step may cause cognitive overloads and an uneven distribution of cognitive resources, but it does not specify the impact of these cognitive-related factors on learning stages and behaviors. In comparison, the COPES model is relatively more comprehensive. It specifically outlines how stages and factors interact and creates possibilities for intervention. It may effectively explain the ineffective learning behaviors of the current study. On the one hand, it details the roles of self-regulated learning stages, cognition, and metacognition, helping us understand the learning process. On the other hand, it indicates the influence of motivation and academic emotions on cognition, metacognition, and learning behavior, which have been extensively discussed in the field of educational psychology.

3.3. MAPS Model

The MAPS model, proposed by Frazier et al., comprises three crucial aspects: possible self, metacognition, and agency [34]. Similar to Markus and Nurius's concept of possible selves, the possible self in the MAPS model refers to the projection of the future—the goals one hopes to accomplish and the outcomes that one is concerned about [53]. These reflect the difference between the current self and the future self. This self-difference is a crucial motivation or resource for self-regulation and behavioral change. However, it does not inherently lead to behavioral change, but requires the implementation of intention to activate metacognition. Metacognition consists of metacognitive monitoring, metacognitive knowledge, metacognitive control, and metacognitive experience, where metacognitive control guides individual behavior, allowing individuals to adopt appropriate metacognitive strategies to achieve behavior control, all under the umbrella of metacognitive monitoring. Frazier et al. described these thought processes, motivations, and behaviors as a sense of agency, which receives internal perceptions of metacognitive monitoring for process attribution, outcome feedback, and attribution, thereby adjusting metacognition, behavior, and feeding back to the self-concept [34].

There may be two aspects of the MAPS model that lead to the failure of goal-directed behavior. One is related to metacognition, such as execution defects and the irrationality of metacognitive strategies [54,55]. For example, students who wheel-spin might maintain a behavior of unproductive persistence, due to the use of irrational metacognitive strategies. Despite the agency receiving and providing relevant information to the self-concept, the behavioral change may fail due to execution defects. Gaming the system is more related to motivation, and one possible reason for gaming is that students do not have the implementation intention to narrow their self-difference, resulting in non-activation of metacognition. The other aspect is related to agency, including agency perception and cognitive bias [56]. Gaming the system may also be a way for learners to sacrifice knowledge mastery for a sense of control over the learning task. For instance, the study by Bucknoff and Metcalfe indicated that participants were willing to trade less reward for more control [57]. Help avoidance and help abuse may be a result of students perceiving their agency as lower or higher than reality, leading to ineffective learning behaviors. However, this point deviates slightly from the MAPS theory; Frazier et al. believed that even if individuals overestimate their actual control level, it can still promote effective self-regulation [34].

In conclusion, the difference between the MAPS theory and the ABR framework and COPES theory lies in their emphasis on metacognition. The MAPS theory suggests that self-regulation does not revolve around metacognition but unfolds as regulatory activities based on self-concept and self-control, where individual behavioral performance stems from the possible self. The challenge lies in the macroscopic nature of the self-concept. It is unclear which experiences that learners gain during each self-regulation activity can update the possible self-state and how this state is manifested. Additionally, the MAPS model cannot focus on each self-regulation activity in every task process. It is challenging to determine when learners successfully update the self-state during self-regulation activities, and whether the updated self-difference prompts self-regulation to approach or move away from the current task. If learners do not update the self-state, does this mean that this self-regulation activity has failed? After failure, what coping strategies should learners adopt?

4. Limitations and Prospects

In summary, researchers have identified various ineffective learning behaviors among children and adolescents in online learning environments, such as help avoidance, help abuse, wheel-spinning, and gaming the system. These ineffective learning behaviors not only occur frequently but also show a moderate and significant negative correlation with students' transfer learning, future learning readiness, and reduced test scores [17,58]. It is evident that students engaging in online learning face significant challenges in their metacognition, which we consider a crucial factor leading to the poor effectiveness of online learning.

Although previous studies have suggested a close connection between ineffective learning behaviors and metacognitive monitoring/regulation [12], there has been little research delving into the underlying psychological mechanisms. Moreover, online learning platforms have demonstrated its effectiveness to improve students' academic performance. Exploring how to leverage these platforms to train learners' metacognitive abilities is worth further investigation. This review detailed influential theories of self-regulated learning, explored the relationship between ineffective learning behaviors and metacognition, and attempted to integrate theory and practice, providing theoretical support for modeling and intervention studies. Several limitations also exist in this narrative review. Firstly, the ineffective learning behaviors reviewed herein primarily relied on empirical studies utilizing microanalytic measures of temporal processes (i.e., event measures). In other words, the analysis of these behaviors is entirely reliant on granular log data from online learning systems, closely associated with self-regulated learning. Consequently, our review perspective leant towards the analysis of micro-behaviors, and the theories included are more inclined towards process-oriented explanations. As a result, we may have overlooked a macro-theoretical perspective, such as neglecting the theoretical viewpoints of self-directed learning and the community of inquiry framework [59]. For example, the temporal and spatial separation between teaching and learning in online learning environments may lead to the absence of social presence and teaching presence, which could be one of the causes of ineffective learning behaviors in online learning. This highlights the importance for educators intentionally establishing social presence, teaching presence, and cognitive presence in online learning. Secondly, due to the reliance on studies using granular log data from online learning systems, there was limited attention given to Bloom's higher-order taxonomy. Empirical research in the field finds it challenging to model students' higher-order abilities using granular log data. Thirdly, given that this study provides a comprehensive discussion on ineffective learning behaviors with a relative broad scope, it is worth noting that this research is only a narrative review. Consequently, there might have been biases in the selection of literature, as the review lacked explicit inclusion and exclusion criteria and rigorous evaluation methods typically found in systematic reviews or meta-analysis.

Future studies should strengthen interdisciplinary research to consolidate and enrich cognitive psychology theories through educational data mining research, addressing the shortcomings of the low ecological validity in cognitive psychology [60]. Conversely, cognitive psychology experiments could compensate for the drawbacks of practicality over theory in educational data mining research, particularly in cases where the design of online learning platforms lacks support from cognitive psychology theories. The COPES model holds the potential to explain the ineffective learning behaviors among children and adolescents in online learning, but future research should investigate its applicability in intelligent tutoring environments, utilizing real instructional materials, log data from online platforms, and experimental techniques from cognitive psychology. Finally, regarding machine learning studies on ineffective learning behaviors, previous researchers have mostly considered learners' cognitive and behavioral features [58,61–63], relatively neglecting metacognition, which may affect the predictive accuracy of machine learning models. Future research could shift the focus of feature engineering onto metacognition, combined with physiological indicators from psychology, such as EEG and eye-tracking, aiming to enhance the model performance of ineffective learning behaviors and lay a solid foundation for personalized interventions.

Author Contributions: Conceptualization, L.F. and X.W.; validation, J.X. and X.W.; resources, X.W.; writing—original draft preparation, J.L., Y.L. and L.F.; writing—review and editing, J.L., L.F., Y.L. and

J.X.; visualization, Y.L. and J.X.; supervision, X.W.; funding acquisition, X.W. All authors have read and agreed to the published version of the manuscript.

Funding: This research was funded by Institute of Psychology, CAS, grant number GJ202011, Chengdu Philosophy and Social Science Planning Office, grant number 2022CZ083 and Sichuan Provincial Center for Educational Informationziation and Big Data, grant number DSJ2022050.

Institutional Review Board Statement: Not applicable.

Informed Consent Statement: Not applicable.

Data Availability Statement: Not applicable.

Conflicts of Interest: The authors declare no conflicts of interest.

References

1. Mihova, P.; Stankova, M.; Andonov, F.; Tsoukka, K.; Proedrou, A.; Tsetsila, E.; Alshawesh, H.; Mavrothanasi, M.; Stoyanov, S. Parental attitudes towards online learning—Data from four countries. In *Smart Education and E-Learning—Smart Pedagogy*; Uskov, V.L., Howlett, R.J., Jain, L.C., Eds.; Springer Nature: Singapore, 2022; pp. 508–517.
2. Dong, C.; Cao, S.; Li, H. Young children's online learning during COVID-19 pandemic: Chinese parents' beliefs and attitudes. *Child. Youth Serv. Rev.* **2020**, *118*, 105440. [CrossRef] [PubMed]
3. Wang, F.; Yang, X.; Huang, H. Research summary on meta-cognitive theory and practice of China. *Res. Pract. High. Educ.* **2022**, *3*, 7–13. (In Chinese)
4. Butler, G.; McManus, F. *Child Psychology: A Very Short Introduction*, 2nd ed.; OUP Oxford: Oxford, UK, 2014.
5. Dunning, D.; Griffin, D.W.; Milojkovic, J.D.; Ross, L. The overconfidence effect in social prediction. *J. Personal. Soc. Psychol.* **1990**, *58*, 568–581. [CrossRef] [PubMed]
6. Carvalho, D.V.; Pereira, E.M.; Cardoso, J.S. Machine learning interpretability: A survey on methods and metrics. *Electronics* **2019**, *8*, 832. [CrossRef]
7. Molennar, I.; Horvers, A.; Dikstra, R.; Baker, R. Designing dashboards to support learners' self-regulated learning. In Proceedings of the 9th International Conference on Learning Analytics and Knowledge, Tempe, AZ, USA, 4–8 March 2019; ACM: Phoenix, AZ, USA, 2019.
8. Huang, R.; Yang, J.; Hu, Y. From digital to smart: The evolution and trends of learning environment. *Open Educ. Res.* **2012**, *18*, 75–84. (In Chinese)
9. Liang, Y.; Liu, C. The application status, typical characteristic and development trends of artificial intelligence in education. *China Educ. Technol.* **2018**, *3*, 24–30. (In Chinese)
10. Gao, H.; Long, Z.; Liu, K.; Xu, S.; Cai, Z.; Hu, X. AutoTutor: Theories, technologies, applications and potential impacts. *Open Educ. Res.* **2016**, *22*, 96–103. (In Chinese)
11. Beck, J.; Rodrigo, M.; Mercedes, T. Understanding wheel spinning in the context of affective factors. In *Intelligent Tutoring Systems, Proceedings of the 12th International Conference on Intelligent Tutoring Systems, Honolulu, HI, USA, 5–9 June 2014*; Springer: Cham, Switzerland, 2014.
12. Baker, R.S.; Corbett, A.T.; Roll, I.; Koedinger, K.R.; Aleven, V.; Cocea, M.; Hershkovitz, A.; de Caravalho, A.M.; Mitrovic, A.; Mathews, M. Modeling and studying gaming the system with educational data mining. In *International Handbook of Metacognition and Learning Technologies*, 1st ed.; Azevedo, R., Aleven, V., Eds.; Springer: New York, NY, USA, 2013; pp. 97–115.
13. Razzaq, L.; Heffernan, N.T. Scaffolding vs. hints in the Assistment system. In *Intelligent Tutoring Systems*; Ikeda, M., Ashley, K.D., Chan, T.W., Eds.; Springer: Berlin/Heidelberg, Germany, 2006; pp. 635–644.
14. Duong, H.; Zhu, L.; Wang, Y.; Heffernan, N.T. A prediction model that uses the sequence of attempts and hints to better predict knowledge: "Better to attempt the problem first, rather than ask for a hint". In Proceedings of the 7th International Conference on Educational Data Mining, London, UK, 4–7 July 2014.
15. Price, T.W.; Liu, Z.; Cateté, V.; Barnes, T. Factors influencing students' help–seeking behavior while programming with human and computer tutors. In Proceedings of the 2017 ACM Conference on International Computing Education Research, Washington, DC, USA, 18–20 August 2017.
16. Aleven, V.; McLaren, B.; Roll, I.; Koedinger, K. Toward meta–cognitive tutoring: A model of help seeking with a Cognitive Tutor. *Int. J. Artif. Intell. Educ.* **2006**, *16*, 101–128.
17. Almeda, V.; Baker, R.; Corbett, A. Help avoidance: When students should seek help, and the consequences of failing to do so. *Teach. Coll. Rec.* **2017**, *119*, 1–24. [CrossRef]
18. Kai, S.; Almeda, M.V.; Baker, R.S.; Heffernan, C.; Heffernan, N. Decision tree modeling of wheel–spinning and productive persistence in skill builders. *J. Educ. Data Min.* **2018**, *10*, 36–71.
19. Credé, M.; Tynan, M.C.; Harms, P.D. Much ado about grit: A meta-analytic synthesis of the grit literature. *J. Personal. Soc. Psychol.* **2017**, *113*, 492–511. [CrossRef] [PubMed]

20. Beck, J.E.; Gong, Y. Wheel–spinning: Students who fail to master a skill. In *International Conference on Artificial Intelligence in Education, Proceedings of the 16th International Conference of Artificial Intelligence in Education, Memphis, TN, USA, 9–13 July 2013*; Springer: Cham, Switzerland, 2013.

21. Matsuda, N.; Chandrasekaran, S.; Stamper, J. How quickly can wheel spinning be detected. In Proceedings of the 9th International Conference on Educational Data Mining, Raleigh, NC, USA, 29 June–2 July 2016.

22. Schneider, M.; Preckel, F. Variables associated with achievement in higher education: A systematic review of meta-analyses. *Psychol. Bull.* **2017**, *143*, 565–600. [CrossRef] [PubMed]

23. Flores, R.M.; Rodrigo, M.M.T. Wheel–Spinning Models in a Novice Programming Context. *J. Educ. Comput. Res.* **2020**, *58*, 1101–1120. [CrossRef]

24. Palaoag, T.D.; Rodrigo, M.M.T.; Andres, J.M.L.; Andres, J.M.A.L.; Beck, J.E. Wheel-spinning in a game-based learning environment for physics. In Proceedings of the 13th International Conference on Intelligent Tutoring Systems, Zagreb, Croatia, 7–10 June 2016.

25. Owen, V.E.; Roy, M.H.; Thai, K.P.; Burnett, V.; Jacobs, D.; Keylor, E.; Baker, R.S. Detecting Wheel-Spinning and Productive Persistence in Educational Games. In Proceedings of the 12th International Conference on Educational Data Mining, Montreal, QC, Canada, 2–5 July 2019.

26. Nunes, T.M.; Bittencourt, I.I.; Isotani, S.; Jaques, P.A. Discouraging gaming the system through interventions of an animated pedagogical agent. In Proceedings of the 11th European Conference on Technology Enhanced Learning, Lyon, France, 13–16 September 2016.

27. Cheng, R.; Vassileva, J. Adaptive reward mechanism for sustainable online learning community. In Proceedings of the 12th International Conference on Artificial Intelligence in Education, Amsterdam, The Netherlands, 18–22 July 2005.

28. Paquette, L.; Baker, R.S.; Moskal, M. A system–general model for the detection of gaming the system behavior in CTAT and LearnSphere. In Proceedings of the International Conference on Artificial Intelligence in Education, London, UK, 27–30 June 2018.

29. Baker, R.S.; Corbett, A.T.; Koedinger, K.R.; Wagner, A.Z. Off-task behavior in the cognitive tutor classroom: When students "game the system". In Proceedings of the ACM CHI 2004 Conference on Human Factors in Computing Systems, Vienna, Austria, 24–29 April 2004.

30. Rus, V.; Banjade, R.; Niraula, N.; Gire, E.; Franceschetti, D. A study on two hint-level policies in conversational intelligent tutoring systems. In *Innovations in Smart Learning*, 1st ed.; Popescu, E., Kinshuk, Khribi, M.K., Huang, R., Jemni, M., Chen, N.-S., Sampson, D.G., Eds.; Springer: Singapore, 2017; pp. 175–176.

31. Ocumpaugh, J.; Andres, J.M.; Baker, R.; DeFalco, J.; Paquette, L.; Rowe, J.; Mott, B.; Lester, J.; Georgoulas, V.; Brawner, K.; et al. Affect dynamics in military trainees using vMedic: From engaged concentration to boredom to confusion. In Proceedings of the 18th International Conference on Artificial Intelligence in Education, Wuhan, China, 28 June–1 July 2017.

32. Dunlosky, J.; Ariel, R. Self-regulated learning and the allocation of study time. *Psychol. Learn. Motiv.* **2011**, *54*, 103–140.

33. Winne, P.H.; Hadwin, A.F. Studying as self-regulated learning. In *Metacognition in Educational Theory and Practice*; Dunlosky, H., Dunlosky, J., Graesser, A., Eds.; Routledge: Newark, NJ, USA, 1998; pp. 277–304.

34. Frazier, L.D.; Schwartz, B.L.; Metcalfe, J. The MAPS model of self-regulation: Integrating metacognition, agency, and possible selves. *Metacognit. Learn.* **2021**, *16*, 297–318. [CrossRef] [PubMed]

35. Dunlosky, J.; Hertzog, C. Training programs to improve learning in later adulthood: Helping older adults educate themselves. In *Metacognition in Educational Theory and Practice*; Dunlosky, H., Dunlosky, J., Graesser, A., Eds.; Routledge: Newark, NJ, USA, 1998; pp. 249–275.

36. Thiede, K.W.; Dunlosky, J. Toward a general model of self–regulated study: An analysis of selection of items for study and self-paced study time. *J. Exp. Psychol. Learn. Mem. Cogn.* **1999**, *25*, 1024–1037. [CrossRef]

37. Metcalfe, J. Metacognitive judgments and control of study. *Curr. Dir. Psychol. Sci.* **2009**, *18*, 159–163. [CrossRef] [PubMed]

38. Liu, X.; Fang, G.; Yang, X. The review of the studies about allocation of study time overseas. *Adv. Psychol. Sci.* **2004**, *12*, 524–535. (In Chinese)

39. Morehead, K.; Dunlosky, J.; Foster, N.L. Do people use category-learning judgments to regulate their learning of natural categories. *Mem. Cogn.* **2017**, *45*, 1253–1269. [CrossRef]

40. Li, P.; Zhang, Y.; Li, W.; Li, X. Age-related differences in effectiveness of item restudy choices: The role of value. *Aging Neuropsychol. Cogn.* **2018**, *25*, 122–131. [CrossRef]

41. Roll, I.; Baker, R.S.; Aleven, V.; Koedinger, K.R. On the benefits of seeking (and avoiding) help in online problem-solving environments. *J. Learn. Sci.* **2014**, *23*, 537–560. [CrossRef]

42. Chen, F.; Li, F.; Li, W. Effects of perceptual cues on metamemory monitoring and control. *Adv. Psychol. Sci.* **2016**, *24*, 494–500. (In Chinese) [CrossRef]

43. Winne, P.H. Modeling self-regulated learning as learners doing learning science: How trace data and learning analytics help develop skills for self-regulated learning. *Metacognit. Learn.* **2022**, *17*, 773–791. [CrossRef]

44. Zimmerman, B.J. Attaining self-regulation: A social cognitive perspective. In *Handbook of Self-Regulation*; Boekaerts, M., Pintrich, P., Zeidnerm, M., Eds.; Academic Press: New York, NY, USA, 2000; pp. 13–39.

45. Zimmerman, B.J. Theories of self-regulated learning and academic achievement: An overview and analysis. In *Self-Regulated Learning and Academic Achievement: Theoretical Perspectives*, 2nd ed.; Zimmerman, B.J., Schunk, D., Eds.; Lawrence Erlbaum: Mahwah, NJ, USA, 2001; pp. 1–38.

46. Winne, P.H. Cognition and metacognition within self-regulated learning. In *Handbook of Self-Regulation of Learning and Performance*; Zimmerman, B.J., Schunk, D.H., Eds.; Routledge: New York, NY, USA, 2017; pp. 36–48.
47. Schuster, C.; Stebner, F.; Leutner, D.; Wirth, J. Transfer of metacognitive skills in self-regulated learning: An experimental training study. *Metacognit. Learn.* **2020**, *15*, 455–477. [CrossRef]
48. Leopold, C.; Leutner, D. Improving students' science text comprehension through metacognitive self-regulation when applying learning strategies. *Metacognit. Learn.* **2015**, *10*, 313–346. [CrossRef]
49. Winne, P.H. Self–regulated learning viewed from models of information processing. In *Self-Regulated Learning and Academic Achievement: Theoretical Perspectives*, 2nd ed.; Zimmerman, B.J., Schunk, D.H., Eds.; Lawrence Erlbaum: Mahwah, NJ, USA, 2001; pp. 153–189.
50. Miller, T.M.; Geraci, L. Improving metacognitive accuracy: How failing to retrieve practice items reduces overconfidence. *Conscious. Cogn.* **2014**, *29*, 131–140. [CrossRef] [PubMed]
51. Engelschalk, T.; Steuer, G.; Dresel, M. Effectiveness of motivational regulation: Dependence on specific motivational problems. *Learn. Individ. Differ.* **2016**, *52*, 72–78. [CrossRef]
52. Karabenick, S.A. Perceived achievement goal structure and college student help seeking. *J. Educ. Psychol.* **2004**, *96*, 569–581. [CrossRef]
53. Markus, H.; Nurius, P. Possible selves. *Am. Psychol.* **1986**, *41*, 954–969. [CrossRef]
54. Metcalfe, J. "Knowing" that the self is the agent. In *Agency and Joint Attention*; Metcalfe, J., Herberts, T., Eds.; Oxford University Press: New York, NY, USA, 2013; pp. 238–255.
55. Metcalfe, J.; Mischel, W. A hot/cool-system analysis of delay of gratification: Dynamics of willpower. *Psychol. Rev.* **1999**, *106*, 3–19. [CrossRef]
56. Zalla, T.; Miele, D.; Leboyer, M.; Metcalfe, J. Metacognition of agency and theory of mind in adults with high functioning autism. *Conscious. Cogn.* **2015**, *31*, 126–138. [CrossRef]
57. Bucknoff, Z.J.; Metcalfe, J. Memory under the SEA (Subjective Experience of Agency). In *Memory Quirks*; Cleary, A., Schwartz, B., Eds.; Routledge: New York, NY, USA, 2020; pp. 197–206.
58. Baker, R.S.; Andrew, W.B.; Sujith, M.G.; Zhang, S.; Hawn, A. Predicting k-12 dropout. *J. Educ. Stud. Placed Risk (JESPAR)* **2020**, *25*, 28–54. [CrossRef]
59. Garrison, D.R.; Arbaugh, J.B. Researching the community of inquiry framework: Review, issues, and future directions. *Internet High. Educ.* **2007**, *10*, 157–172. [CrossRef]
60. Hatfield, G. Psychology, philosophy, and cognitive science: Reflections on the history and philosophy of experimental psychology. *Mind Lang.* **2002**, *17*, 207–232. [CrossRef]
61. Crossley, S.A.; Karumbaiah, S.; Ocumpaugh, J.; Labrum, M.J.; Baker, R.S. Predicting math identity through language and click-stream patterns in a blended learning mathematics program for elementary students. *J. Learn. Anal.* **2020**, *7*, 19–37. [CrossRef]
62. Zhang, J.; Andres, J.; Hutt, S.; Baker, R.S.; Ocumpaugh, J.; Nasiar, N.; Mills, C.; Brooks, J.; Sethuaman, S.; Young, T. Using machine learning to detect smart model cognitive operations in mathematical problem-solving process. *J. Educ. Data Mining* **2022**, *14*, 76–108.
63. Hutt, S.; Wong, A.; Papoutsaki, A.; Baker, R.S.; Gold, J.I.; Mills, C. Webcam-based eye tracking to detect mind wandering and comprehension errors. *Behav. Res. Methods* **2024**, *56*, 1–17. [CrossRef]

MDPI AG
Grosspeteranlage 5
4052 Basel
Switzerland
Tel.: +41 61 683 77 34

Behavioral Sciences Editorial Office
E-mail: behavsci@mdpi.com
www.mdpi.com/journal/behavsci

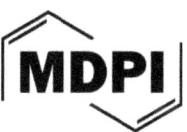

www.ingramcontent.com/pod-product-compliance
Lightning Source LLC
LaVergne TN
LVHW070623100526
838202LV00012B/710